pilates FOR rehab

A GUIDEBOOK TO INTEGRATING PILATES IN PATIENT CARE

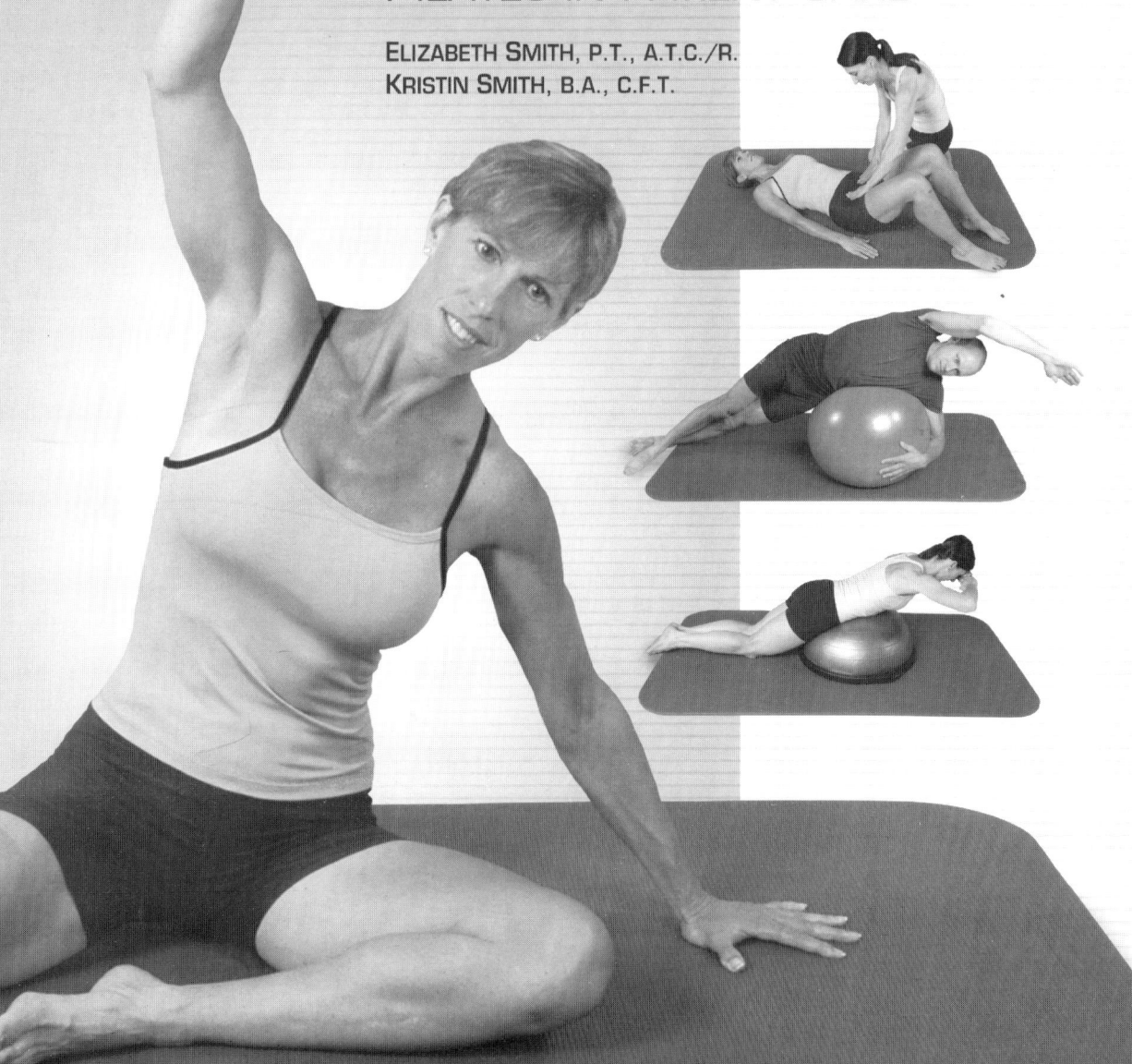

Elizabeth Smith, P.T., A.T.C./R.
Kristin Smith, B.A., C.F.T.

Table of Contents

<u>Chapter</u>

1. Putting Pilates in a Rehabilitation Context 1

2. A Clinical Foundation for Applying Pilates in Rehabilitation 9

3. Designing and Progressing Traditional Rehabilitation Programs Using Pilates 19

4. The Pilates Principles: Creating the Framework for Movement 35

5. Core Stabilization Strategies: Breathing, Transversus Abdominis, Neutral Pelvis 55

6. Fundamental Exercises: The Principles in Action 69

7. The Exercises 91
   - Spinal Flexion and Articulation 93
   - Spinal Extension, Mobility, and Stability 107
   - Torso: Stabilization, Rotation, and Lateral Flexion 111
   - Hips: Joint Mobilization and Muscle Strengthening 119
   - Upper Body Strengthening and Stabilization 132

8. Using Equipment to Teach and Challenge 135
   - Spinal/Thoracic Flexion 148
   - Spinal/Thoracic Extension 152
   - Torso: Stabilization, Rotation, and Lateral Flexion 155
   - Hips: Joint Mobilization and Strengthening 158
   - Upper Extremity Strengthening and Mobilization 164

9. The Art of Teaching 167

10. Using Imagery to Improve Movement: A Framework for Physical Therapists 173

11. Patient Focus: Case Studies of Pilates Application in Rehabilitation 189

12. Fitness Training for Athletes: Rehabilitation and Return to Play 209

13. References and Resources 221

Preface

The goals of therapeutic rehabilitation are similar to those of Pilates. Restored muscle function, balance, and range of motion are among the many shared objectives of these two movement-based therapies. No wonder rehabilitation specialists are increasingly integrating Pilates-based methodology with rehabilitation strategies.

The evolution of this practitioner guide stems from our work with rehabilitation specialists that began four years ago. Early in our Pilates training we understood the value of many of the Pilates-based principles and exercises to fitness and rehabilitation practice. Concepts that include torso stabilization in wide-ranging movement activities and stability before mobility seemed appropriate content for continuing education courses designed for such movement educators as physical and occupational therapists, fitness trainers, athletic trainers, and physical medicine physicians.

Since getting our feet wet as course instructors we've observed the power of Pilates-based methodology in improving patient outcomes and the provider experience in helping patients return to activities of daily living, work, and athletics.

Based on our clinical and fitness experience, we've tailored our approach to Pilates to introduce perspectives that may be more clinically relevant. Too, we've tapped the respected works of rehabilitation and exercise science resources that include Valdmir Janda, Diane Lee, Paul Hodges, Shirley Sahrmann, and Stuart McGill.

Beyond this, Pilates has fundamentally changed our approach to movement. As ever-growing students of this methodology, we apply Pilates' work in all facets of patient treatment, education, and fitness instruction. We apply it in our personal lives, changing how we sit at our desk, ride a bike, lift a child, or work in the garden. It's changed the lives of the people who live and train with us.

Our hope is that the content presented here will pique your interest to pursue further education and training. Expand your therapeutic toolbox and use this guide as a resource for discovery and growth in all facets of your life.

E. Smith
K. Smith

Acknowledgments

The development of this guidebook would not have been possible without the contributions and input of many Pilates instructors and trainers, Pilates education centers, clinicians, patients, and clients. We thank STOTT Pilates and the PhysicalMind Institute for providing an excellent foundation and training ground and applaud them for their continuing commitment to improving and expanding the Pilates repertoire.

We thank the many instructors who have unknowingly helped us realize new ways of presenting the work or who have opened the door to our current understanding. We thank the clinicians who have taken our courses out of idle interest and have given of themselves wholeheartedly in embracing the methodology and, in asking questions, have challenged us to expand our knowledge. Nothing has been more fulfilling than hearing from clinicians who are using Pilates clinically for the first time and seeing results.

We thank our clients and fitness students who have been the subjects of intense scrutiny in identifying faulty movement patterns and compensations and tolerated our experimentation. Last, we thank our families for their unending patience and encouragement in moving this book from simply a course manual to something that may impact the health and well-being of others.

chapter 1

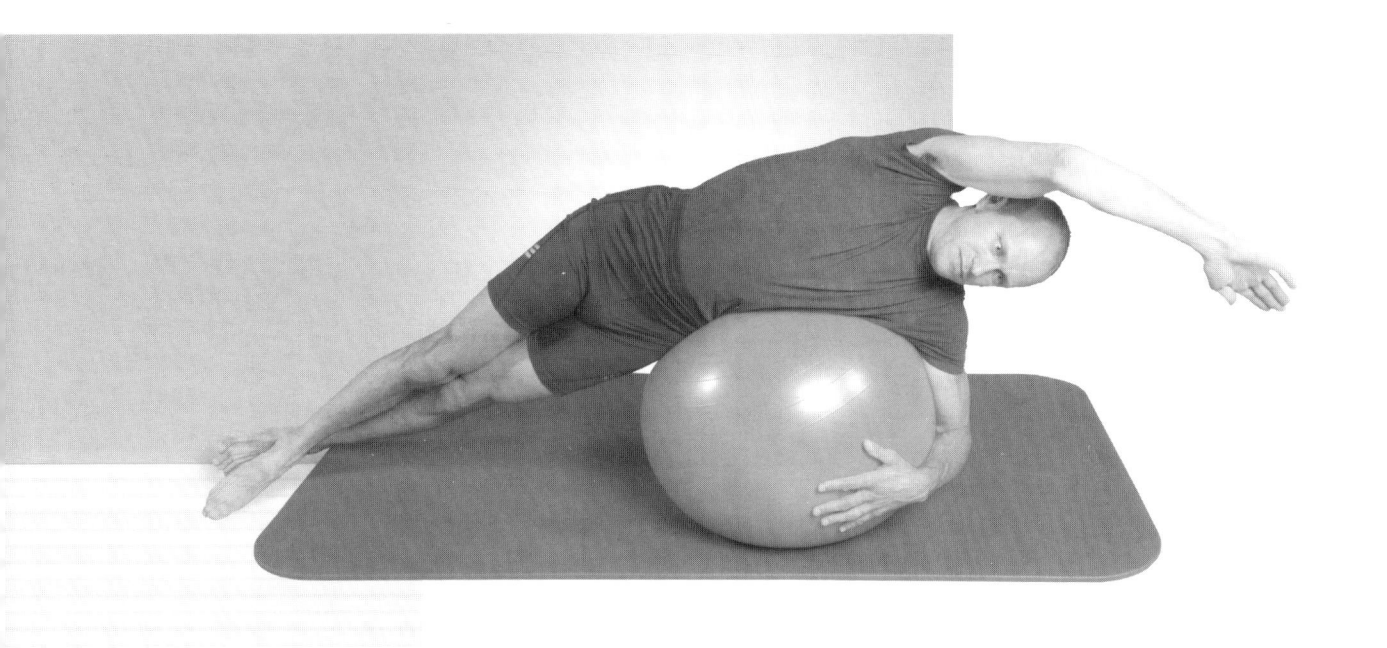

PUTTING PILATES
IN A
REHABILITATION
CONTEXT

What Is Pilates?

It is a rare practitioner who hasn't been asked about Pilates by a patient or physician. What is your response? In our experience, many practitioners have an idea of Pilates; some have taken a class or workshop. Most are unprepared to respond succinctly to questions that include:

- What is Pilates?
- Is it safe for my patient?
- Can I return to my Pilates class after rehabilitation?
- What books, videos, or DVDs do you recommend?
- Can Pilates help me?

It's hard to formulate a response if you haven't exposed yourself to Pilates through a community course or more formalized training, or given thought to how you might respond when asked. In this chapter and throughout this guidebook, we hope to better prepare you to respond to these queries with confidence.

What is Pilates (Pu-la-tees)? Practitioners describe it as a unique method of body conditioning that combines muscle strengthening and lengthening with breathing to develop "the powerhouse" of the body or the trunk and restore muscle balance to the musculoskeletal system.

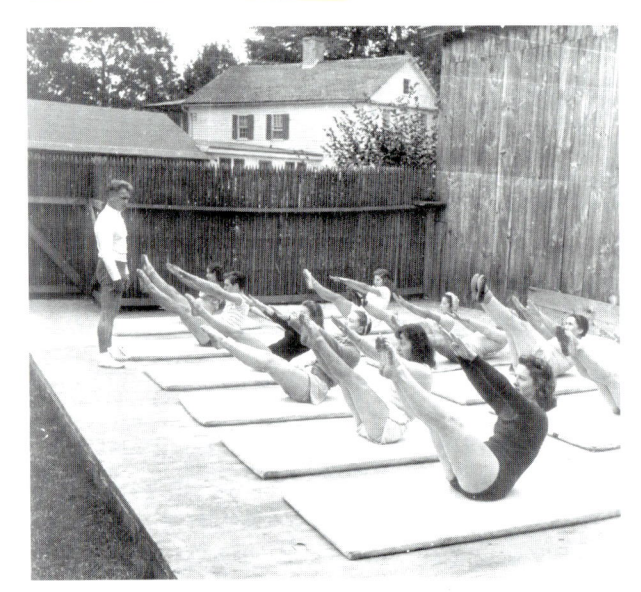

Permission to reprint photos granted by Jacob's Pillow Dance.

Joseph Pilates at 60 years old, 1941

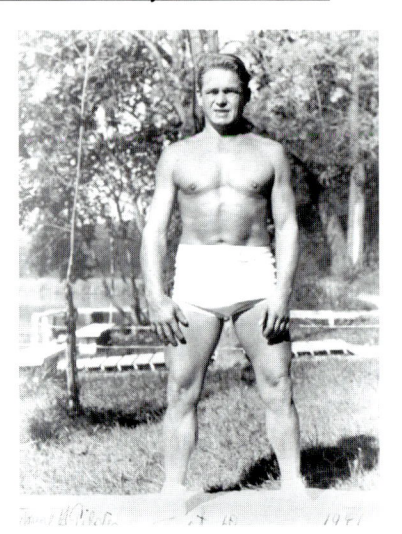

Joseph Hubertus Pilates developed the Pilates method in Germany more than 85 years ago to overcome such physical maladies as asthma and rickets. Extremely concerned about the impact of "technology" on the spine, posture, and breathing, he sampled from diverse movement regimens and therapies that included Eastern-based yoga, self-defense, weight training, and gymnastics to develop his method of "Contrology" or conscious muscle control. He first used Pilates to help World War I interns recover from injury and illness more quickly and to help rehabilitate nonambulatory patients (1). Latter-day enthusiasts included dancers and movement educators such as Martha Graham and George Balanchine.

"I invented all these machines. Began back in Germany, was there until 1925 - used to exercise rheumatic patients. Look, you see it resists your movements in just the right way so those inner muscles really have to work against it. That way you can concentrate on the movement. You must always do that (1)."

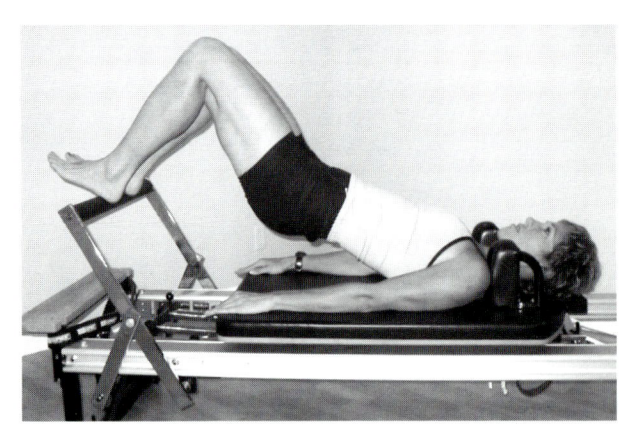

Contrology was coined by Pilates to describe his method of conscious, intentional control of all movement and the correct use of gravity, equilibrium, and leverage principles of the musculoskeletal system. He believed that Contrology led to a balance of mind, body, and spirit: neither took priority over the others. Further, he believed that the role of the spine was long misunderstood, leading to ill health. According to Pilates, one only needs to learn proper breathing and posture to eliminate the need for "artificial" exercise and prevent such everyday ailments as obesity, asthma, and heart disease.

Defining the modern-day powerhouse or "core" is no easy task; a number of fitness and rehabilitation perspectives appear in the literature (2). Our definition is evidence-based and generally refers to the muscles that span from the rib cage to the base of the pelvis. The core includes but is not limited to such muscles as the transversus abdominis (TrA), internal (IO) and external obliques (EO), lumbar multifidus (LM), pelvic floor (PF), and diaphragm, as well as the gluteus maximus and medius and the quadratus lumborum. Muscles that contribute to core stability via a neurophysiologic connection include the hip adductors (3).

Core stabilization also occurs via muscles that stabilize the scapulae and are commonly termed "secondary stabilizers" of the core. The body of research in this arena is ever-changing, and practitioners and patients alike can look forward to benefiting from this work as the evidence base continues to expand.

A Clinical Perspective

From a clinical perspective, Pilates comprises multiple muscle synergies that include isometric, concentric, and eccentric muscle contractions and co-contractions (1,3). Pilates emphasizes lumbo-pelvic stability, segmental mobilization of the spine, mobilization of the shoulder, hip, and other extremity joints, joint stability, precision, muscle stamina, coordination, and balance.

Pilates breathing is performed as an inhale through the nose and an exhale through pursed lips. Different from yoga, and more akin to the breath patterns used by singers, Pilates breathing occurs via rib cage excursion posterior and laterally. Such breathing facilitates extremity motion and natural movements of the spine on inhalation and exhalation. It also helps to prevent Valsalva, promote relaxation, and encourage concentration.

Pilates consists of more than 500 beginning to advanced exercises that are performed on mats or machines in supine, prone, sidelying, four-point, kneeling, and standing positions. On the mat, the extremities and torso provide resistance. Some of the most popular machines are the Universal Reformer, the stability chair, and the Cadillac, which rely on a system of cables and springs to provide resistance and guide range of motion.

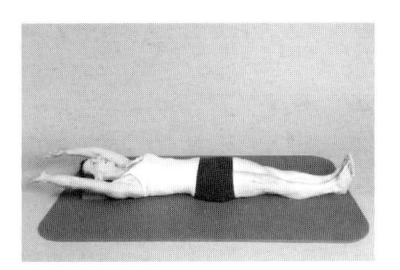

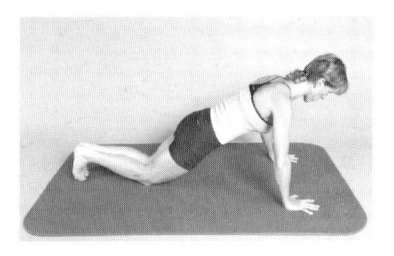

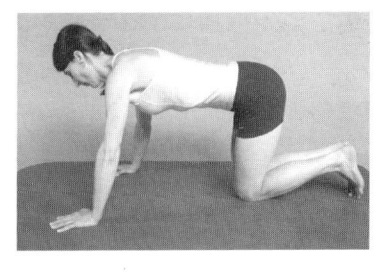

Fundamental Pilates exercises emphasize stability while advanced exercises build on stability to promote mobility, balance, coordination, and muscle stamina. In recent years, Pilates mat exercises have been introduced with equipment that includes stability balls, small balls, exercise bands, wooden dowels, balance boards, and foam rollers.

Equipment such as exercise bands, foam rollers, and stability balls can increase exercise challenge and reinforce fundamental Pilates principles of movement awareness.

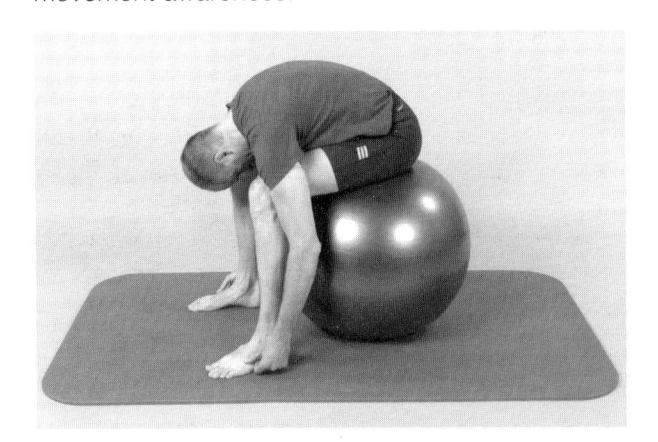

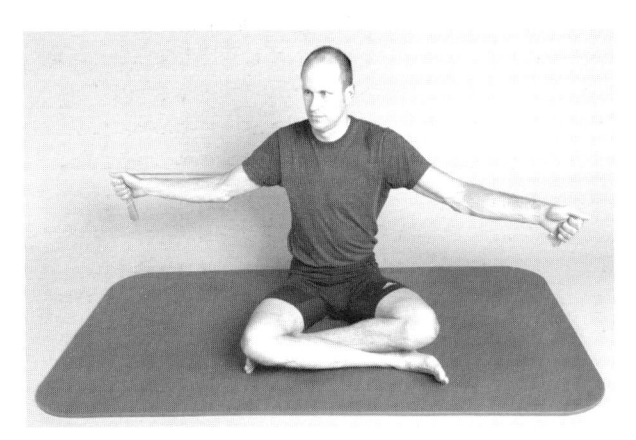

An Evolution in Thinking

Since its inception and coinciding with improved science of movement, Pilates has evolved. Today, Pilates training and education centers across the country have developed their unique approach to the work, while other schools of thought adhere to the classic Pilates teachings. Some instructors use Pilates as a method of torso stability training and as an adjunct to functional training. Others adhere to a therapeutic approach, while still others maintain a technique-driven, dynamic movement methodology.

The position of the pelvis during exercises is a differentiating point among the many methodologies. While Pilates' original intent of spinal and joint mobility remains, some newer methods emphasize a neutral spine and pelvis alignment in all exercises, while others encourage a posterior tilt or a combination of both (4). Some schools of thought promote early TrA pre-contraction in preparation for movement.

Canada-based STOTT Pilates and Florida-based Polestar Education in particular have developed "principles of core stabilization" that emphasize proper alignment of the cervical, thoracic, and lumbar spine as well as scapular and rib cage positioning. Doing so suggests enhanced kinesthetic awareness and encourages appropriate neuromuscular training, which has implications for functional movement (4).

Whatever the philosophy or style, it is important to remember that Pilates is meant to complement fitness and rehabilitation programs, invigorate the body, and stimulate the mind, as Joseph Pilates originally intended. Practitioners must find a methodology that works best for those who are in their care and reflects the latest in research-supported exercise techniques. We present an evidence base in later chapters and propose an approach for you.

There are many training centers, schools, and resources that can help you expand your knowledge and use of Pilates in a rehabilitation setting. Here are a few to get you started:

Pilates Method Alliance™:
  www.pilatesmethodalliance.com
Polestar Education®: www.polestareducation.com
STOTT Pilates™: www.stottpilates.com
PhysicalMind Institute®:
  www.themethodpilates.com

Pilates for Strengthening, Musculoskeletal Awareness

Pilates is a departure from traditional rehabilitation programs where the focus is muscular isolation. Most Pilates exercises integrate the entire body, training several areas of the body at one time through stabilization and mobilization.

Each Pilates exercise has a muscular focus (mobilization, stability, stamina, balance) that is supported by the rest of the musculoskeletal system. Repetitions are low, usually six to 10. This, in juxtaposition to traditional, therapeutic, isolative, high-repetition strengthening, has implications for increased compliance as well as transfer to functional activities where the musculoskeletal system is an integrated chain spanning foot to head (4).

Pilates emphasizes quality over quantity. Precision and control contribute to quality of movement. With this emphasis on quality of motion and technique, muscles are worked to fatigue in less time and with less repetition.

Pilates offers patients other benefits, including accessibility and safety. Resistance and machines are not required to perform Pilates exercise, which may help patients who lack the confidence or strength to use resistance or who may not have access to traditional weight training tools such as free weights, resistance tubing, and cable/pulley systems (4).

Perhaps most important, Pilates introduces rehabilitation professionals and their patients to a methodology that emphasizes movement awareness. Broken down to fundamental movement patterns, Pilates can help your patients learn how to move with proper form, efficiency, and safety.

Pilates as Core Training

As an exercise regimen that is also recognized as core training or torso stabilization, many Pilates methods focus on training the spine and pelvis to neutral, the body's strongest position. Neutral positioning helps minimize strain on soft tissues and the spine and ultimately helps the body work more effectively and safely. To this end, Pilates strengthens and lengthens the muscles of the core so that they can support the spine and pelvis. People who perform Pilates exercises can apply the principles of core training to everyday movements of life, work, and athletics.

Stability to Mobility

From our experience, contemporary approaches to Pilates seek to stabilize the pelvis, spine, and shoulder girdle in single planes of natural, flowing motion. Beginner exercises are usually performed supine or prone. The torso remains still via the core stabilizers while the arms and legs move in patterns.

Once torso stabilization and control of the body is mastered, exercises then advance to multiplanar, multi-articular movements that increase dynamically in effort by integrating the upper and lower body without compromising form. Lumbo-pelvic stability is challenged by taking away stability points, such as a leg or arm, or by performing exercises in sidelying, kneeling, and upright positions. The concept of stability before mobility will be addressed further in Chapter 3.

Pilates exercises challenge stability by removing stability points and encouraging proper form and alignment.

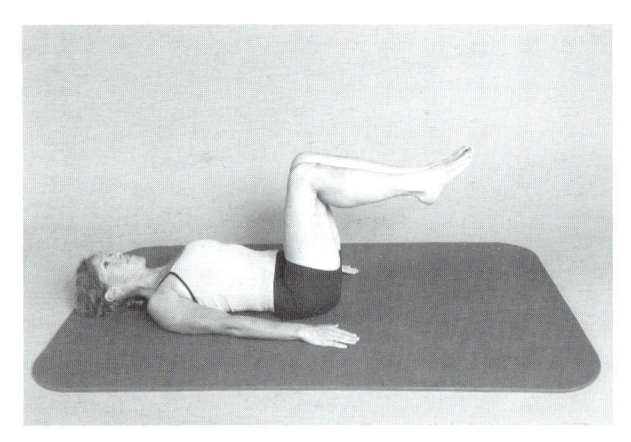

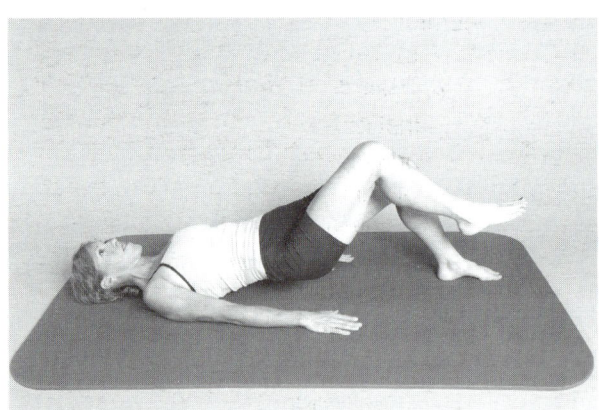

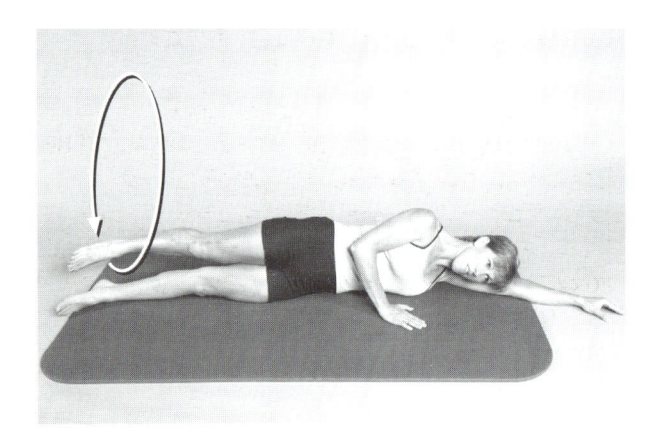

A Mind-Body Challenge

Concentration is a central Pilates tenet, bringing together mind and body to create an overall regime that complements traditional rehabilitation therapies and strength and cardiovascular training. For some, Pilates practice is meditative: the combination of breath and flowing motion is relaxing. For others, the mind-body connection comes from the challenge of coordinating complex neuromuscular patterns, requiring significant concentration. Still others are physically challenged to work the body intensely, necessitating mental preparation.

Pilates: What Can It Do for You and Your Patients?

Let us count the ways Pilates can be beneficial: Improved posture and kinesthetic awareness. Compliance. Concentration. Enhanced strength. Improved movement and breathing. Increased coordination. Neuromuscular reeducation. Pilates is all this and more, benefiting people young and old and from all walks of life.

Most people need three to five practice sessions to determine if Pilates is a fit for them. Initially, Pilates can seem fairly technical. Coupled with breathing, the new terminology and mechanics of moving in a coordinated fashion can be overwhelming.

The same can be said for rehabilitation specialists who see value in Pilates personally but cannot imagine incorporating it into traditional rehabilitation therapies. It is being done with success! The key is to understand the fundamental philosophies behind the mechanics of Pilates and apply those philosophies to the rehabilitation mission: to restore function.

Pilates mastery comes with practice, commitment, patience, and the ongoing discovery of many deep muscles that help patients perform activities of daily living (ADLs), work, and sports. In time, your patients can expect to feel stronger, more self-aware, and hopefully be on the road to healing.

Using This Guidebook

While the Pilates methodology and principles can be applied to all traditional rehabilitation programs, many Pilates exercises are not appropriate or are contraindicated for patients who are recovering from injury or have an existing health condition.

We've teased out specific Pilates exercises you can easily incorporate into a rehabilitation setting. Most are simple to perform and remember, helping to increase patient compliance. Many provide a foundation on which to layer other exercises. Some may resemble exercises you already use, and the difference will be in the application of Pilates-based principles. Others will be unlike anything you've seen before.

To tailor your rehabilitation program, look at the clinical application and patient populations for each exercise. It is not inclusive but will give you a starting point from which to work.

Early book chapters provide an overview of Pilates from the eye of a rehabilitation specialist and suggest fundamental exercises and principles that, ideally, patients will master before advancing to more challenging exercises. Later chapters address specific exercises for the upper and lower extremities and give you ideas for using equipment that you already have at your disposal.

Use this book as a reference guide to adding Pilates exercises to your patient's rehabilitation program. We've also included information we hope you'll find useful in your practice, such as how to use visual imagery to enhance

Tips for Integrating Pilates into a Rehabilitation Program

The beauty of Pilates is that it can be customized to the needs and conditions of your patients and can be practiced at home. With or without equipment, Pilates offers rehabilitation specialists wide-ranging exercises that can expand the therapeutic repertoire.

That said, there are a couple of things to note about introducing Pilates into a rehabilitation program.

- Pilates exercises are usually performed without shoes and socks. Sensory feedback from the feet helps patients to more fully experience the movement. Some patients may be reluctant to remove socks, and we generally accommodate their wishes.
- For anyone starting to explore the world of Pilates, it's normal to experience neck tension and calf or foot cramping, often the result of muscles unaccustomed to this type of movement or improper technique. More than 70 percent of Pilates exercises are performed with the head elevated off the floor, which can lead to neck discomfort in some patients. Teaching patients how to "reach or lengthen" from the hip and shoulder, instead of from the knee or elbow, is something that can benefit your populations. Modify appropriately (see next bullet).
- Relative to neck tension, retrained muscles will soon be sufficiently strengthened to tolerate Pilates-based movement patterns. Rehabilitation therapists should suggest movement modifications or variations based on faulty recruitment patterns of the deep neck flexors or faulty cervical spine alignment, such as keeping the head on the floor, using a hand for support, or using towels and pillows to help relieve tension.
- Some patients initially may experience headaches or nausea. This can be prevented by encouraging patients to start slowly and by avoiding breathing patterns that can lead to hyperventilation. Some patients will find it helpful to come to therapy with a semi-empty stomach and to support the head with a small pillow or towel.

Chapter References

1. Gallagher, S.P., Kryzanowska, R. 2000. *The Complete Writings of Joseph H. Pilates.* Philadelphia, PA: Bain Bridge Books.

2. Vogel, A. 2001. Core Conditioning Takes Center Stage. *Idea Health & Fitness Source*, March, pp. 32-38.

3. Hulme, J.A. 1999. Beyond Kegels: Assessment and Treatment of Incontinence, Course Manual, Minneapolis, MN, February 19-20, p. 13.

4. Anderson, B.D., Spector, A. 2000. Introduction to Pilates-Based Rehabilitation. *Orthopaedic Physical Therapy Clinics of North America* 9(3): 395-410.

chapter 2

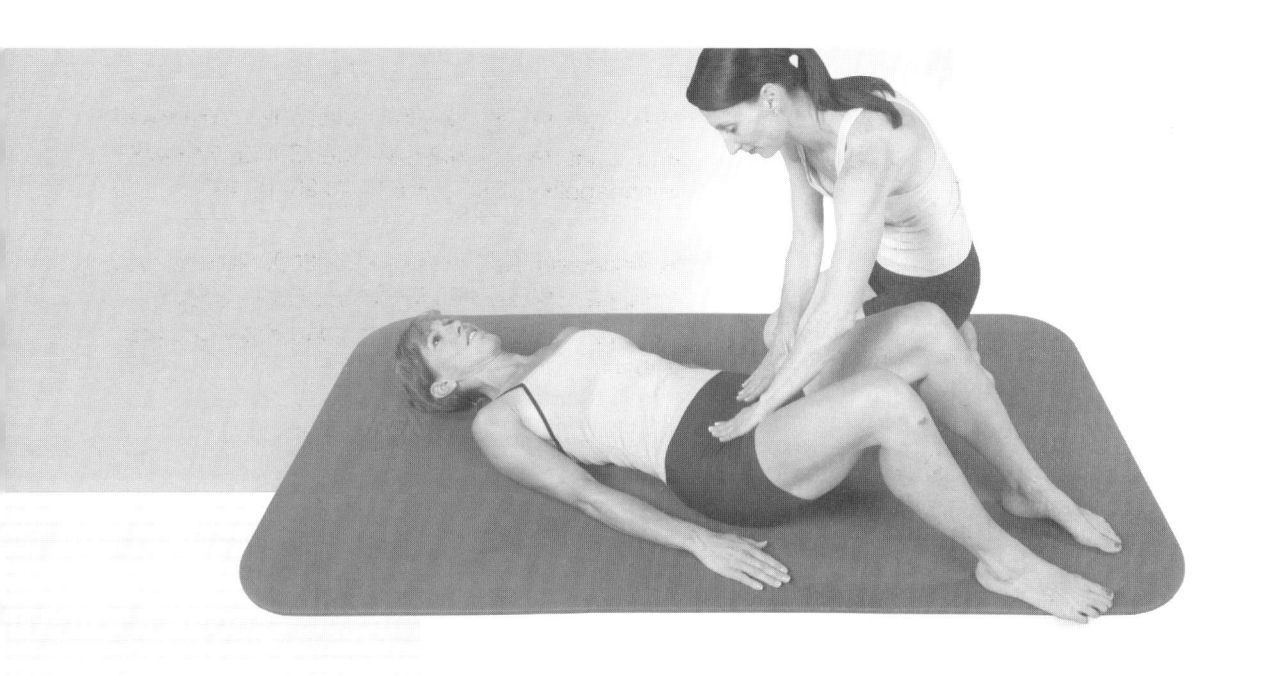

A Clinical Foundation for Applying Pilates in Rehabilitation

Rehabilitation professionals are increasingly taking advantage of core strengthening and torso stabilization exercises to treat many types of musculoskeletal dysfunctions. From a Pilates perspective, it's important that rehabilitation professionals understand the clinical value of the regimen as a core-strengthening regimen and as a method of restoring muscle balance and function, proprioception, and proper joint function. Key is education about its appropriate clinical use (1).

Our early Pilates training defined the "powerhouse" of the body as the abdominals, low back muscles, gluteals, and hamstrings. After much discussion and frequent reviews of current literature, we now refer to the powerhouse as the abdominals, erector spinae, pelvic floor, diaphragm, multifidus, quadratus lumborum, and gluteus maximus and medius. Muscles that support the powerhouse include the hip adductors and the scapulae stabilizers. These muscles work together in an integrated fashion to support the spine and safe, efficient movement patterns.

Although there is no significant research supporting Pilates, there are conceptual frameworks and a plethora of research in the literature that lays a clinical foundation for Pilates-based exercise. We encourage you to develop your own thoughts about this practice based on current, leading-edge thinking and advocate for increased research efforts into this important work.

Spinal and Pelvic Stabilization: The Conceptualized Framework

Panjabi created the conceptual framework for spinal stabilization, defining it as a system that could be delineated into specific subsystems that are interdependent: passive, active, and neural (2). To keep the spine in equilibrium, the spinal ligaments, articulations, and bones of the passive subsystem work with the active subsystem, which includes muscles and tendons, and the neural subsystem, which is composed of the central nervous system and nerves. When there is dysfunction in one of the subsystems, stabilization of the spine is affected secondary to adaptations in one or both of the other subsystems (2).

How does Pilates dovetail with Panjabi's thought process? There is coordination of the active and neural systems with Pilates-based training, minimizing stress on the passive subsystem. In other words, the focus is restoration of neutral spine.

Panjabi also provided evidence that the spine's neutral zone exists when an area of normal intervertebral motion occurs; there is minimal stress to the passive subsystem and the spine is in equilibrium. He hypothesized that clinical instability occurs when there is an increase in the neutral zone and an inability to maintain normal intervertebral motion with spinal dysfunction (3).

There was supporting evidence for his theory with an increase in neutral zone leading to spinal injury, disc degeneration, and muscle weakness, but it was not conclusive (3). It was also hypothesized that increasing trunk muscle strength when clinical instability exists could help restore normal intervertebral motion in the neutral zone, but further research is warranted (3). This supports Pilates as it relates to restoration of spinal stability.

Since then, other conceptual models for pelvic girdle stabilization have been introduced. For example, Snijders and Vleeming identified a pelvic girdle stabilization model of the sacroiliac joint that included components of the osteo-ligamentous and muscle systems to provide stability through form and force closure mechanisms (4,5).

Spinal stabilization can also be defined from a muscular perspective and continues to be an area of debate as to what particular muscles are core stabilizers. Bergmark defined the muscles of spinal stabilization as either local or global systems according to anatomical location and function (6). Under his definition, muscles of the local system include the transversus abdominis (TrA), lumbar multifidus, interspinal, intertransverse, internal oblique (IO) via thoracolumbar fascia attachments, and lumbar portions of the iliocostalis and longissimus muscles, which contribute to intervertebral stiffness and regulation of intervertebral motion for spinal stabilization (6). The global muscles are spinal mobilizers and trunk stabilizers that consist of the lateral portion of the quadratus lumborum, thoracic portions of the iliocostalis and longissimus, rectus abdominis, and external and internal oblique muscles (6). They assist with force transference between the ribs and the pelvis (6).

Richardson and Hodges et al. identified a conceptual model for teaching lumbo-pelvic stabilization with focus on the musculofascial complex spanning from ribs to pelvis (7,8). Muscles of this model are categorized as the inner or outer unit (7,8). Muscles of the inner unit include the transversus abdominis, pelvic floor, diaphragm, and multifidus and provide lumbar segmental stabilization through their synergistic action as evidenced in the literature (7,8). Outer unit muscles contribute to general trunk stabilization and should be trained after the inner unit. Lee also performs training per this model but defines the outer unit, also known as the global system, as composed of four systems that have fascial and muscular components of the lumbo-pelvic-hip complex that contribute to general trunk stabilization (9,10).

Trunk Muscle Strengthening

Trunk muscle strengthening, also referred to as core strengthening, torso stability, abdominal bracing, motor control training, and dynamic stabilization, has historically been applied to spinal injury rehabilitation. Such strengthening is now more mainstream as therapeutic consideration shifts to applying stabilization training to extremity rehabilitation. Clinically, torso stability or core training is increasingly turned to today as an adjunct to conventional therapies for reducing the occurrence and recurrence of injury and improving functional movement, proprioception, coordination, and balance (1).

Core strengthening is purported to reduce injury rates and risk and lead to more efficient, powerful movement, particularly in athletes. There are few studies supporting these assertions (11), but research has demonstrated that neuromuscular control of the torso can impact balance, joint stability, and proprioception training via muscle co-contractions (12).

Kavcic, Grenier, and McGill looked at several muscles that contribute to spinal stability with trunk strengthening exercises. They found that no one specific muscle was superior in contributing to lumbo-pelvic stability and that the role of core stabilizing muscles changed depending on the movement pattern (13,14).

Modern-day thinking generally defines the powerhouse or "core" as muscles of the lumbo-pelvic and thoracic regions. Our definition is evidence-based and generally refers to the muscles that span from the rib cage to the lumbo-pelvic-hip complex. The core includes but is not limited to such muscles as the transversus abdominis, lumbar multifidus, pelvic floor, and diaphragm (local muscles), as well as the rectus abdominis, internal and external obliques, gluteus maximus and medius, and hip adductors, quadratus lumborum, and erector spinae (global muscles). The ability to stabilize the torso depends on the ability of the local and global muscles to work together synergistically in all planes of movement.

Global Muscles

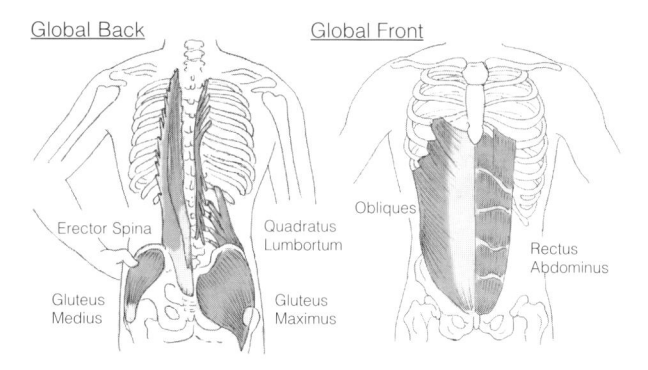

Global Back — Erector Spina, Quadratus Lumbortum, Gluteus Medius

Global Front — Obliques, Rectus Abdominus, Gluteus Maximus

Local Muscles

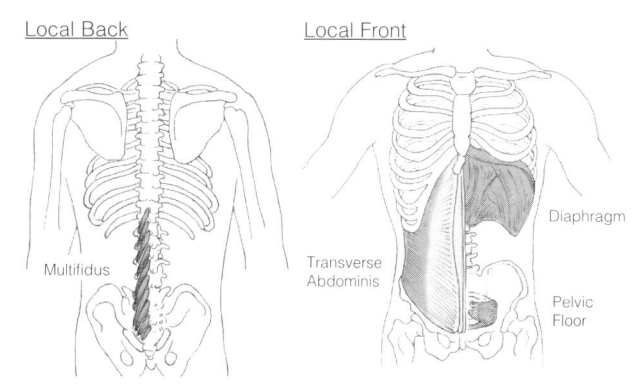

Local Back — Multifidus

Local Front — Diaphragm, Transverse Abdominis, Pelvic Floor

Evidence Base to Support Pilates-Based Rehabilitation

With today's emphasis on evidence-based research in clinical practice, it is crucial for clinicians to familiarize themselves with core stabilization and Pilates-based research as well as evolving research in both areas to support the use of Pilates in rehabilitation. It can also help to educate physicians, other medical professionals, and patients.

Research in the area of core stabilization draws from various areas that include anatomy, biomechanics, low back dysfunction, and exercise (11). Among researchers who are contributing to the body of knowledge about core stabilization and training in musculoskeletal rehabilitation are Panjabi, McGill, Hodges, Vleeming, Sapsford, Richardson, and O'Sullivan.

McGill's work supports abdominal bracing or fixing the rib cage over the pelvis with co-activation patterns of the abdominals and the spinal extensors. Relative to low back dysfunction, Hodges and Richardson et al. and others have demonstrated that neuromuscular reeducation of the TrA is an effective treatment strategy for low back pain (7-10,15,16).

Listed here is a sampling of evidence-based research in the area of core stabilization that supports Pilates-based training with rehabilitation of musculoskeletal dysfunction. We've selected research that focuses on various areas contributing to spinal stabilization and efficient transfer of energy to the full kinetic chain in preparation for movement. Use this information as a starting point and continue to examine the research as it evolves, especially in the area of Pilates-based training for musculoskeletal dysfunction.

Transversus Abdominis (TrA)

Literature supporting the role of the TrA as a contributor to lumbo-pelvic stabilization at a segmental level is vast (17).

- The TrA is recruited prior to other abdominals with external forces on the trunk without anticipation or force application with anticipation, indicating that TrA contraction may be volitional (18);
- TrA facilitation is not dependent on trunk movement and remains active irrespective of trunk motion (19);
- TrA contraction occurs before other trunk muscles irrespective of upper (20) or lower (21) limb movement, indicating feedforward muscle activation of the TrA; and
- TrA activation is not dependent on directional changes of upper (20) or lower limb movement (21).

There is little discussion in Pilates' writings about the role of the TrA as a contributor to the method. Some Pilates training centers are increasing their emphasis on TrA activation in exercise performance, but practitioner training methods are wide ranging, and some researchers in this area are questioning the appropriateness of this type of training.

What does the research demonstrate? The TrA is a muscle that contributes to local spine stabilization and assists other large muscle groups in force transference through the spine. It does not perform rotary movements, nor is its function to flex or extend the spine, but it performs a stabilization role in these movement patterns. Global trunk muscles that include the erector spinae, obliques, rectus abdominis and quadratus lumborum work hard to stabilize the spine in the three planes of motion. The strongest spine is one that recruits many muscles, not just a few.

Reeducation of the TrA is appropriate as a corrective exercise for low back dysfunction where lumbo-pelvic stability is compromised, as demonstrated by Hodges, Richardson, and others. Further research in weight-bearing, functional movement patterns is needed. Training the TrA for voluntary contraction when it is already functioning normally may be inappropriate and could lead to low back dysfunction (13). We encourage consideration of the current literature and your therapeutic judgment in working with your patient.

Lumbar Multifidus (LM)

Research shows that the lumbar multifidus (LM) contributes to lumbar stability via segmental stiffening. In a biomechanical study, Wilkes et al. demonstrated that the LM increased intervertebral stiffness by more than two-thirds at the L4-L5 segments with contraction (22). Further evidence of the multifidus' role as a spinal stabilizer was noted by Moseley et al. where intervertebral movement was controlled via the deep fibers of the multifidus (23).

Pelvic Floor (PF)

The pelvic floor has a unique contribution to spinal stabilization via its neurophysiologic connection to the TrA, as evidenced by Sapsford, Richardson, and others (24,25). Lee indicates that initial research by Sapsford et al. examining the relationship between the pelvic floor and abdominals demonstrates a natural co-activation pattern between the abdominals and pelvic floor with volitional activation of the abdominals. It was hypothesized that selective activation of the TrA co-activated the pubococcygeus, but further research was needed (9).

These early findings were later substantiated by Sapsford et al., who explored co-activation of the pelvic floor muscles with volitional submaximal abdominal activation in either a hollowing or bracing manner, with or without breath. Abdominal bracing without breath showed the greatest increase in pubococcygeus activity (24).

Sapsford et al. also showed evidence that supports a co-activation pattern of the abdominals with maximal pelvic floor contraction regardless of pelvic position. External oblique activity was greatest when the pelvis was in a posterior tilt; TrA activity increased over other abdominals with the pelvis tilted anteriorly and a submaximal PF contraction (24). Although further research is needed, it suggests a preprogrammed abdominal response that occurs independent of pelvic position. The evidence is limited secondary to the size of the study and the lack of statistical support by Sapsford suggesting that volitional submaximal pelvic floor contraction selectively facilitates the TrA regardless of pelvic position (24). Later research by Sapsford and Hodges did provide evidence that pelvic floor muscles are co-activated with a conscious abdominal contraction (25).

What is the clinical relevance of this research? The pelvic floor can be used as a method of TrA reeducation when TrA dysfunction exists. A submaximal pelvic floor contraction is recommended to selectively activate TrA (8).

Diaphragm

There is growing evidence that the diaphragm contributes to more than just breathing. In fact, evidence suggests that the diaphragm is important to spinal stabilization via an increase in intra-abdominal pressure (IAP). Early experimental research by Cresswell et al. found that TrA activation increased IAP with isometric trunk loading and demonstrated potential contributions to trunk stabilization (19). Research by Hodges et al. evaluated diaphragmic contraction with postural adjustments (26). Findings showed a simultaneous pre-anticipatory activation of the diaphragm and TrA prior to upper limb movement, indicating this may be a preprogrammed action to help with torso stabilization (26). Further research by Hodges and Gandevia showed that the TrA and the diaphragm continually work to control trunk movement and the breathing cycle during movement of the extremities (27).

Breathing

Breathing is a fundamental Pilates principle. Pilates endorsed active inhalation and exhalation from a perspective of cleansing the lungs, but today's research goes far beyond this, demonstrating a link between breathing and torso stability. Research also questions the appropriateness of active inhalation, suggesting that such a pattern of active exhalation can lead to early and overrecruitment of the external obliques (7).

Hip

Research also demonstrates that the muscles of the hip are key to torso stabilization and in force transference from the legs to the trunk in daily activity (28). In vivo research by Van Windergerden and Vleeming showed that muscles of the lumbo-pelvic-hip complex consisting of the biceps femoris, gluteus maximus, and erector spinae contribute to sacroiliac joint stability via force closure mechanisms and supports current thinking about force transference from hip to spine (29).

Thoracolumbar Fascia

The thoracolumbar fascia also has unique contributions to stabilization of the spine, pelvis, and the kinetic chain. In particular, the muscle fibers of the TrA have multiple attachments to the lumbar vertebrae via the middle and posterior layers of the thoracolumbar fascia. Hodges and Richardson found evidence that TrA facilitation contributed to spinal stiffness with increasing thoracolumbar tightening and intra-abdominal pressure (30). Evidence has also shown that the thoracolumbar fascia may contribute to lumbar and pelvic girdle stabilization to move force from the pelvis to the lower extremities efficiently (31).

Musculoskeletal Dysfunction and Spinal Stability

Most of the research exploring musculoskeletal dysfunction and core stabilization centers around low back pain. For example, research indicates that TrA recruitment is delayed and can affect motor and postural control (30, 32-34).

Research is starting to focus on other areas that include the hip and proprioception relative to spinal stabilization. Cowan et al. showed that delayed TrA muscle recruitment occurs with long-standing groin pain, but further research is warranted (35).

Research by Mok et al. provided initial evidence that lack of postural control at the hip occurs as a result of compromised balance and muscle control in subjects with low back pain (36).

As stated earlier, reeducation of the TrA is appropriate as a corrective exercise for low back pain where lumbo-pelvic stability may be compromised due to a faulty recruitment pattern (7-10, 15,16). Further research in weight-bearing, functional movement patterns is needed. Training the TrA for voluntary contraction when it is already functioning normally may be inappropriate and could lead to spinal muscle imbalances (13).

Postural Retraining
Clinicians work with patients to retrain proper posture for ADLs, work, and sport during the rehabilitation process, but is there really carryover? Short term? Long term?

Research by O'Sullivan et al. demonstrated that core stabilizing muscles consisting of the erector spinae, superficial multifidus, and internal obliques increased firing with neutral spine in standing and sitting alignment and decreased firing with swayback posture and slumped sitting (37). How do these findings relate to Pilates-based training? Pilates-based training enhances postural retraining through restoration of normal postural alignment by neuromuscular reeducation of muscle imbalances and core strength to support posture with stationary and mobile positions. Furthermore, postural retraining occurs with each Pilates-based movement pattern to some degree, enhancing spinal elongation and kinesthetic awareness. There is conscious control. Is there carryover to changes in posture? The answer is yes.

In general, the individual that performs Pilates-based training consistently will note changes in posture as early as six to eight weeks after starting a program. The key to this change is compliance. If you do not use it, you will lose it.

Training the Core
Some of the best positions for initially teaching patients to develop core muscles include supine, prone, quadruped, and sidelying positions while maintaining neutral spine and pelvis. Doing so has been shown to best demonstrate neuromuscular reeducation of the TrA, reduce tension of overactive muscles around the lumbo-pelvic area, and maximize movement patterning in the extremities (8).

Because functional movement generally occurs in gravity-based positions such as standing or sitting and moves the spine through neutral to nonneutral positions, it is important to transition patients to weight-bearing positions once the local and global muscles have been appropriately trained and recruited and patients have been taught to stabilize the spine in more stable positions. Transitioning from prone and supine positions to weight-bearing is a logical progression once stability is mastered.

Core Strength Training in the Aging Adult
A handful of studies examining older adults and trunk muscle strength, stability, gait, and posture do not focus on core strengthening as a movement prescription or for reducing injury risk. In one of the few to examine trunk muscle strength in older adults and its relationship to osteoporosis, fractures, and falls, Pfeifer et al. showed that osteoporosis in postmenopausal women is associated with trunk muscle strength and bone mineral density, where trunk muscles were defined as the abdominal flexors and lumbar extensors (1,40). The same study established body sway as a fall risk factor.

Increasing core strength may help reduce the impact of muscle- and joint-related changes associated with age: torso stability and strength, posture, balance, reaction time, gait, and coordination. Although research is needed, a strong core may transfer to increased efficient use of the lower and upper extremities and increased balance, which are crucial elements for traditional strength training, ADL instruction, and injury prevention in older adults (1).

A Theoretical Framework for Using Pilates to Develop Core Strength

From a theoretical perspective, integrating Pilates-based fundamental movement patterns and exercises that emphasize proper alignment and torso stability into rehabilitation programs can complement treatment plans in a number of ways for patients young to old, athlete to nonathlete, sedentary worker to manual laborer.

- Normalize and enhance muscle recruitment patterns
- Identify and correct faulty movement pattern(s)
- Increase segmental spinal stabilization
- Use as an adjunct to manual therapy to improve mobility and neuromuscular control of hypomobile segment(s)
- Improve postural alignment
- Develop kinesthetic awareness
- Restore or reteach hip and shoulder movement independent of pelvic or spinal motion
- Improve breathing mechanics
- Improve functional movement, proprioception, and balance through neuromuscular reeducation
- Enhance stabilization with traditional strength training and flexibility exercises

Lumbo-pelvic stability in single-joint and single-planar exercises and breathing technique should be emphasized first, with progression to multijoint and multiplanar movement patterns that stretch and strengthen muscles.

A Motor Learning Framework

Pilates-based training can enhance motor learning and sensory-motor development through specific exercise goals that challenge stability, coordination, balance, and muscle stamina.

According to accepted motor development theory, motor learning coordinates with sensory processes of the nervous system that include tactile, proprioceptive, and vestibular. Sensory integration is the ability of the brain to process and organize sensory stimulation through touch, vision, sound, movement, and body position in space, facilitating motor planning or the body's adaptive response to movement (38). This adaptive response, also known as motor learning, generally progresses in three phases or stages: the cognitive, associative, and automatic learning phases (39). This model has been used successfully to manage patients with chronic low back pain where the focus is lumbo-pelvic stabilization for spinal stability (39).

<u>Cognitive Phase:</u> In the cognitive or early learning phase, the overall goal is to gain understanding of the movement or skill and, through trial and error, develop strategies that allow for successful mastery of the movement pattern. Movement is typically disorganized and clumsy. Learning is visual, and repetition is necessary to stimulate sensory-motor components. The length of this phase is about three to six weeks (39).

Associative Phase: Movement in the associative phase is more coordinated and is performed with less clumsiness. Patients are more kinesthetically adept, are able to respond more quickly to tactile cues, and are able to focus on movement performance rather than on what movement to perform. Learning in this phase often depends on the nature of the exercise, the motivation and experience of the patient, and the teaching strategies of the rehabilitation therapist. The length of this stage varies from eight weeks to four months (39).

Autonomous Phase: In this phase, movement is highly coordinated and very refined. Movements are now "automatic," and the patient doesn't have to concentrate to perform a movement pattern, regardless of environment (39).

Applying the Motor Learning Framework to Pilates

Motor learning concepts and motor patterns can be applied within the framework of Pilates.

Cognitive Phase: Patients focus on developing breathing skills, learning gross movement patterns, and targeting key muscles while isolating the movement of the hips and shoulders independent of the lumbo-pelvic area.

For patients to develop movement isolation skills or dissociation, they must understand the purpose and benefit of the movement: Why am I doing this? How will this help me? The role of the clinician is to observe quality of movement and make modifications with emphasis on visual imagery and hands-on cueing. The principles of stabilization in Chapter 4 and the fundamental exercises in Chapter 6 are best suited to the cognitive phase of learning.

Associative Phase: Patients master breathing and such isolation skills as abdominal bracing and pelvic positioning with a focus on refining gross movement patterns and coordinating isolated movement patterns.

The key components of this stage include identifying compensatory movement pattern(s) in the exercise and breaking down faulty movement into smaller components to train isolated movement. Patients must be able to proprioceptively sense compensatory or faulty movement patterns and, once they have mastered the isolated skill, coordinate it with others. The exercises in Chapters 7 and 8 are best suited to the associative phase of motor learning.

Autonomous Phase: Patients require a low degree of attention to correct performance of the motor task and demonstrate the ability to master fine movement patterns. Most are able to perform dynamic, functional movements that emphasize coordination of the upper and lower extremities while maintaining core stability. The exercises in Chapters 7 and 8 are best suited to this phase of motor learning.

In summary, moving forward, the challenge for Pilates practitioners is to initiate and publish research supporting Pilates not only as a viable methodology for rehabilitation, but for core stability training. An excellent research foundation exists, and we are missing an opportunity to expand the knowledge base leading to improved patient outcomes if we do not.

Chapter References

1. Smith, K.A., and Smith, E. 2005. Integrating Pilates-based core strengthening into older adult fitness programs: Implications for practice. *Topics in Geriatric Rehabilitation* 21(1): 57-67.

2. Panjabi, M.M. 1992. The stabilizing system of the spine. Part I. Function, dysfunction, adaptation and enhancement. *J Spinal Disord* 5(4): 383-389.

3. Panjabi, M.M. 1992. The stabilizing system of the spine. Part II. Neutral zone and instability hypothesis. *J Spinal Disord* 5(4): 390-397.

4. Snijders, C.J., Vleeming, A., Stoeckart, R. 1993a. Transfer of lumbosacral load to iliac bones and legs. 1: Biomechanics of self-bracing of the sacroiliac joints and its significance for treatment and exercise. *Clinical Biomechanics* 8: 285-294.

5. Snijders, C.J., Vleeming, A., Stoeckart, R. 1993b. Transfer of lumbosacral load to iliac bones and legs. 2: Loading of the sacroiliac joints when lifting in a stooped posture. *Clinical Biomechanics* 8: 295-301.

6. Bergmark, A. 1989. The local and the global systems. *Acta Orthop Scand 6* (suppl. 230): 20-24.

7. Richardson, C., Jull, G., Hodges, P., Hides, J. 1999. *Therapeutic Exercise for Spinal Segmental Stabilization in Low Back Pain: Scientific Basis and Clinical Approach.* Edinburgh, U.K.: Churchill Livingstone.

8. Hodges, P. 2002. Science of Stability: Clinical Application to Assessment and Treatment of Segmental Spinal Stabilization for Low Back Pain, Course Manual. Bloomington, MN, October 4-5.

9. Lee, D. 1999. *The Pelvic Girdle: An Approach to the Examination and Treatment of the Lumbo-Pelvic-Hip Region.* Edinburgh, U.K.: Churchill Livingstone.

10. Lee, D. 2003. The Pelvis—Bridging the Gap Between the Science and the Clinic, Course Manual. Edina, MN, October 4-5.

11. Akuthota, V., Nadler, S.F. 2004. Core strengthening. *Arch Phys Med Rehabil* 85(3 Suppl. 1): S86-92.

12. Caraffa, A., Cerulli, G., Projetti, M., Aisa, G., Rizzo, A. 1996. Prevention of anterior cruciate ligament injuries in soccer. A prospective controlled study of proprioceptive training. *Knee Surg Sports Traumatol Arthrosc* 4: 19-21.

13. McGill, S. 2004. *Ultimate Back Fitness and Performance.* Waterloo, Ontario, Canada: Wabuno Publishers.

14. Kavcic, N., Grenier, S., McGill, S.M. 2004. Determining the stabilizing role of individual torso muscles during rehabilitation exercises. *Spine* 29(11): 1254-1265.

15. O'Sullivan, P.B., Twomey, L.T., Allison, G.T. 1997. Evaluation of specific stabilizing exercise in the treatment of chronic low back pain with radiologic diagnosis of spondylolysis or spondylolisthesis. *Spine* 22(24): 2959-2967.

16. Richardson, C.A., Snijders, C.J., Hides, J.A., Damen, L., Pas, M.S., Storm, J. 2002. The relation between the transversus abdominis muscles, sacroiliac joint mechanics, and low back pain. *Spine* 27(4): 399-405.

17. Hodges, P. 1999. Is there a role for transversus abdominis in lumbo-pelvic stability? *Manual Therapy* 4(2): 74-86.

18. Cresswell, A.G., Oddsson, L., Thorstensson, A. 1994. The influence of sudden perturbations on trunk muscle activity and intra-abdominal pressure while standing. *Exp Brain Res* 98: 336-341.

19. Cresswell, A.G., Grundstrom, H., Thorstensson, A. 1992. Observations on intra-abdominal pressure and patterns of abdominal intra-muscular activity in man. *Acta Physiol Scand* 144: 409-418.

20. Hodges, P.W., Richardson, C.A. 1997. Feedforward contraction of transversus abdominis is not influenced by the direction of arm movement. *Exp Brain Res* 114: 362-370.

21. Hodges, P.W., Richardson, C.A. 1997. Contraction of the abdominal muscles associated with movement of the lower limb. *Physical Therapy* 77(2): 132-143.

22. Wilke, H.J., Wolf, S., Claes, L.E., Arand, M., Wiesend, A. 1995. Stability increase of the lumbar spine with different muscle groups: A biomechanical in vitro study. *Spine* 20(2): 192-198.

23. Moseley, G.L., Hodges, P.W., Gandevia, S.C. 2002. Deep and superficial fibers of the lumbar multifidus muscle are differentially active during voluntary arm movements. *Spine* 27(2): E29-36.

24. Sapsford, R.R., Hodges, P.W., Richardson, C.A., Cooper, D.H., Markwell, S.J., Jull, G.A. 2001. Co-activation of the abdominal and pelvic floor muscles during voluntary exercises. *Neurourology and Urodynamics* 20: 31-42.

25. Sapsford, R.R., Hodges, P.W. 2001. Contraction of the pelvic floor muscles during abdominal maneuvers. *Arch Phys Med Rehabil* 82: 1081-1088.

26. Hodges, P.W., Butler, J.E., McKenzie, D.K., Gandevia, S.C. 1997. Contraction of the human diaphragm during rapid postural adjustments. *Journal of Physiology* 505(2): 539-548.

27. Hodges, P.W., Gandevia, S.C. 2000. Changes in intra-abdominal pressure during postural and respiratory activation of the human diaphragm. *J Appl Physiol* 89: 967-976.

28. Lyons, K., Perry, J., Gronley, J.K., Barnes, L., Antonelli, D. 1983. Timing and relative intensity of hip extensor and abductor muscle action during level and stair ambulation: An EMG study. *Phys Ther* 63: 1597-605.

29. Van Wingerden, J.P., Vleeming, A., Buyruk, H.M., Raissadat, K. 2004. Stabilization of the sacroiliac joint in vivo: Verification of muscular contribution to force closure of the pelvis. *Eur Spine J* 13: 199-205.

30. Hodges, P., Richardson, C. 1996. Inefficient muscular stabilization of the lumbar spine associated with low back pain: A motor control evaluation of transversus abdominis. *Spine* 21(22): 2640-2650.

31. Vleeming, A., Pool-Goudzwaard, A.L., Stoeckart, R., Van Windgerden, J.P., Snijders, C.J. 1995. The posterior layer of the thoracolumbar fascia: Its function in load transfer from spine to legs. *Spine* 20(7): 753-758.

32. Ferreira, P.H., Ferreira, M.L., Hodges, P.W. 2004. Changes in recruitment of the abdominal muscles in people with low back pain: Ultrasound measurement of muscle activity. *Spine* 29(22): 2560-2566.

33. Hodges, P.W., Richardson, C.A. 1998. Delayed postural contraction of transversus abdominis in low back pain associated with movement of the lower limb. *Journal of Spinal Disorders* 11(1): 46-56.

34. Hodges, P.W., Richardson, C.A. 1999. Altered trunk muscle recruitment in people with low back pain with upper limb movement at different speeds. *Arch Phys Med Rehabil* 80: 1005-1012.

35. Cowan, S., Schache, A.G., Brukner, P., Bennell, K., Hodges, P.W., Coburn, P., Crossley, K.M. 2004. Delayed onset of transversus abdominis in long-standing groin pain. *Med Sci Sports Exerc* 36(12): 2040-2045.

36. Mok, N.W., Brauer, S.G., Hodges, P.W. 2004. Hip strategy for balance control in quiet standing is reduced in people with low back pain. *Spine* 29(6): E107-E112.

37. O'Sullivan, P.B., Grahamslaw, K.M., Kendell, M., Lapenskie, S.C., Moller, N.E., Richards, K.V. 2002. The effect of different standing and sitting postures on trunk muscle activity in a pain-free population. *Spine* 27(11): 1238-1244.

38. Sensory Integration International. 1991. A Parent's Guide to Understanding Sensory Integration. Torrance, CA: Author.

39. O'Sullivan, P.B. 2000. Lumbar segmental 'instability' clinical presentation and specific stabilizing exercise management. *Manual Therapy* 5(1): 2-12.

40. Pfeifer, M., Bergerow, B., Minne, H.W., Scholtthauer, T., Pospeschill, M. 2001. Vitamin D status, trunk muscle strength, body sway, falls, and fractures among 237 postmenopausal women with osteoporosis. *Exp Clin Endocrinol Diabetes* 109(2): 87-92.

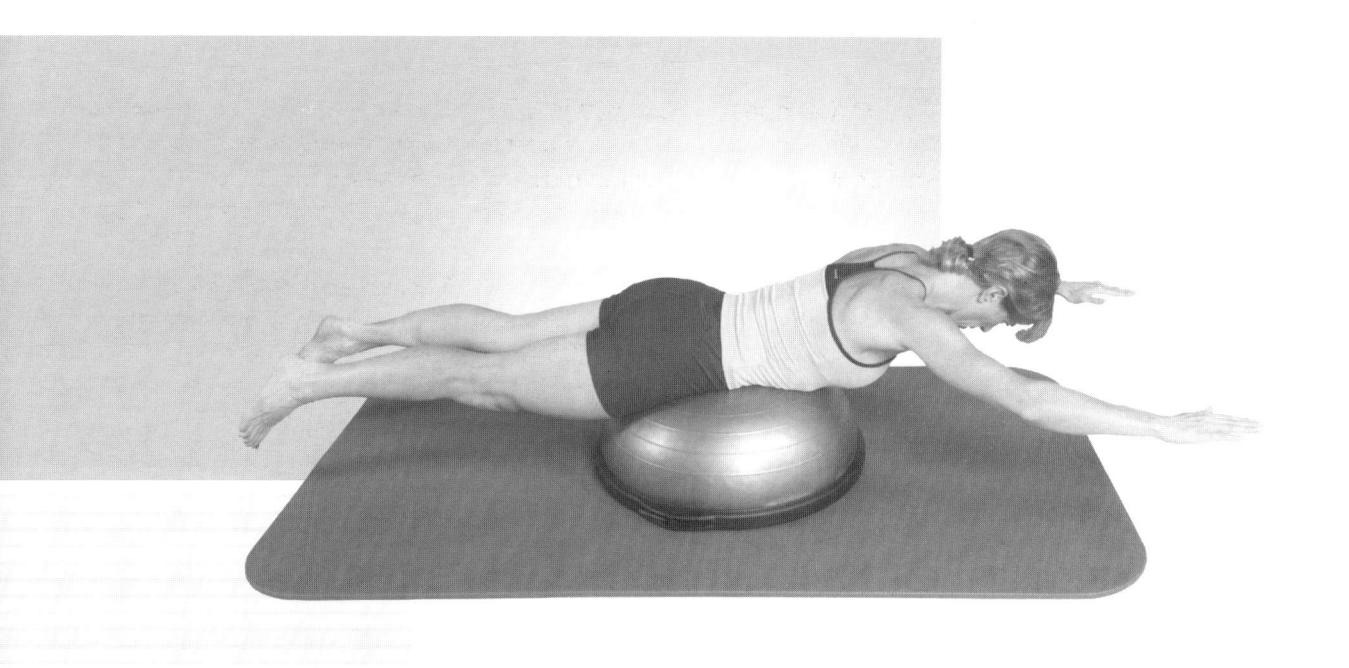

chapter 3

DESIGNING AND
PROGRESSING
TRADITIONAL
REHABILITATION
PROGRAMS USING
PILATES

The Pilates principles and many Pilates-based exercises are great tools for any clinician's toolbox and provide an excellent foundation for corrective exercises meeting your patient's long- and short-term goals. This is particularly true when you first design your patient's rehabilitation program and then progress it when he or she is ready.

The key is knowing what Pilates exercises to use and when and how to progress the patient.

We generally begin by gaining a holistic orthopaedic perspective of our patient, leading to a treatment blueprint. Following are common questions to consider:

- What does the patient's medical history and posture tell you about the quality of movement?
- What muscle imbalances are present and contributing to dysfunction?
- How do identified muscle imbalances correlate with your musculoskeletal evaluation?
- How does the patient move when performing such activities as walking, sitting or standing, or stair climbing?
- Does the patient have sufficient balance? If not, does he or she demonstrate compensatory strategies that might contribute to injury?
- Overall, what is the patient's level of movement awareness?

From Pilates' perspective, you must first know what is incorrect before you can begin to suggest what is correct. Once you've gathered this information, use Pilates as one of many tools to enhance your patient's treatment outcomes, increase home exercise compliance, and decrease the chances of reinjury.

Getting Started: The Medical History

Most clinicians are familiar with the medical history and already complete it as part of routine patient charting. Current and past health status are among the many pieces of information that contribute to the larger rehabilitation puzzle. Screen for risk- or health-related factors that signal red flags and refer your patient to an appropriate medical professional for further assessment. Identify such medical conditions as osteoporosis, spinal stenosis, osteoarthritis, disc degeneration, or Scheuermann's disease that can influence the type of exercises you select to create your patient's custom program.

Other less obvious pieces of information that you might have previously overlooked or discarded as "nonfactors" in your treatment plan can shed light on musculoskeletal dysfunctions.

Such data warrants further evaluation and includes a history of recurring or chronic low back pain, scoliosis, abdominal scarring as the result of a C-section, appendectomy, or hysterectomy, urinary incontinence, pelvic pain, or torso injuries that occurred several years ago (cracked/fractured ribs, etc.). This information can be relevant to your treatment plan because surgery, chronic pain, and other such conditions can affect muscle recruitment patterns in deep stabilizing muscles such as the transversus abdominis.

Common questions in the medical history include, but are not limited to:

- Do you experience urinary "leaking" or dribbling?
- If you have children, were they delivered vaginally or by C-section?
- Have you had surgery of any kind that occurred in the abdominal or low back areas?
- Do you have a history of high blood pressure?

Answers to these questions can provide important clues to creating a blueprint that can help you successfully incorporate Pilates-based principles and exercises into your patient's rehabilitation program.

Musculoskeletal, Posture, and Movement Assessments

Following the medical history, we usually conduct musculoskeletal and movement assessments. Doing so ensures that we are creating a program specific to our patient's needs and abilities.

Muscle imbalances often lie at the heart of musculoskeletal dysfunctions and injuries. Considering that most people's postures are well developed by three years of age, physical therapists and other rehabilitation specialists have a tough but not insurmountable task of helping to restore muscle balance and function.

A successful rehabilitation program begins with understanding your patient's muscle imbalances and the multifactorial causes that may contribute to changes in his or her musculoskeletal system. After all, these muscle imbalances may have contributed to your patient's dysfunction and will certainly be evident in activities of daily living.

What is a muscle imbalance? A muscle imbalance is characterized by changes in the muscle length-tension relationship resulting in changes in muscle force production, faulty muscle recruitment patterns, and weakness, or tightness of specific muscles surrounding a joint. Physical therapy legend Florence Kendall (1) defines muscle imbalances as:

"When disharmony occurs in the tension relationship of muscles acting around a joint. A muscle maintained in a lengthened position becomes weak while the muscle in a shortened positioned becomes stronger than normal."

What are the causes? There are many reasons, among them faulty posture (structural as well as functional), lifestyle, sport and occupational demands, disease, psychological causes, trauma, heredity, and pain associated with joint dysfunction (2).

Will these imbalances respond to musculoskeletal rehabilitation programs? Many do over time. Pilates documented improved posture, breathing, movement control, and more in subjects who practiced his exercise regimen with regularity.

Musculoskeletal Assessment: Building the Blueprint

Most practitioners start with a comprehensive musculoskeletal assessment, head to toe, that focuses on the area of dysfunction and the joints above and below it. Rehabilitation specialists use a variety of assessment tools to identify baseline orthopaedic function:

- Postural alignment
- Joint range of motion
- Muscle strength
- Flexibility
- Joint accessory movement
- Neurological status

- Special tests
- Palpation
- Functional movement testing

The posture assessment is the first step in creating your orthopaedic blueprint. Combine the data you collect here with the objective findings from other areas of your evaluation and look for correlations.

- Does manual muscle testing support your posture assessment findings?
- Are there other reasons for muscle imbalances? Consider excessive joint mobility or lack of joint mobility, requiring a focus on stability of the unstable segment(s) or neuromuscular reeducation of the hypomobile segment(s).
- Look for relationships between the posture and movement assessments and other conventional therapeutic tests.

The posture assessment tool in this manual is based on the work of Florence Kendall, where imbalances present as muscles in an elongated/weak or strong/shortened position. Kendall identified muscle imbalances associated with scoliosis and four primary postures (3):

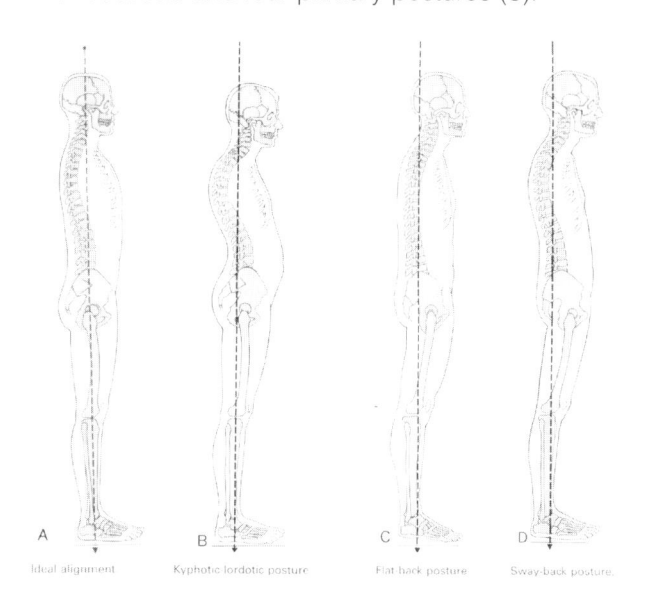

A. Ideal alignment B. Kyphotic-lordotic posture C. Flat-back posture D. Sway-back posture

Permission to reprint photo granted by Lippincott, Williams & Wilkins.

Ideal, Kyphosis-lordosis, flat back, Sway-back

*For purposes of this guide, we are not addressing military posture because it isn't as prevalent as the other faulty postural alignments.

Pilates was focused on using Contrology to correct faulty posture and malalignment that contributed to improper breathing, fatigue, and disrupted sleep, among many human concerns. Pilates asserted that proper posture came only when attention was paid to controlled quality of movement that required just 25 percent of one's total energy expenditure.

Helpful tip: While the alignment of the body in standing or moving positions can indicate specific muscle problems, a definitive assessment should not be made on the basis of the disturbance of alignment alone (1).

The Posture Assessment Tool: An Example

Our posture assessment tool is a variation on many that are available in both rehabilitation and fitness settings. Findings from the assessment help us determine which Pilates exercises we might use as an adjunct to traditional therapies to help restore function and balance. Use this tool as a guide to developing your own version.

Practitioner's note: The following posture assessment is a crucial starting point in creating your rehabilitation program. If and when time allows, complete a functional movement assessment as listed on the following pages to complete your holistic orthopaedic blueprint.

Posterior View (Circle selection)

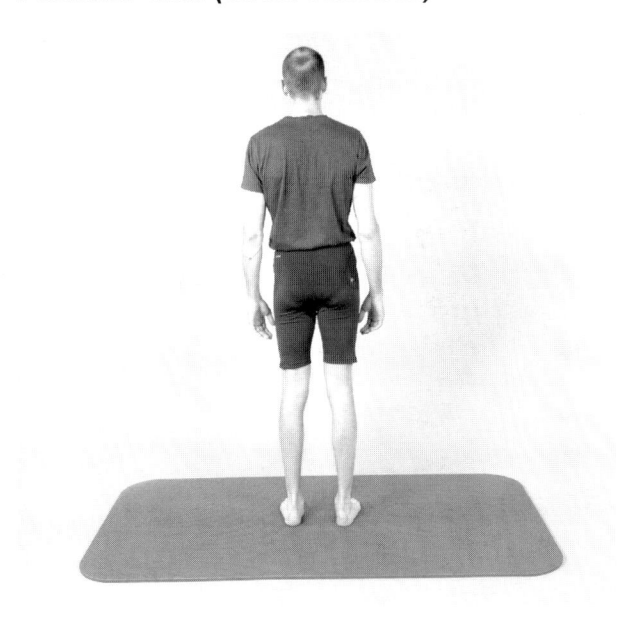

Head	Neutral	Side Bent R/L	Rotated R/L
Shoulders	Level	Asymmetrical	
Scapula Position	Normal	Abducted	Elevated
Spine	Normal	C-Curve	S-Curve
Rib Cage	Normal	Rotated	
Pelvis	Level	Asymmetrical	
Calcaneal Position	Neutral	Varus	Valgus

Trunk Forward Bend—Note: (Quality of movement, spinal asymmetries, etc.)

_____
_____

Side View

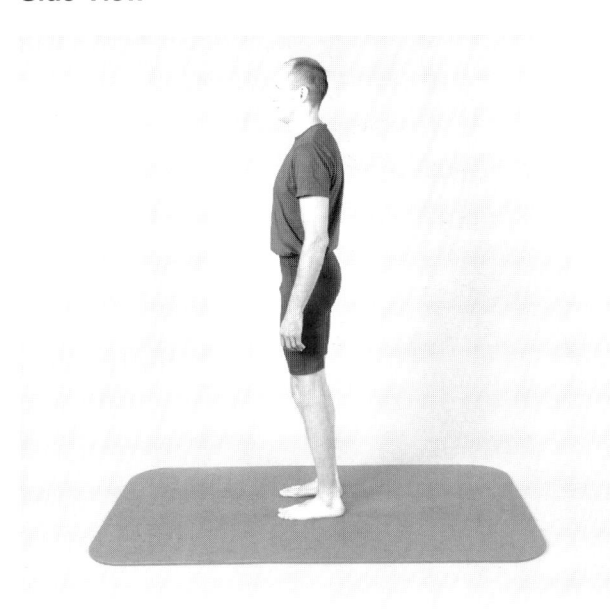

Head	Neutral	Forward	
Cervical Spine	Normal	Hyperextension	Flat
Thoracic Spine	Normal	Kyphosis	Flat
Lumbar Spine	Normal	Lordosis	Flat
Pelvis	Neutral	Anterior Tilt	Posterior Tilt
Knees	Neutral	Genu Recurvatum	Flexed
Ankle Joint	Neutral	Plantar flexed	Dorsiflexed

Additional Observations: _____

Front View

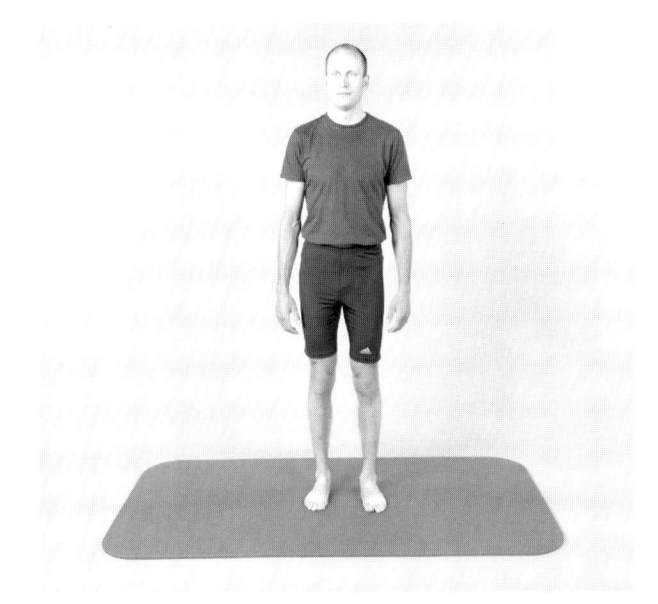

Humerus Position	Normal	Rotation (medial/lateral)	
Knees	Normal	Genu Valgus	Genu Varum
Feet	Normal	Pronated	Supinated

Additional Observations: _____

Breathing Assessment: Another area that is crucial to include in musculoskeletal exam is evaluation of the breath pattern. (Refer to Chapter 5 for further information.)

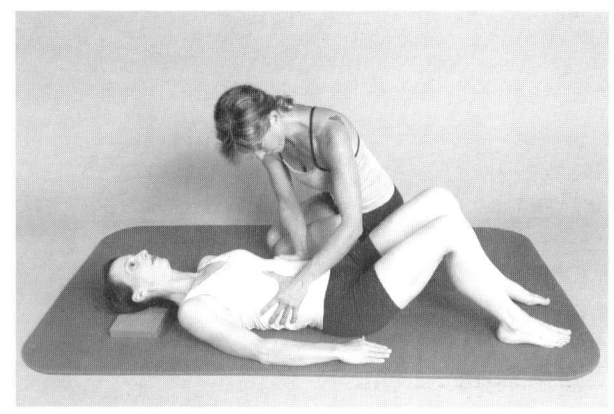

Breathing	Normal (Abdominal/ diaphragmatic)	Abdominal	Chest
Inhalation/ Exhalation Ratio	Normal (1:1)	Abnormal	
Breath depth	Normal	Shallow	
Breaths per minute	Normal	Abnormal	
Rib cage excursion	Normal	Decreased	
Rib cage mobility	Restrictive	Unrestrictive	

Additional Observations: _____

(Refer to Chapter 5 for further detail.)

Functional Movement Assessment Tool

Like the posture assessment, a functional movement assessment contributes to creating the orthopaedic picture of your patient. Defined here, our assessment gives us information that may support or disprove our suspicions of muscle imbalances, altered muscle recruitment patterns, etc.

Specifically, we are observing the impact of suspected muscle imbalances in movement, particularly as it relates to core stabilization and performance of activities of daily living, work, and/or sport. From a Pilates perspective, the entire body is an integrated, connected chain. Dysfunction or movement restrictions in one part of the body influence another. Before offering corrective exercises, we must first know what to correct.

The goals of the movement assessment are to:

- Evaluate the quality and tenor of movement in your patient's activities of daily living (walking, climbing stairs, sit-to-stand transition, body mechanics), work, sport, and in exercises common to the rehabilitation setting (squats, leg raises, abdominal curls);
- Evaluate muscle balance, strength, and endurance;
- Evaluate torso stabilization, with and without cueing;
- Evaluate the primary and secondary stabilizers, with and without cueing;
- Identify faulty movement patterns or compensations due to muscle imbalances with observation and other assessment tools.

The results of your movement assessment will guide you in integrating Pilates principles and exercises into rehabilitation to help restore normal function to your patient.

Helpful tip: Many practitioners don't have the luxury of time! Today's health care environment barely allows time for provider-prescribed protocols, much less other potentially helpful therapies or prescriptions.

If you can't complete a functional assessment in the first visit, try to complete it in the second or third. Pick the tests we've outlined here that are most appropriate for your patient or observe the quality of movement in exercises you've given them. Choose movement patterns with consideration of the musculoskeletal dysfunction you are treating.

If you never have the chance to complete an assessment, use your skills to observe your patient as they walk from their car to your practice, stand at the desk, walk to the treatment area, sit, or stand. Listen for footfall and gait emphasis. You'll be surprised what you can learn about your patient's quality of movement.

Sample Functional Movement Assessment Tool

The following functional assessment tool is a variation on many that are available in both rehabilitation and fitness settings. Use this movement assessment in conjunction with your other tools to identify faulty movement patterns and compensatory strategies. Observe movement in all planes of motion and from anterior, posterior, and side views to gain a comprehensive picture of overall movement quality.

We often ask patients to perform the following with little direction to observe initial movement quality, followed by cueing to ascertain proprioceptive and self-correction skills. Use the *Additional Observations* section in this tool to detail other dysfunctions.

Movement Assessment Form

Walking

Purpose of Assessment: To observe movement quality in the entire chain with specific focus on identifying dysfunction at the thoracic spine, pelvis, hip, knee, ankle, or foot during a fundamental activity of daily living. Evaluate your patient's ability to control his or her torso and extremities. Listen for changes in the gait cycle and observe weight transfer.

Thoracic spine	Normal	Abnormal
Pelvis	Normal	Trendelenburg
		(Compensated/True)
Hip	Normal	Abnormal
Knee	Normal	Hyperextended
	Genu Valgus	Genu Varus
Ankle	Normal	Limited ROM
Foot	Normal	Pronated Supinated

Additional Observations: _____

Stairs (Evaluate descent/ascent)

Purpose of Assessment: To observe movement quality and/or dysfunction at the pelvis, hip, knee, ankle, and foot during a fundamental activity of daily living. Listen for changes in the gait cycle and observe weight transfer. Where does movement initiate? As your patient descends, observe which joints are initiating movement. Are the hip, knee, and ankle joints moving in synchronicity, or are there compensatory strategies?

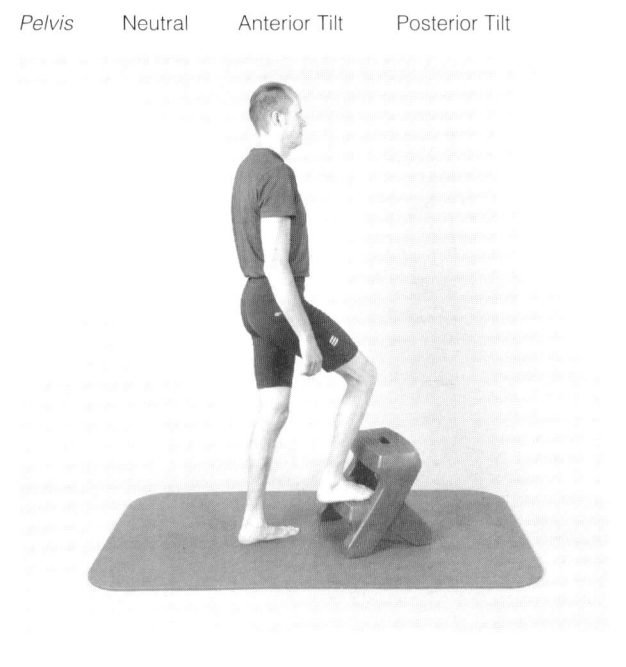

Pelvis   Neutral   Anterior Tilt   Posterior Tilt

			Lateral Tilt
Knee	Normal	Genu Valgus	Genu Varus
Ankle	Normal	Limited ROM	
Foot	Normal	Pronation	Supination

Additional Observations: _____

Squat*

Purpose of Assessment: To observe movement quality and/or dysfunction at the pelvis, hip, knee, ankle, foot, and shoulder during a fundamental movement pattern for such activities of daily living as transitioning from sitting to standing and reaching overhead. What does the patient feel when squatting? Are the gluteals firing appropriately? Are the hamstrings dominant with hip extension? Observe weight transfer or excessive loading to one side, as well as how the movement changes when the shoulders are flexed forward or overhead.

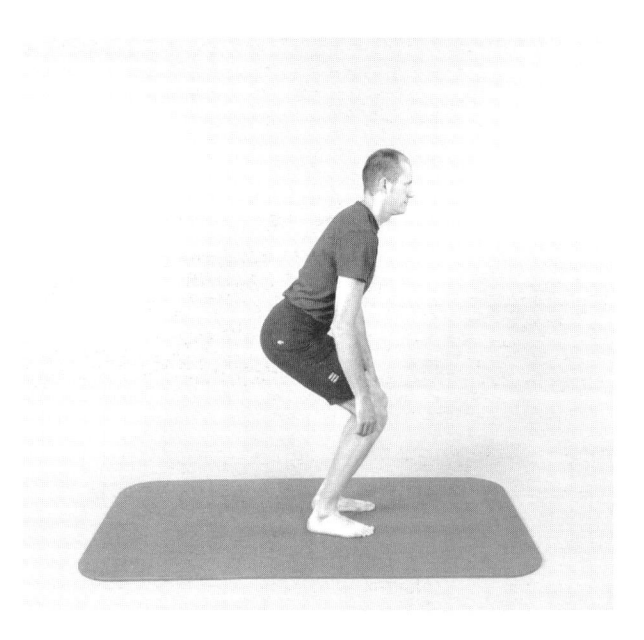

*Observing what occurs at the pelvis and hip with shoulder flexion can provide additional clues to faulty movement patterns such as a compensatory anterior pelvic tilt due to tight latissimus dorsi.

Pelvis	Neutral	Anterior Tilt R/L/Rotation	Posterior Tilt R/L/Tilt
Disassociation Femur from Pelvis	Normal	Abnormal	
Hips	Normal	Internally rotated	Externally rotated
Quads/Ham/Glut Maximus Recruitment Pattern	Normal	Abnormal	
Knee Concentric/ Eccentric Quad Control	Normal Normal	Genu Valgus Abnormal	Genu Varus
Ankle	Normal	Limited ROM	
Foot	Pronation	Supination	
Weight Load	Forward on Toes	Central	Back to Heels
Squat with Shoulder Flexion	Pelvis Neutral ROM Normal	Anterior Tilt ROM Abnormal	Posterior Tilt

Additional Observations: _____

Stationary Lunge*

Purpose of Assessment: To observe balance and movement quality and/or dysfunction at the pelvis, hip, knee, ankle, foot, and shoulder during a fundamental movement pattern for such activities of daily living as standing from a chair, getting out of a car, and stair climbing, or athletic activities that require asymmetrical lower extremity movement, such as running, lunging, and jumping. Observe weight transfer or excessive loading to one side.

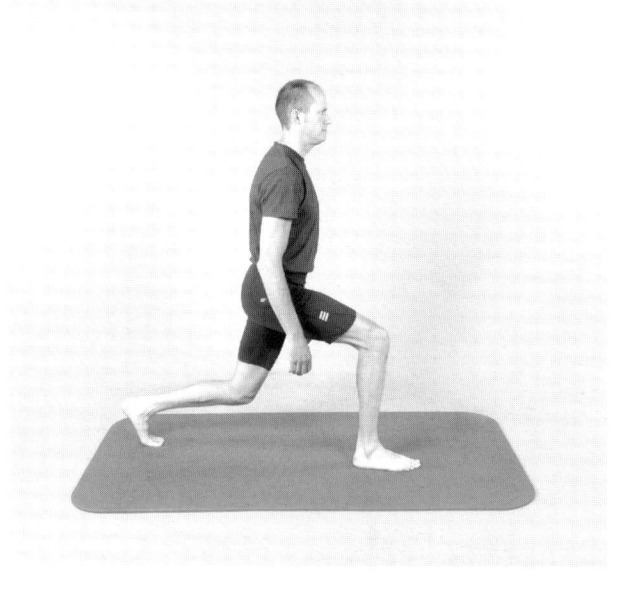

Pelvis	Neutral	Anterior Tilt R/L/Rotation	Posterior Tilt R/L/Tilt
Hips	Normal	Internal Rotation	External Rotation
Quads/Ham/ Glut Maximus Recruitment Pattern	Normal	Abnormal	
Knee	Normal	Genu Valgus	Genu Varus
Ankle ROM	Normal	Limited ROM	
Foot	Normal	Pronation	Supination
MTP Joint Ext	Normal	Abnormal	
Weight Load	Forward Leg	Back Leg	

Additional Observations: _____

*Following stationary observation, add a mobile lunge as an option and repeat observation.

Standing One-Leg Balance (evaluate the following with hip flexion at 90 degrees)

Purpose of Assessment: To observe balance, quality of movement, and/or dysfunction at the pelvis, hip, knee, foot, and ankle when a stability point is removed. Use hip flexion to 90 degrees to assess ADLs such as stair climbing, ergonomic-related activities that require climbing a ladder, and sports that demand momentary balance on one leg, such as tennis, soccer, and basketball. If balance is poor, assess the patient's ability to flex the hip in supine position. (See Single-Leg Tabletop in Chapter 6.)

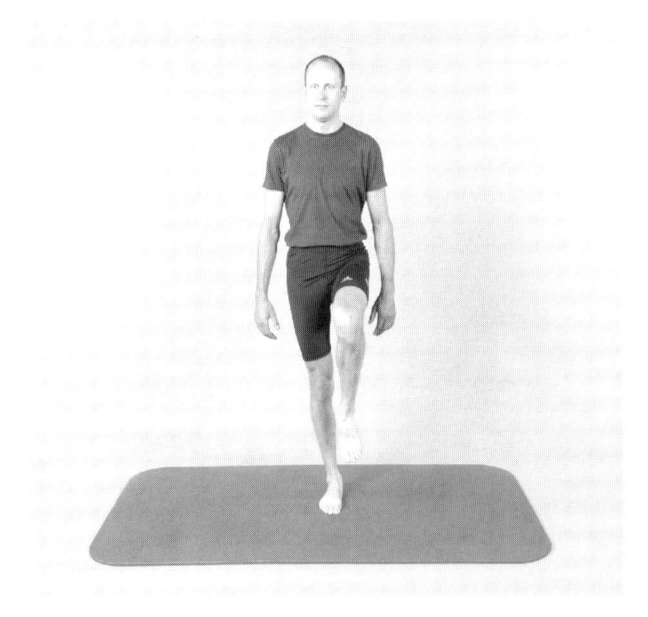

Stance Loading	Normal	Lateral Sway	
Pelvis	Neutral	Anterior Tilt R/L/Rotation	Posterior Tilt R/L/Tilt
Hips	Normal	Internal Rotation	External Rotation
Knee	Normal	Hyperextended	
Foot	Normal	Pronation	Supination

Additional Observations: _____

Bridge

Purpose of Assessment: This assessment's purpose is threefold: To observe quality of movement during hip extension, which is essential to performing such movements as walking, standing, and squatting; to observe the ability to stabilize the torso with hip extension and flexion and when stability points are removed; to observe breathing mechanics in less stable positions. Also observe the following: Are the gluteals firing appropriately? Are the hamstrings dominant with hip extension?

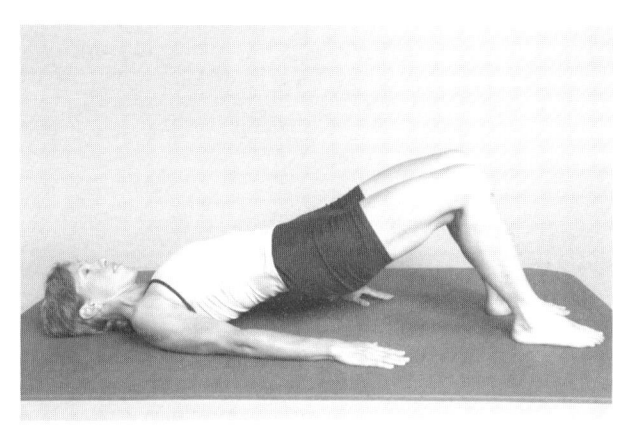

Loading Bilaterally	Normal	Unequal R/L	
Pelvis	Neutral	Anterior Tilt R/L/Rotation	Posterior Tilt R/L/Tilt
Torso Stability	Normal	Abnormal	
One-Leg Lift	Normal	Abnormal Weight Transfer	
Breathing Abd Assessment	Normal	Abdominal Bulging	

Additional Observations: _____

Sitting Rotation Right and Left with Shoulder Abduction (also refer to Chapter 6, Spine Twist with Legs Crossed)

Purpose of Assessment: To observe quality of movement and/or dysfunction in rotary movement with lumbo-pelvic stabilization and to assess normal/abnormal muscle recruitment patterns. This is a fundamental movement pattern for walking, running, ergonomic training, and sports. Where does the rotary movement occur? Can your patient control pelvic motion?

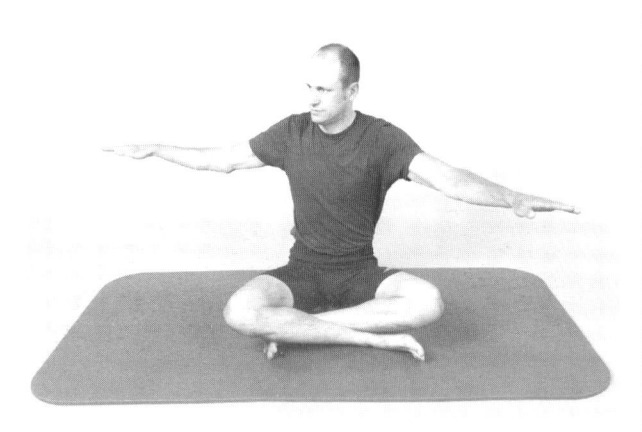

Loading Ischial Tuberosities	Equal	Unequal Loading R/L	
Pelvis	Neutral	Anterior Tilt R/L/Rotation	Posterior Tilt R/L/Tilt
Hip External Rotation	Normal	Limited	
Thoracic Rotation Sequential Articulation/Restriction	Normal	Abnormal	
Oblique Recruitment	Normal	Abnormal	
Trunk	Neutral	Side Bend	
Cervical Spine	Neutral	Protracted	Retracted

Additional Observations: _____

Seated Bilateral Shoulder Flexion to 180 Degrees

Purpose of Assessment: To observe quality of movement and/or dysfunction at, above, and below the shoulder and to observe movement mechanics of the torso and lower extremities with shoulder flexion. This is a fundamental movement pattern for reaching overhead or sports that require overhead motion.

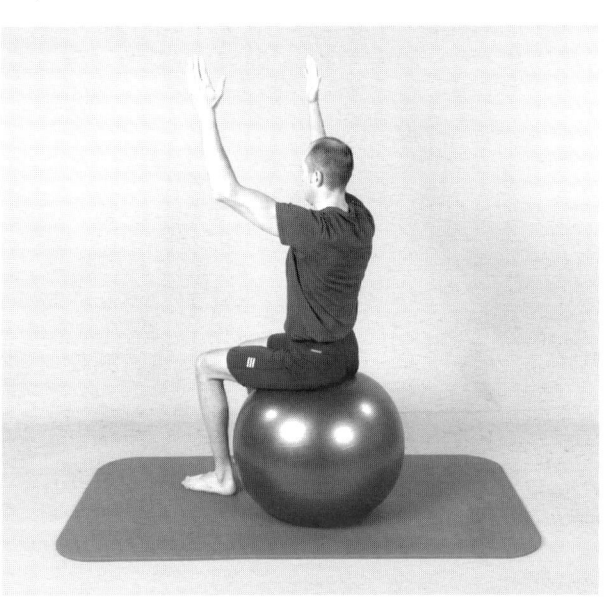

Scapulohumeral Rhythm	Normal	Abnormal
Thoracic Alignment	Normal	Abnormal
Lumbar Alignment	Normal	Abnormal

Additional Observations: _____

Pushup (Semi-plank or Plank)

Purpose of Assessment: To observe quality of movement and/or dysfunction of the upper extremities and to observe torso stability with shoulder/elbow flexion and extension. If scapular stability is not adequate, choose an alternative movement pattern such as wall pushups with emphasis on starting alignment. If scapular stabilization is demonstrated in the semi-plank/plank position, continue the exercise to assess with these watch-points in mind: stability and/or stability and mobility.

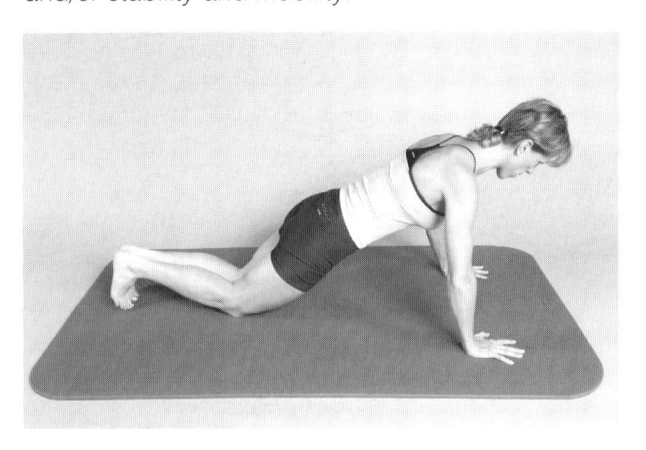

Pelvis	Neutral	Anterior Tilt	Posterior Tilt
R/L/Rotation	R/L/Tilt		
Cervical Spine	Neutral	Protracted	Retracted
Scapular Position	Normal	Retracted	Elevated
Torso Stability	Poor	Good	Excellent
Elbow	Normal	Hyperextension	

Additional Observations: _____

Quarter Rollup with Neutral Pelvis (also see Chapter 7)

Purpose of Assessment: To observe quality of movement or dysfunction head to tailbone with spine flexion while keeping the pelvis in neutral and the feet fixed on a stable surface. To observe breathing mechanics with spinal flexion. Look for faulty movement patterns, such as using the gluteals to posteriorly tip the pelvis, gripping with the hip flexors or abdominal bulging.

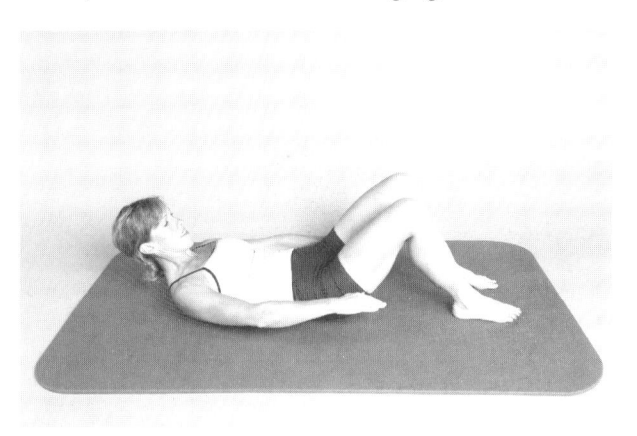

Pelvis	Neutral	Anterior Tilt	Posterior Tilt
Cervical Spine	Neutral	Hyperflexion	Hyperextended
Scapular Position	Normal	Protracted	Elevated
Breathing/ Abd Assessment	Bulging	Flattening	

Additional Observations: _____

Trunk Extension with Neutral Pelvis

Purpose of Assessment: To observe quality of movement and/or dysfunction at the lumbo-pelvic area with trunk extension. Look for faulty movement patterns, such as anterior pelvic tilt, and encourage co-contraction of the abdominals and gluteals to stabilize the pelvis.

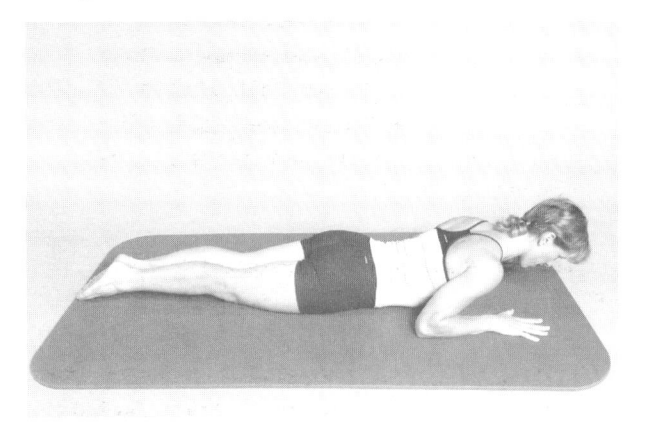

Pelvis	Neutral	Anterior Tilt	Posterior Tilt
Erector Spinae Recruitment	Normal	R/L/Bilateral	Tonic
Gluteal Recruitment	Normal	Abnormal	

Additional Observations: _____

Pulling It All Together: Fitting Pilates into Your Rehabilitation Program

Once your assessments are completed, progress with treatment planning. Begin by asking these questions:

1. What are your patient's short- and long-term goals? Initially, the treatment goal(s) may focus on decreasing pain, restoring range of motion, and/or reducing swelling, depending on the nature of the dysfunction. While goals differ from patient to patient, there is a common thread for each: functional movement. The foundation for reintroducing or improving functional movement starts at the center of the body—the core—and that begins with the principles of core stabilization. Refer to Chapter 6 for detailed information.

2. What muscle imbalances are present based on your musculoskeletal and functional movement assessments? Pilates-based exercises should initially be selected based on either strengthening a long muscle by working in it's shortened range and emphasizing concentric contractions or lengthening a tight muscle with emphasis on working in the muscle's elongated range to restore balance to the muscles surrounding the joint.

3. If there is low back dysfunction, can the patient voluntarily contract the TrA? Is the contraction symmetrical/asymmetrical? Phasic/tonic? Is the TrA recruitment pattern altered or absent? If yes, normal firing mechanics need to be restored first with initial core training for lumbo-pelvic stabilization, regardless of the patient's diagnosis. Once this corrective exercise is successful in reeducating TrA muscle recruitment, progress to abdominal bracing with core strength training.

Helpful tip: There is an exception to the rule with initial neuromuscular reeducation of the TrA when faulty pelvic and/or lumbar mechanics are present. Refer to Chapter 10, The Art of Teaching.

4. Is a disease process present? Selected Pilates-based exercises or the timing of their use may need to be modified or avoided completely. Exercises that involve spinal flexion and rotation are contraindicated with osteoporosis secondary to risk of vertebral fracture. If respiratory disease is present, such as asthma, TrA muscle recruitment may be affected. According to Hodges, where there is a high respiratory demand, some patients may be not able to use those muscles for stability and therefore need to exercise when respiratory demand is low (4).

Once these questions are answered, keep the following exercise guidelines in mind:

- Introduce Pilates-based principles or exercises that start in the most stable positions, such as supine or prone. An essential component to advancing your patient is his or her understanding and demonstration of the principles with each exercise. Help your patient get there: Ask your patient what muscles he or she is feeling with movement. Examine the movement. Are faulty movement patterns present? Rib cage popping? Abdominal breathing?

- If compensatory strategies are present, avoid progressing your patient until core stabilization is mastered in the most stable exercise positions

- Break faulty movement patterns down into smaller components and layer movements one on top of another as you progress your patient

- Each Pilates principle and exercise has a goal or purpose. Does the exercise match your patient's goals? An exercise may focus on key muscles and types of contractions, joint mobilizations, balance, coordination, stamina, stability (static/dynamic positioning of the body), and/or initiation of movement. The goals for your patient should match those of the exercise.

Ideas for Integrating Pilates and Conventional Therapies

Example a: Lack of joint mobility (i.e., anterior hip capsule tightness) or faulty pelvic mechanics (i.e., altered TrA recruitment pattern with anterior innominate). In both instances, the first goal is to restore normal joint and pelvic mechanics with manual therapy techniques, reassess muscle strength and recruitment patterns, and then introduce appropriate Pilates-based exercises as an adjunct to treatment.

Example b: If excessive joint mobility is present, such as excessive anterior glenohumeral capsule mobility, what muscle imbalances present? What is the treatment focus? Restoration of joint stability is initially the primary focus of the rehabilitation program for an unstable shoulder with emphasis on closed chain training. However, the foundation for the program begins with the principles of core stability training, and that is where Pilates can be helpful. Once principles are mastered, integrate them into closed chain exercises, open chain exercises, and such techniques as proprioceptive neuromuscular facilitation (PNF).

Example c: Can the hip or shoulder move independently from the pelvis and spine with movement (for example, the squat, pushup, or transitional movements, such as from sit to stand)? If the hip or shoulder is not moving independently from the lumbo-pelvic region with movements ranging from a heel slide or shoulder elevation to a squat, pushup, or sit to stand, the focus should begin with the Pilates principles related to core stabilization.

A Word About Progressing Patients

"Is my patient ready for more?" is a common question among rehabilitation and fitness practitioners. The answer to progressing is not without its complexities. We have all seen patients or clients who have not mastered the basics of quality movement: injuries have occurred or recurred, they are not healing, desired results have not been attained. The question is why.

From the patients' perspective, they may feel they are not being challenged enough with the fundamentals and require more from you before they are truly ready. Compliance or boredom may also be an issue, and you may feel it necessary to respond by offering more advanced exercises.

Knowing when and how to add more complexity or challenge to a patient's program comes with fine-tuned observational skills, experience, and intuition. Ask this question: Has the patient's basic movement patterns that include squatting, hip extension, or rotation improved from your baseline assessment? Time is key and often at the crux of the matter, given today's health care marketplace.

An answer may lie in the genius of Joseph Pilates and those who have advanced his work by offering variations and modifications to the host of original exercises. Today's options include exercises for the beginner, intermediate, and advanced patient. Most of the exercises progress from static to dynamic stabilization, addressing:

- Muscle synergies: co-contractions, isometric, eccentric, concentric
- Symmetrical to asymmetrical movement patterns of the upper and lower extremities
- Uniplanar to multiplanar patterns; single-joint to multiarticular
- Stability and motor control with movement of the arms and legs

From our experience, it is essential that your patient understand and demonstrate the Pilates principles and fundamentals of stabilization before progressing. There are any number of strategies to introduce and reinforce this early learning, helping to ensure compliance and stave off boredom. As general rules of thumb:

1. Ask your patient what muscles he or she is feeling with movement.

2. Observe the movement. Are faulty movement patterns present? Rib cage popping? Abdominal breathing? Refer to Chapter 5.

3. Avoid progressing your patient until core stabilization is mastered. Break down the movement pattern into smaller components and build from there.

4. Introduce Pilates-based exercises that emphasize single-joint and uniplanar movements first. Fundamental exercises that emphasize stability are generally those where the body has the most contact with the mat (supine/prone) and/or where movement is uniplanar.

5. Choose exercise patterns that challenge stability, muscle stamina, coordination, and mobility once simpler exercises are mastered without faulty movement patterns. Progress to less stable positions such as sidelying, quadruped, or standing, or use equipment. You can also introduce multiplanar movement patterns of the upper and lower extremities to challenge coordination and mobility.

6. Incorporate principles into functional training movements such as squats and lunges, single-leg balance, riding a stationary bike, resistance training, sport-specific drills (i.e., swinging a bat), ADLs (transitioning from sit to stand), and closed/open kinetic chain training.

Chapter References

1. Kendall, F.P., McCreary, E.K. 1983. *Muscles, Testing and Function*, Third Edition. Baltimore, MD: Williams and Wilkins.

2. Franke, B., Bauman, S. 1992. *Treatment of Muscle Imbalances*. Course Manual, Health Forum, Institute for Athletic Medicine, Saint Paul, MN, November.

3. Kendall, F.P., McCreary, E.K., Provance, P.G. 1993. *Muscles, Testing and Function, Posture and Pain,* Fourth Edition. Baltimore, MD: Williams and Wilkins.

4. Hodges, P.W. 2002. *Science of Stability: Clinical Application to Assessment and Treatment of Segmental Spinal Stabilization for Low Back Pain.* Course Manual, Supplementary Notes, October. Bloomington, MN: Northeast Seminars.

chapter 4

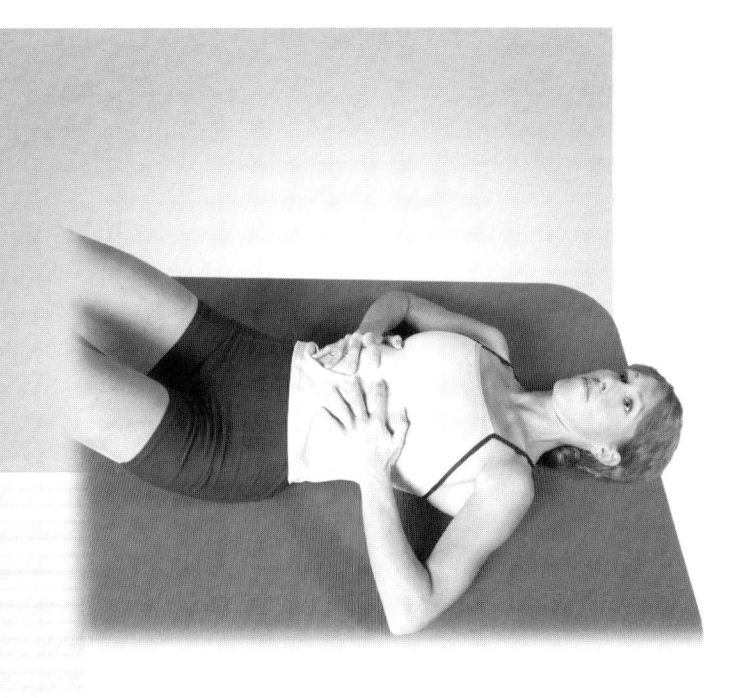

THE PILATES
PRINCIPLES:
CREATING THE
FRAMEWORK FOR
MOVEMENT

Pilates-based principles create the framework for performing the 500-plus and growing number of Pilates exercises. Their development has been evolutionary, with many schools of thought and perspectives collectively contributing to the evolution.

Classical Pilates methodologies identify up to nine principles that range from breathing and concentration to flow and precision. More contemporary approaches identify principles that are biomechanically based. We have selectively pulled from a number of these philosophies and perspectives and respectively acknowledge our training in STOTT Pilates and the Physicalmind Institute. We urge you to consider the principles presented here and add them to your rehabilitation toolbox to support conventional strength training programs, ADL instruction, functional training, and postoperative protocols.

It's also important to note that modern science has advanced the Pilates exercise regimen to a degree that Pilates himself likely never anticipated. Pilates developed his method with a focus on spinal mobility, posture, breathing, and flexibility.

While his intent remains true to modern-day practice, newer concepts and language such as "neutral pelvis," "core stabilization," and "scapular and rib cage positioning" are examples of concepts that tend to reflect today's rehabilitation and exercise scientific study and concern for safety. Pilates' original exercise descriptions include directions to "keep the knees locked," the body "tense," and "the chin touching the chest," emphasizing cervical flexion—all examples of movements that today's rehabilitation and exercise scientists do not endorse. As you advance your Pilates training, consider a balance between classic methodology and today's evidence base.

Why the Principles?

These Pilates-based principles serve two purposes. First, they can be used as an education tool to teach kinesthetic awareness and movement quality. When applied, they help strengthen the powerhouse of the body to support the spine and pelvis in neutral before introducing more challenging movements and patterns. In the following pages, we divide the principles into two categories, some with greater detail.

- Musculoskeletal Principles: breathing, positioning of the pelvis, scapula, rib cage, head and neck, motor coordination, and isolated integration
- Mind-Body Principles: centering and concentration

Guidelines for Practicing the Principles

We provide review of the principles and, when appropriate, variations, clinical application and faulty movement patterns. We also suggest some easy ways to practice them.

Initially, training is performed supine without shoes and socks to enhance sensory feedback throughout the kinetic chain. Neutral alignment of the cervical spine may need to be supported by a towel or padding.

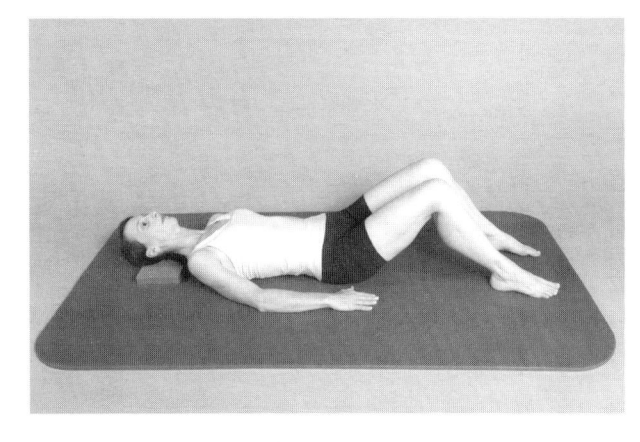

Once the principles are mastered alone and in combination with each other, progress your patient to sitting, sidelying, and four-point positions, followed by standing, walking, and other activities of daily living. Doing so can help enhance your patient's understanding of his or her body when moving in less stable positions.

Use your own creativity to find ways to illustrate and demonstrate the principles to your patient. Observe the quality and tenor of the movement, looking for compensatory strategies as listed in this guidebook.

Musculoskeletal Principles
Breathing

Correct breathing is the foundation of all Pilates exercises. Pilates believed that most people needed to be taught how to breathe correctly: drawing in long, deep breaths to expand the rib cage to its fullest capacity, followed by full exhalation to deflate the lungs. Doing so helped to cleanse the lungs of impurities and restore normal posture. He introduced the concept of mental dominance—or intention—to facilitate correct breathing, leading to a normal, natural posture and a reenergized circulatory system (1).

In practice, rolling exercises and spinal flexion in particular allow the lungs to be "cleansed" by forcing impure air from them.

A Clinical Perspective on Pilates Breathing

Most Pilates methods advocate inhaling through the nose and exhaling through the mouth using pursed lips, and we subscribe to this practice with the modifications noted in the *Teaching tips* section.

Inhalation serves to expand the ribs posterolaterally, naturally mobilizing the ribs upward and outward and slightly extending the spine, as opposed to the upper chest or abdominal breathing common to many mind-body practices such as yoga. Inhalation helps open the body, an important consideration in that many of our patients sit, stand, and perform ADLs in a spine-flexed position. What does this do for their breathing mechanics? For oxygenating the body?

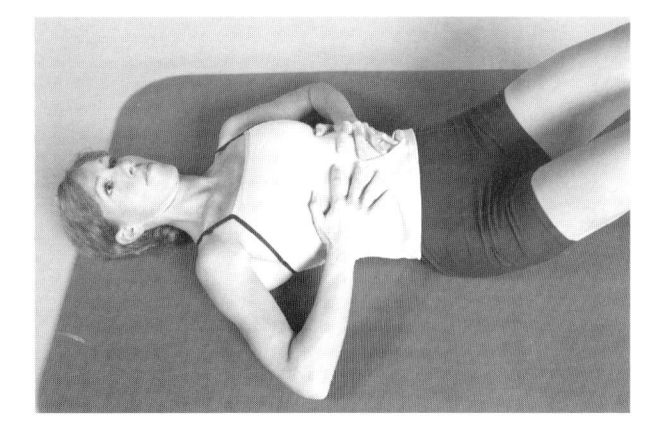

On exhalation through pursed lips, the intercostals and obliques contract along the anterior, lateral, and posterior portions of the ribs, mobilizing the ribs down and inward, facilitating spinal flexion.

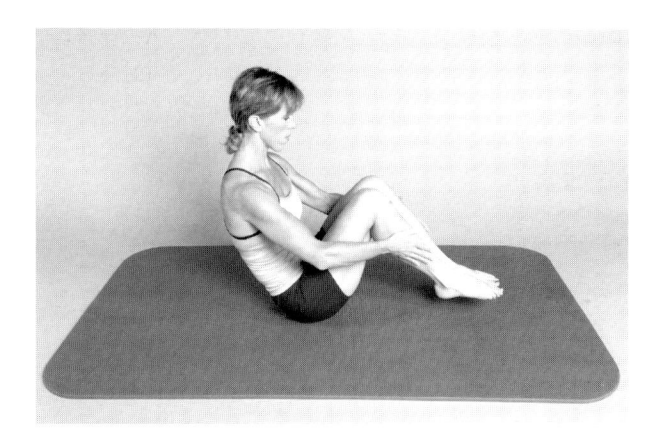

Rolling Like a Ball is an example of a Pilates exercise that incorporates "rolling" along the spine to help force impurities from the lungs (see Chapter 6).

Teaching tips:

1. *Each Pilates exercise has a specific breathing pattern. Breathing is a skill, and coordinating breath with a movement pattern can be frustrating for some patients. To enhance learning, teach your patient to exhale on the "work effort," which generally occurs during spinal flexion, and inhale on spine extension. If this emphasis still proves frustrating, change the focus to motor control only or reverse the breathing. With patience and practice, the breathing will come.*

2. *Overexaggeration of the breath pattern is a common symptom with reeducation of breathing. Encourage natural breathing and kinesthetic awareness, feeling the ribs slightly draw apart and together. You may need to start with a smaller breath to establish a normal breathing pattern.*

3. *Be aware that some forms of Pilates advocate active exhalation. There is growing research to suggest that this practice recruits large respiratory and torso "global" muscles prior to deeper, smaller "local" muscles (see Chapter 5). Remind your patient that the breath should occur naturally—avoid cueing for the forceful, active exhalation common to some Pilates practice.*

Teaching Breathing

There are many ways to teach and practice intentional breathing. For patients, an excellent starting point is in hooklying or supine position with knees bent. This position facilitates proprioceptive feedback to the body via the floor's surface.

Start by finding neutral pelvis and spine, head, and neck alignment. The heels are hip-width apart, arms alongside the body. Spread the hands open and place them bilaterally along the anterior and lateral portions of the rib cage.

Inhale through the nose and breathe into the sides and back of the ribs. Patients should feel the ribs move up and out, leading to slight spinal extension. Exhale, breathing through pursed lips to feel the ribs move down and in, leading to slight spinal flexion.

(Use a towel or small pillow for cervical spine support, if needed. Patients should be in neutral cervical spine.)

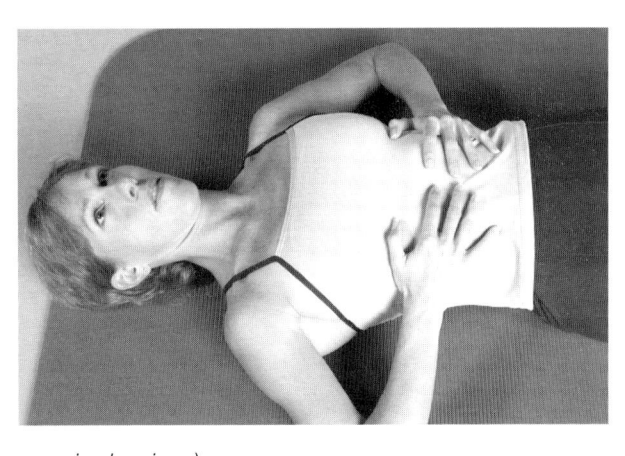

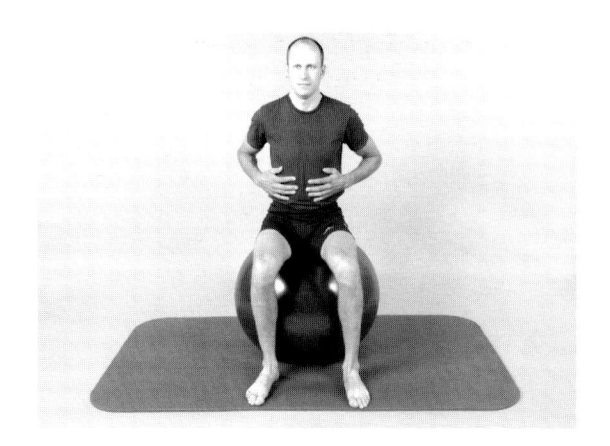

Variations: Once patients have mastered correct breathing in hooklying, advance them to prone, quadruped, seated, and standing positions. Encourage patients to practice proper breathing at work or in the car.

Purpose:

- To teach kinesthetic awareness of the breath pattern while maintaining the natural rhythm of the ribs as they mobilize during inhalation and exhalation
- Natural exhalation stimulates the deep muscles of the body, including the transversus abdominis, the diaphragm, and muscles of the pelvic floor. Contraction of the obliques and intercostals allows the rib cage to move down and in.
- Breath helps to push oxygen to the extremities and reduce tension in the neck, chest, and upper back

Clinical Application:

- Breathing initiates a chain of events that begins with mobilizing the ribs and thoracic spine in the sagittal plane or in a combination of the sagittal and transverse planes, increasing stability through contraction of core muscles and more efficient movement in the extremities
- Breathing helps patients to focus on centering, decreases the likelihood of Valsalva during exercise, and promotes relaxation
- Use breathing to enhance traditional and Pilates-based flexibility/strengthening exercises, transitional movements, activities of daily living, and sport-specific drills

Faulty Movement Patterns: Ribs not sliding down/in with natural exhalation; anterior ribs popping; lateral and posterior ribs not expanding with inhalation (unilateral or bilateral restrictions); too forceful an exhalation (breath remains in the throat); Valsalva; upper chest breathing; shoulder elevation and protraction; not maintaining neutral cervical spine; abdominal popping (abdominal breathing)

Practitioner tips:

1. Patients who are postpartum, who have had surgery, or who are "upper chest or abdominal breathers" typically experience abdominal popping or bulging when first learning Pilates-style breathing. From an onlooker's perspective, it appears as if the abdominal area below the umbilicus is expanding like a balloon. Practitioners should observe a flattening if the breathing technique is done correctly. Patients should have a sensation of muscles tightening like saran wrap or abdominal bracing where there is co-activation of the abdominals and back extensors.

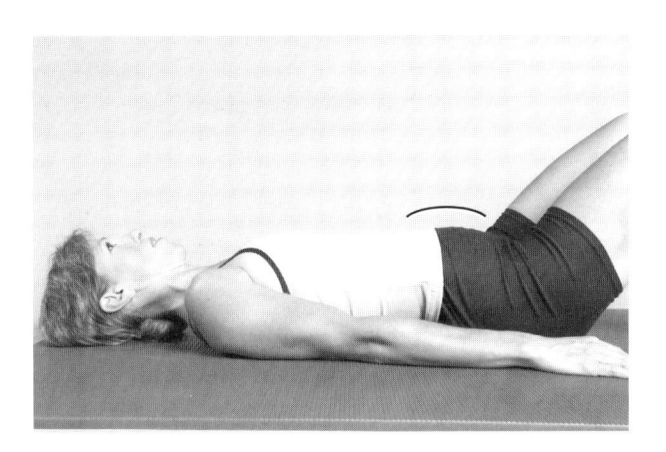

2. A too-common response to initiating Pilates breathing is to draw the abdominals up and in, creating a hollow beneath the inferior portion of the rib cage with contraction of the external obliques, among other muscles. This is incorrect and should be avoided. For further instruction, see Chapter 5.

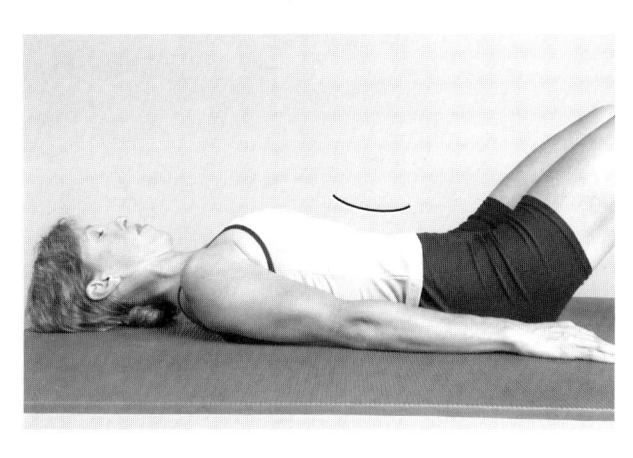

Pelvic Positioning

The pelvis moves in all planes and ranges of motion. Many people are unaware of these ranges, much less how to intentionally "move" the pelvis without employing faulty movement patterns. Teaching the normal movements of the pelvis helps to develop kinesthetic awareness of pelvic mechanics and its relationship to the lumbar spine, hips, and femurs as well as how to maintain stability of the pelvis with movement of the upper and lower extremities.

The position of the pelvis during Pilates practice is debated among Pilates practitioners. Pilates himself performed his exercises with a flat lumbar spine, or a posterior tilt. Many schools of thought continue the method as intended, while others have introduced regimens that advocate neutral pelvis in all exercises or a combination of both.

While Pilates' original intent of spinal and joint mobility is useful to rehabilitation, the training method of a continuous posterior pelvic tilt doesn't serve the wide-ranging needs of most rehabilitation patients, nor does it coincide with the improved science of movement, which demonstrates the spine is at its strongest when in neutral.

As a general rule of thumb, we advocate neutral in closed kinetic chain exercises and a posterior, or imprinted, pelvic tilt when patients are performing open kinetic chain exercises (2) or a combination when segmental articulation is required. As patients progress and become stronger, we move them to neutral pelvis in selected exercises. Our goal: To return patients to life equipped to function at their optimal level. Training to neutral helps to support this goal.

Neutral pelvis when one or both feet are in contact with the floor.

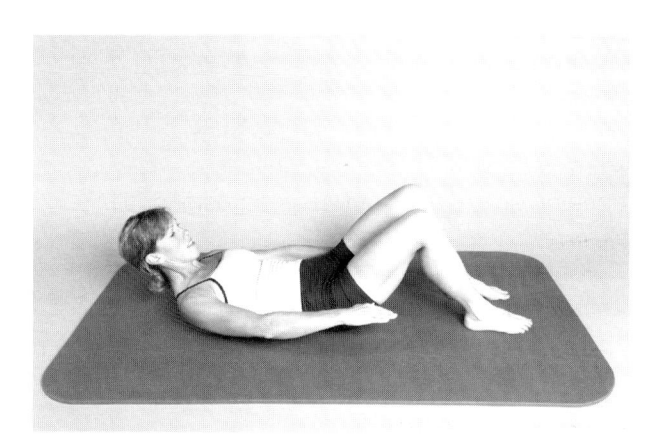

Posterior tilt, or imprinted pelvis, when both feet are not in contact with the surface. Move patients toward neutral spine as they become stronger.

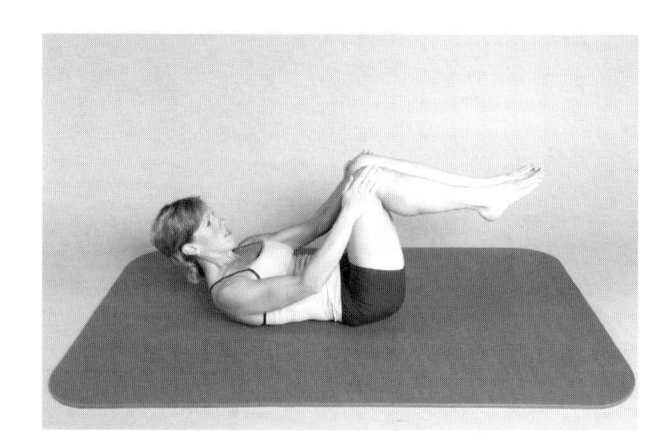

Purpose:

- To develop kinesthetic awareness of pelvic position with the goal of striving toward neutral
- To teach kinesthetic awareness of maintaining neutral with movement isolation at the hip joint
- To create safe and efficient movement through the spine and pelvis

Clinical Application:

- Apply to all types of exercise to reduce faulty movement patterns that can result in acute or overuse injuries and degenerative changes over time
- Neutral pelvis encourages core muscles to work optimally and prepares the lower and upper extremities for more efficient movement
- Imprinted spine, also known as a posterior tilt, initially helps improve abdominal strength and prepares your patient for open chain exercise patterns and patterns that require sequential spinal articulation

Teaching Patients Pelvic Awareness

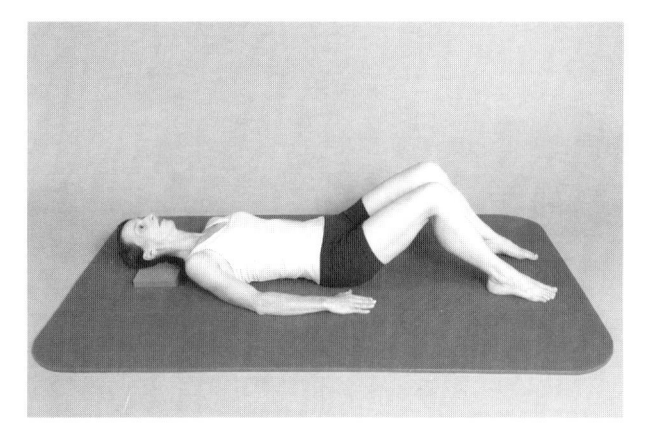

Start in hooklying with neutral spine, head, and neck alignment, heels hip-width apart, arms alongside the body, elbows slightly bent, with the palms facing down on the mat.

Movement Pattern 1: Finding Neutral—Direct Method

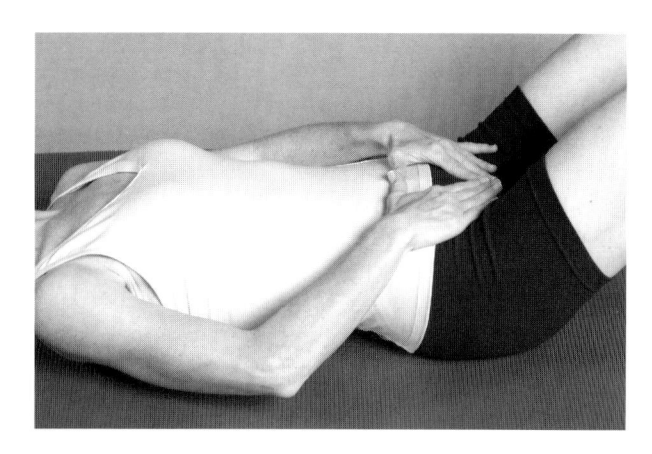

1. Place the heels of the hands (hypothenar eminence) on each anterior superior iliac spine (ASIS) and angle the second fingers toward the midline to form a triangle. Slide the second fingers toward the symphysis pubis, keeping the fingers parallel to the floor.

2. Once the symphysis pubis is located, determine the position of the pelvis. The pelvis will be in one of the following three positions: 1) neutral, where the triangle is parallel to the floor; 2) posterior tilt, also known as imprint; or 3) anterior tilt. If the pelvis is in an anterior or imprint position, move the pelvis to neutral. If low back pain or strain is felt in neutral, back off slightly.

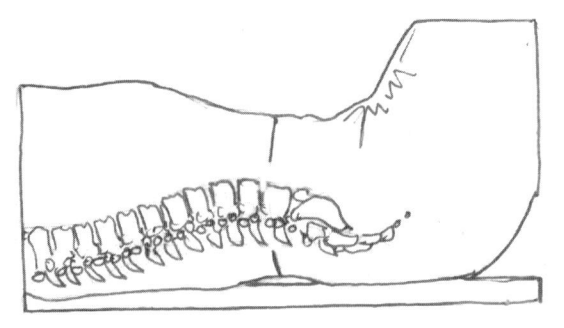

Neutral, where the triangle is parallel to the floor

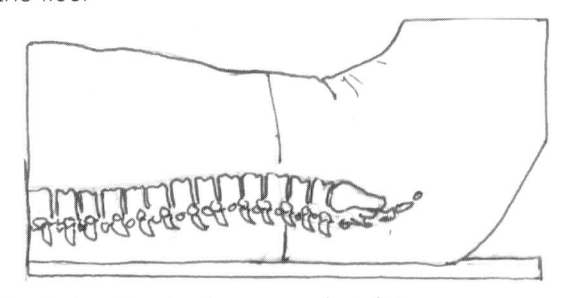

Posterior tilt, also known as imprint

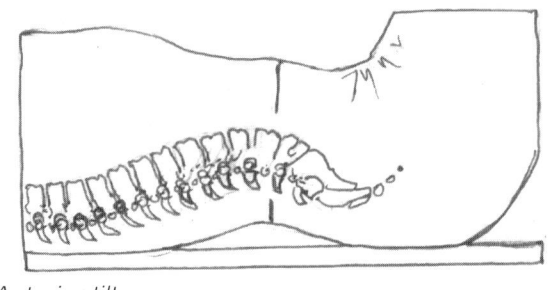

Anterior tilt

Movement Pattern 2: Finding Neutral—Indirect Method

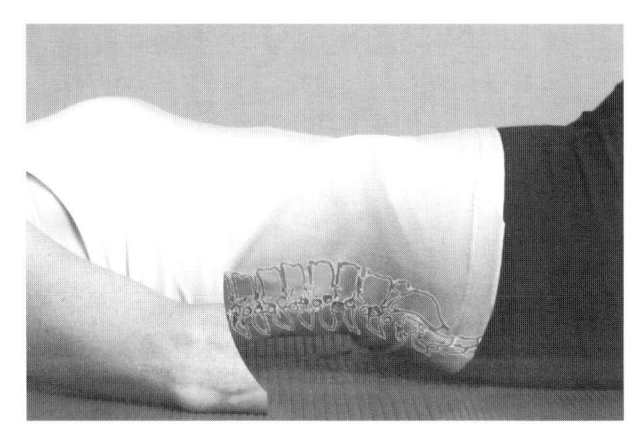

For some patients, finding anatomical landmarks can be frustrating and discouraging as they learn this principle.

Tilt the pelvis posterior by curling the tailbone toward ceiling, then reverse to the starting position. Tilt the pelvis anterior by curling the tailbone toward floor, then reverse to the starting position. To find neutral, feel the movement that occurs between the two ranges and find the midpoint in the range.

Movement Pattern 3: Finding Imprint (also known as a slight posterior tilt)

Inhale through the nose and breathe into the backs and sides of the ribs, maintaining neutral pelvis. Exhale through pursed lips and tip the ASIS bilaterally toward the rib cage, gently flattening the lumbar spine into the floor while keeping the gluteals relaxed. The motion should initiate with the abdominals. Inhale and maintain imprint. Exhale and release to neutral.

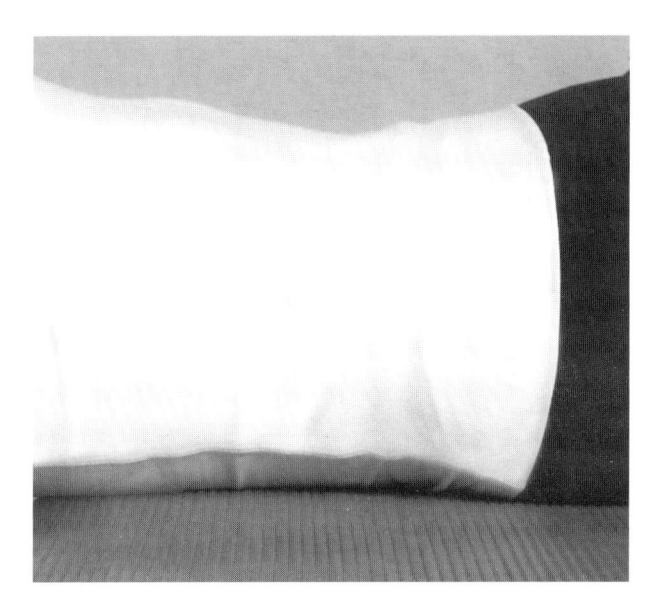

Helpful tip: Avoid overflexing of the lumbar spine, which some patients will verbalize as "it hurts my back." Others will notice their tailbone lifting off the floor. Instead, apply gentle pressure to the floor's surface.

Movement Pattern 4: Finding Imprint

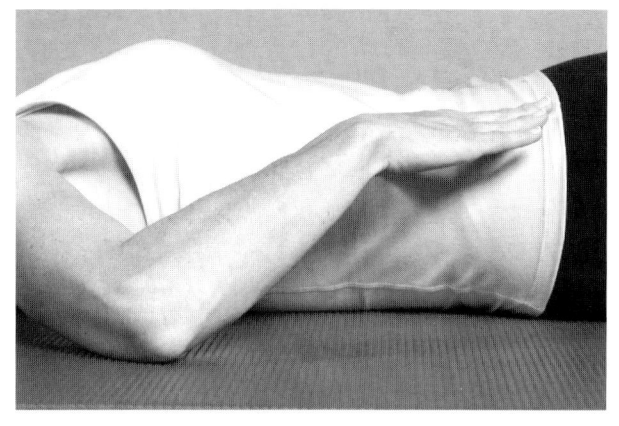

Follow the exercise as described in Movement Pattern 3. Ask patients to place their index finger on the ASIS and their thumbs on the apex of the rib cage. Inhale through the nose and breathe into the backs and sides of the ribs, maintaining the distance between the thumbs and index fingers. Exhale through pursed lips and tip the ASIS bilaterally toward the rib cage, gently flattening the lumbar spine into the floor while keeping the gluteals relaxed. Cue your patients: "Feel your fingers draw closer together and the abdominals tighten." Inhale to stay. Exhale and "Feel the fingers draw apart, returning to their original position of neutral pelvis."

Faulty Movement Patterns: Overactive gluteals; inability to keep the tailbone on the mat/floor; exaggerated posterior pelvic tilt; inability to maintain pelvic position; inability to stabilize the femurs independent of the pelvis; rib cage and/or abdominal popping; upper body tension; weight transfer right or left; sliding of the body along the mat

Scapular Control: Open and Closed Chain Training of the Upper Extremities

The shoulder girdle is composed of the humerus, clavicle, scapulae, and a complex network of muscles, ligaments, and tendons that help support movement of the upper extremities and efficient joint function.

The contributions of the scapulae at the scapulothoracic joint are key to efficient use of the shoulder. Because the scapulae have no direct bony attachment to the shoulder, rib cage, or spine, they are highly mobile. Efficient function of the shoulder is dependent on the scapular muscles as mobilizers and stabilizers.

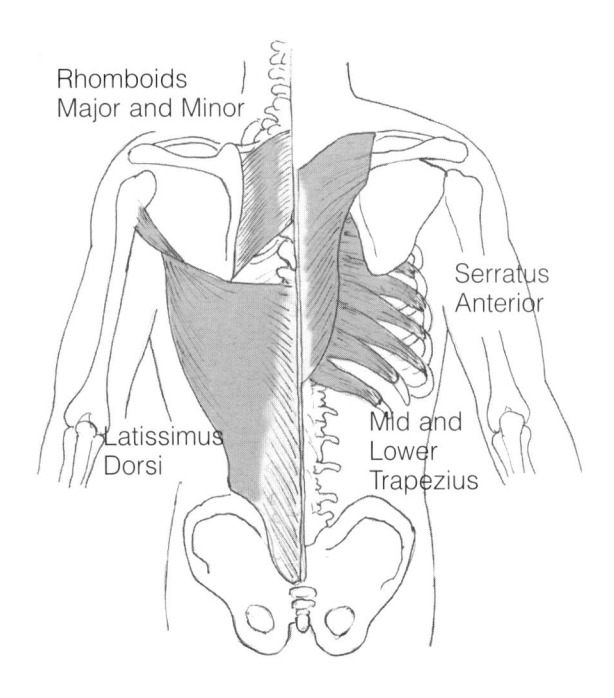

As mobilizers at the scapulothoracic joint, extrinsic muscles have specific roles in enhancing shoulder joint range of motion. As stabilizers, these same extrinsic muscles also have specific roles in stabilizing the scapulae against the rib cage with or without movement of the shoulder.

The serratus anterior, rhomboid major and minor, pectoralis minor, and the middle and lower trapezius have specific contributions to scapular stabilization during open and closed chain upper extremity training.

The latissimus dorsi and the sternal portion of the pectoralis major muscles also contribute to scapular stabilization but have an indirect role.

How does this anatomical review relate to Pilates practice? The link has evolved with time. Pilates was concerned about posture and the impact of technology on it and cites a number of health concerns related to posture that include abdominal obesity and asthma.

It's no secret that Pilates had good reason to red-flag posture. Of today's orthopaedic-related concerns requiring surgical or nonsurgical treatment, shoulder injuries and dysfunctions comprise more than 20 percent. Many treatments might have been reduced or eliminated with attention paid to the position of the scapulae, the muscles that facilitate their movement, and their relationship to proper posture and core strength.

As the third Pilates-based principle, scapular control teaches patients how to properly and safely position the scapulae in open and closed kinetic chain rehabilitation exercises as well as in functional activities and sport. Moreover, this principle can reveal muscle imbalances or restrictions that contribute to one's inability to stabilize the shoulder, leading to injury or dysfunction.

Here we lay the groundwork for shoulder and scapular stabilization in Pilates-based exercises by starting with teaching patients the basic movement mechanics of the scapulae or secondary stabilizers and how these mechanics impact trunk stabilization, and vice versa.

Key is teaching patients how to stabilize the scapulae against the torso and how to reduce the likelihood of faulty movement patterns. Benefits to patients include learning how to reduce tension in the neck, chest, and upper back that can occur with scapular elevation and protraction.

Purpose:

- To teach kinesthetic awareness of the scapular position. For many, this awareness is poor because patients can't see them or sense their positioning on the posterior upper to middle back.

Clinical Application:

- This principle is an essential patient education tool and is applicable to any exercise, Pilates-based or otherwise
- Optimizes torso stabilization through the secondary stabilizers without creating excessive stress in the upper back and neck muscles and reducing the likelihood of faulty movement patterns

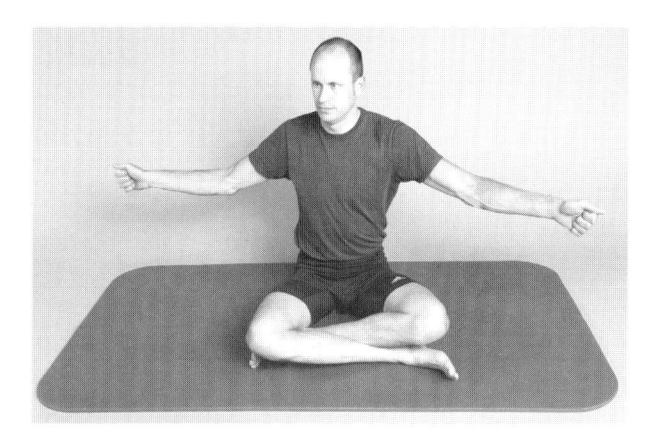

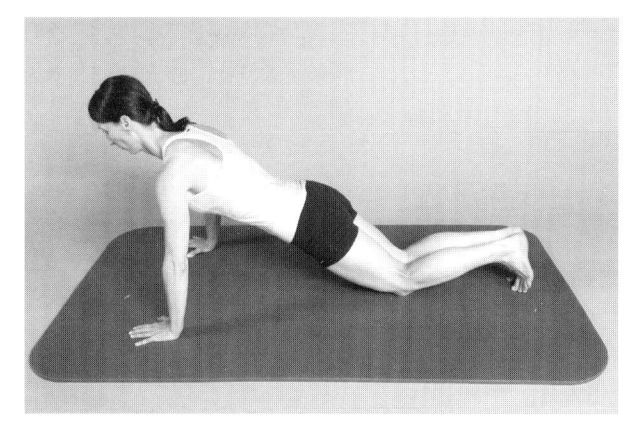

Teaching tip: Generally, in open kinetic chain training, the scapulae are positioned in slight depression and retraction. In closed kinetic chain training, such as in the pushup, the scapulae are slightly depressed and gently protracted. Special consideration should be given to the role of the serratus anterior muscle in stabilizing the scapulae along the ribs.

Open Chain Kinesthetic Awareness Training—Scapular Protraction/Retraction

Start in hooklying with neutral pelvis/spine, head, and neck alignment, the heels hip-width apart, the arms above the shoulders with the palms facing toward the midline.

Scapular Protraction

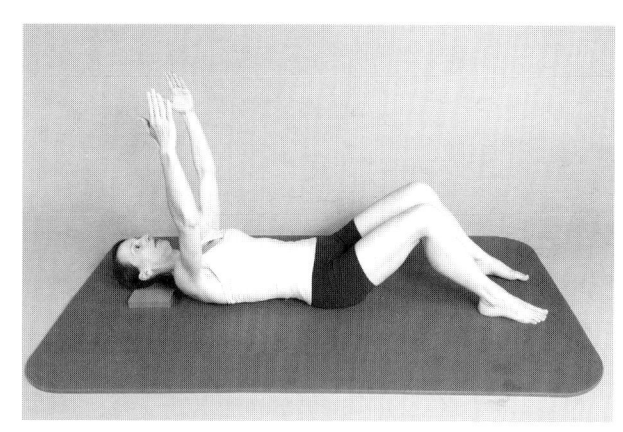

Scapular Retraction

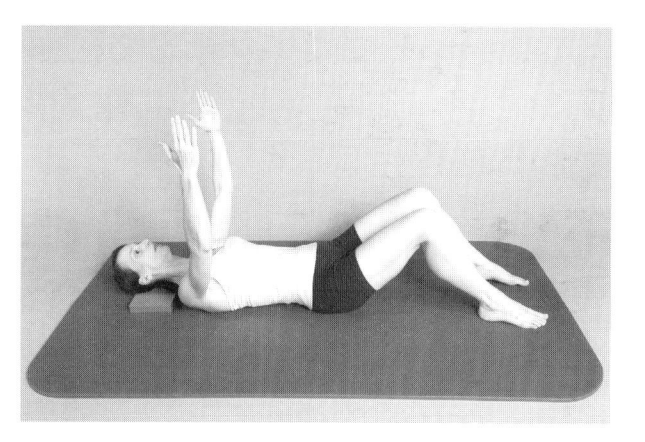

Inhale through the nose and reach the shoulders to the ceiling, drawing the scapulae off the floor (protraction). Exhale through pursed lips, keep the arms long, and pull the shoulders down to the floor, with widening across the chest, anterior shoulder regions (retraction), and upper back.

Place a stability ball, wooden doweling, small ball, or exercise band in your patient's hands to reinforce and/or challenge the secondary stabilizers against slight resistance.

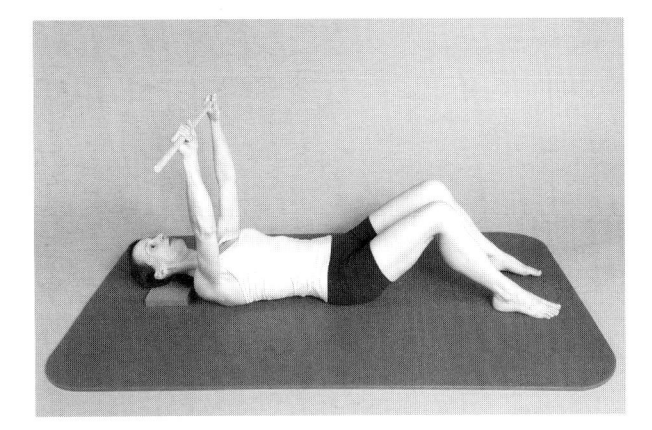

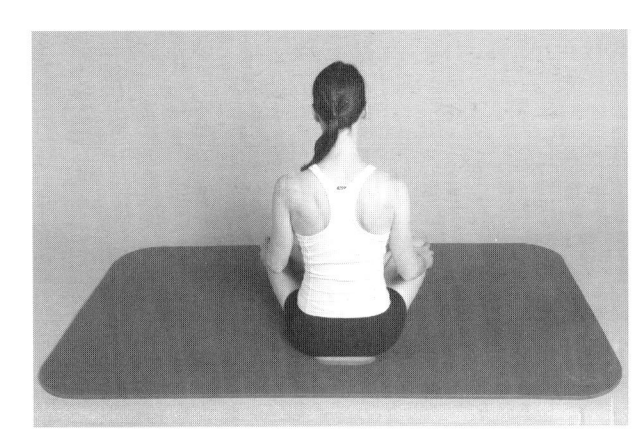

Faulty Movement Patterns: Rib cage popping; tension in the chest, upper back, and neck; hyperextended elbows; increased lumbar lordosis

Open Chain Kinesthetic Awareness Training—Elevation and Depression

Start in hooklying with neutral pelvis, head, and neck alignment, the heels hip-width apart, arms alongside the body, elbows slightly bent, with the palms facing down on the mat.

Inhale and slide the shoulders toward the ears while keeping the arms long, elbows soft. Exhale and naturally slide the shoulders away from the ears.

Faulty Movement Patterns: Excessive scapular depression resulting in increased tension in the upper back and neck muscles; hyperextended elbows

Open Chain Kinesthetic Awareness Training—Depression and Retraction

Start in hooklying with neutral pelvis, head, and neck alignment, the heels hip-width apart, arms alongside the body, elbows slightly bent, with the palms facing down on the mat.

Inhale through the nose and simultaneously depress and retract the scapulae slightly while keeping the arms long. Exhale and release to the starting position.

Helpful tips:

1. *Many patients tend to hyperextend the elbows (in this exercise and many others). To optimize scapular stabilization, cue patients to keep the elbows slightly bent and move from the shoulder. As skills practice, have patients try to stabilize the scapulae with the elbows hyperextended versus slightly bent. Most will find that hyperextended elbows affect the ability to depress and retract the scapulae. This drill also teaches kinesthetic awareness of the elbow and its impact on scapular stabilization.*

2. *Some patients respond better to sitting as an initial position for scapular training. Feedback can be achieved visually through a mirror and/or tactile cueing from the therapist to enhance kinesthetic awareness.*

Faulty Movement Patterns: Rib cage popping; tension in the chest, upper back, and neck; hyperextended elbows; increased lumbar lordosis; scapular elevation/protraction

Closed Chain Kinesthetic Awareness Training—Depression and Protraction

Neutral

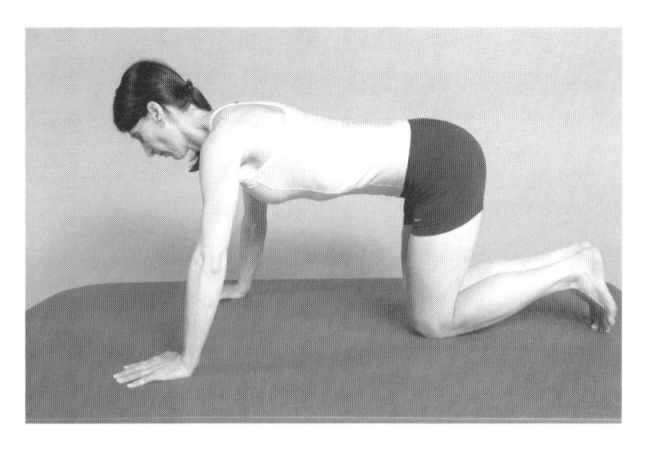

Start in quadruped with the hands aligned outside the shoulders, the elbows slightly bent, and the hips abducted so the knees align under the hips.

Scapular Retraction

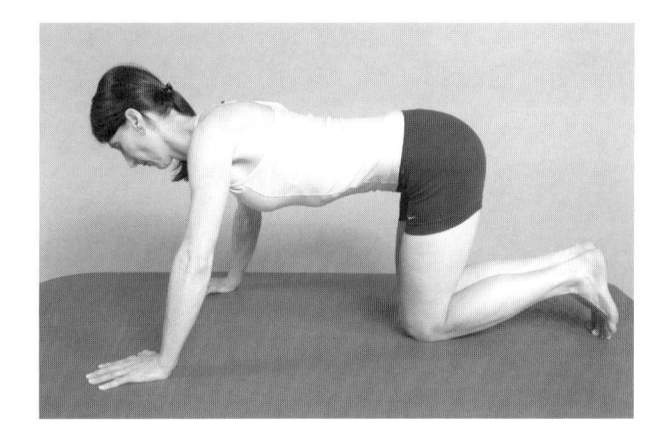

Let the chest "sag" toward the floor, creating scapular retraction. Arch the upper back toward the ceiling to produce scapular protraction. Ask patients to feel the range of motion between the two positions. Find the midpoint between the two end points.

Scapular Protraction

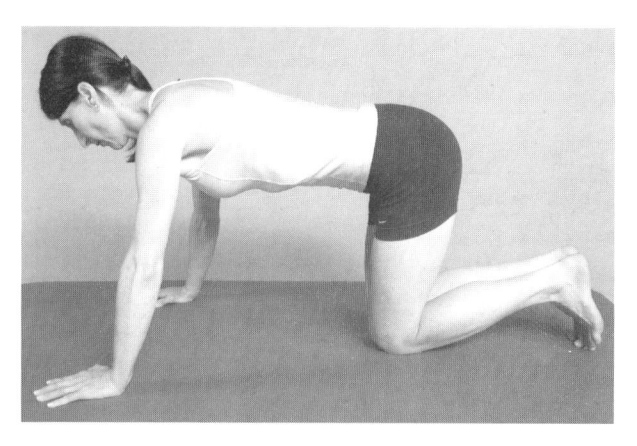

Stabilize the scapulae against the torso through slight protraction and depression.

Helpful tip: Use the wall as an early option if scapular winging presents in four-point position and progress patient to the floor when stabilization is mastered.

Faulty Movement Patterns: Scapular winging; excessive scapular depression resulting in increased tension in the neck and upper back; hyperextended elbows

Rib Cage Positioning

Positioning of the rib cage is just as necessary to torso stabilization as the pelvis, and the relationship between the two is critical. The rib cage is highly mobile, expanding and contracting with every breath, moving inward and out, upward and down. It influences movement of the thoracic spine via its attachments (anterior and posterior articulation to sternum and thoracic vertebra) to the more than 12 muscles that connect to the rib cage, most of them linking to the pelvis or spine.

Why is rib cage positioning important? For one, the abdominals have attachments to the ribs, and to function optimally, the rib cage needs to be aligned over the pelvis with and without movement of the shoulders. When rib cage alignment is not optimal, neutral lumbo-pelvic positioning may be altered and abdominal muscle function affected.

Rib cage positioning can be affected in several ways. Rib cage restrictions or rigidity can have a profound effect(s) on the position of the pelvis and spine, on breathing, and on movement of the upper and lower extremities. The resting position of the ribs can be altered, for example, with hypertonic thoracic erector spinae muscles, resulting in thoracic extension and the ribs positioned anterior to the pelvis. Decreased mobility of the upper thoracic spine and shoulder or tight latissimus dorsi can affect the position of the rib cage with end-range shoulder flexion. Because the rib cage is a central player in torso stabilization, educating patients about proper positioning with or without arm movement is important to performing Pilates-based exercises as well as activities of daily living, work, and/or sport.

Purpose:

- *More than 58 percent of the ribs have an abdominal attachment. To keep the rib cage in proper alignment over the pelvis and the abdominals engaged at optimal length, the ribs should not pop anteriorly in sitting, standing, prone, or supine positions or when the arms raise over the head. When supine, the lower ribs should maintain contact with the mat. Proper breathing mechanics can help stabilize the ribs via the abdominals.*

Clinical Application:

- *This is an essential patient education tool to include with teaching traditional lumbar stabilization exercises and strengthening of the abdominals and upper/lower extremities.*
- *Reteaching breathing mechanics*
- *Reducing the likelihood of faulty movement patterns (i.e., hyperlordotic or kyphotic posture)*

Movement Pattern 1:

To increase kinesthetic awareness of rib cage alignment and positioning with exercises that require lumbo-pelvic neutral, ask your patient to place one hand along the ribs while flexing the opposite shoulder to end range. Rib cage positioning is achieved just prior to feeling the anterior ribs popping forward. Repeat and compare on the opposite side. Ask your patient to practice without tactile feedback of his/her hands to enhance kinesthetic awareness of rib cage alignment.

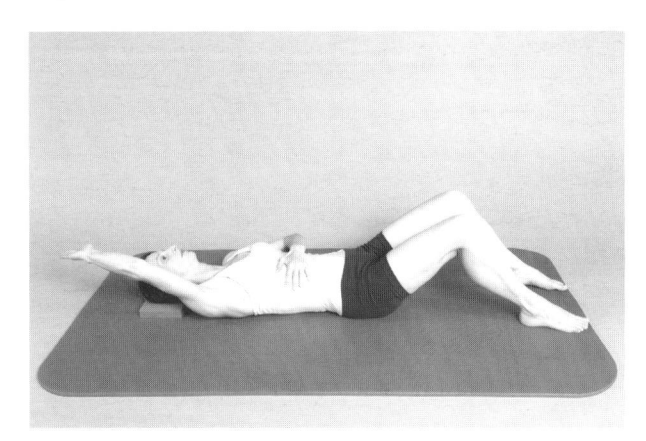

Movement Pattern 2:

Start in hooklying with neutral pelvis, head, and neck alignment, the heels hip-width apart, arms alongside the body, elbows slightly bent, with the palms facing down on the mat. The distal ribs should be in contact with the mat for the normal resting position.

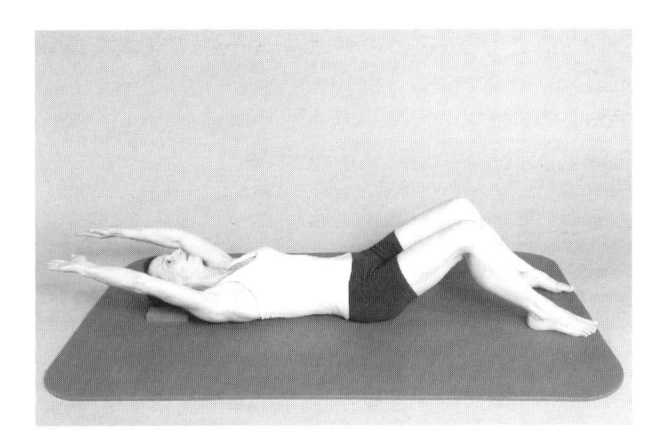

Exhale and move the arms overhead while maintaining abdominal connection and contact of the lower ribs against the mat. Inhale and reverse directions. Feel the difference? Feel the challenge? The movement should be seamless, flowing from one motion to the next.

Helpful tip: If the thoracic erector spinae muscles are hypertonic or thoracic dysfunction is present, relaxation training in the yoga-based "child's pose" position and/or manual therapy techniques applied to the thoracic spine/ribs are recommended to achieve the normal resting position of the ribs before teaching rib cage positioning (3).

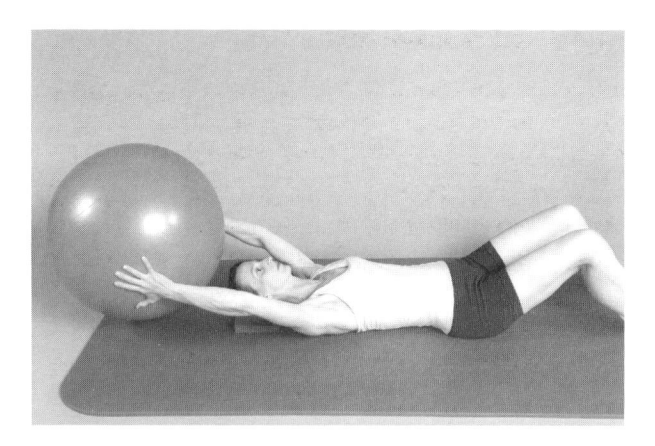

Place a wooden dowel, ball, or exercise band in your patient's hand to assist in maintaining proper alignment or to challenge rib cage positioning with slight resistance. The average stability ball weighs 2 to 3 pounds.

Faulty Movement Patterns: Ribs popping in prone, supine, or sitting, with the arms at rest by the sides or with the arms lifted overhead; low back arching in supine (anterior pelvic tilt) secondary to tight latissimus dorsi, decreased shoulder joint mobility, and/or hypomobility in the upper to mid-thoracic spine (T1-T6); hyperextended elbows; thoracic extension in resting secondary to hypertonic thoracic erector spinae and/or mechanical thoracic spine/rib dysfunction

Teaching tip: Rib cage alignment is controlled by movement of the shoulder into flexion. If there is hypomobility of the upper and mid-thoracic spine (T1-T6), tight latissimus dorsi, and/or restricted joint mobility of the shoulder, the position of the ribs will be affected. If this is the case, instruct patients not to push the most distal ribs to the floor. Rather, they should control the position of the ribs via movement at the shoulder.

Head and Neck Positioning

In classical Pilates, many exercises require excessive neck flexion. Some methods continue this today while others advocate for the cervical spine in neutral. Given the potential of injury and excessive stress to neck muscles, ligaments, and discs, we encourage neutral alignment.

Defined by Kendall, the cervical spine is in a slightly convex anterior position (4). Normal cervical lordosis creates balance for the cervical neck flexors and extensors. When there is not balance, the normal recruitment pattern of the deep neck flexors will be altered, leading to tension of the face, neck, and shoulders—just the opposite of what Pilates intended.

The general rule is to nod the head slightly with emphasis on craniovertebral flexion at C1-C2 and that the cervical spine follows the curvature of the thoracic spine.

For patients who have an excessive thoracic kyphosis, supine and prone positions increase the cervical lordosis. Practitioners should provide support by using either a towel or padding to promote neutral starting alignment. Patients will be appreciative!

In sitting, standing, and quadruped positions, it is just as important to support the cervical spine in neutral. Patients with a forward head position should be repositioned with a slight cervical retraction.

Purpose:

- In many exercises, the cervical nod initiates segmental mobilization of the spine
- The cervical nod reinforces the position of the cervical spine, which should follow the curvature established by the thoracic spine
- Minimizes stress on the cervical spine and facilitates a normal muscle recruitment pattern of the deep neck flexors

Clinical Application:

- This is an essential patient education tool to reinforce proper alignment of the cervical spine and to strengthen the deep neck flexors
- Use to avoid excessive neck strain

Movement Pattern: Cervical Nod

Start in hooklying with neutral pelvis, head, and neck alignment, the heels hip-width apart, arms alongside the body, elbows slightly bent, with the palms facing down on the mat.

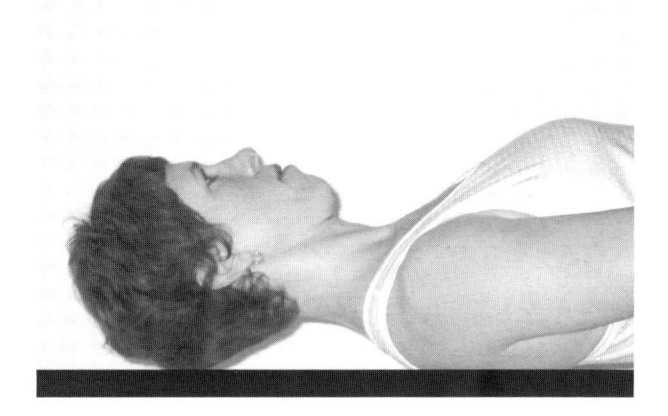

Inhale through the nose and lengthen the back of neck, nodding the head slightly (craniovertebral flexion, C1-C2). Exhale through pursed lips and release.

Teaching tips:

1. Ask your patient to imagine that he or she is nodding to the queen. Or ask the patient to nod the length of the dime to establish range of motion of the upper cervical spine. He or she will note that the movement is extremely small, enhancing kinesthetic awareness with training.

2. Next, ask your patient to place his/her thumbs at the mastoid processes and cradle the head with the hands and the first and second fingers at the base of the occiput. Gently apply a slight manual traction to the occiput to create the nod.

Variation: The seated (gravity-assisted) position is a nice alternative for patients who experience overrecruitment of the superficial neck flexors when performing the cervical nod in supine. Use the seated position initially for neuromuscular reeducation of the deep cervical flexors.

Equipment: Pillow/foam pad, for faulty posture (i.e., forward head)

Faulty Movement Patterns: Excessive cervical flexion; hyperextended cervical spine (i.e., C2-C3 and/or upper cervical spine dysfunction); inability to perform the cervical nod; compensatory firing of the sternocleidomastoid/anterior scalene muscles

Excessive Flexion

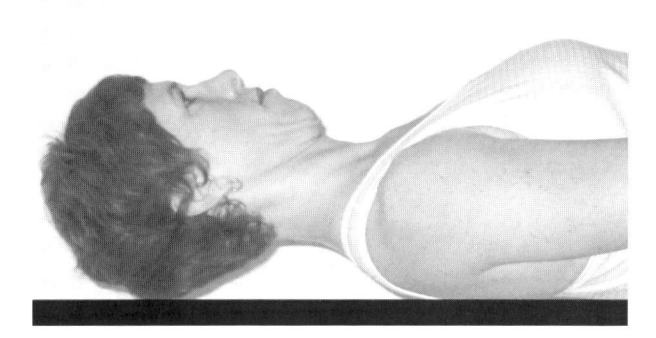

Excessive Extension

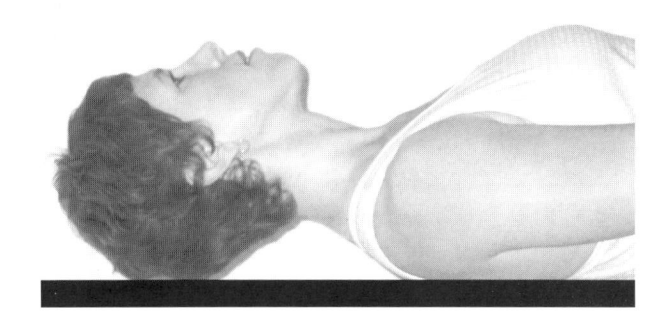

Helpful tips:

1. Generally, the chin should be a fist's distance from the chest. A common Pilates cue is to "draw the chin to the chest." While it's fine to cue "chin to chest," be sure your patient does not thrust the chin forward or overflex the chin to the chest.

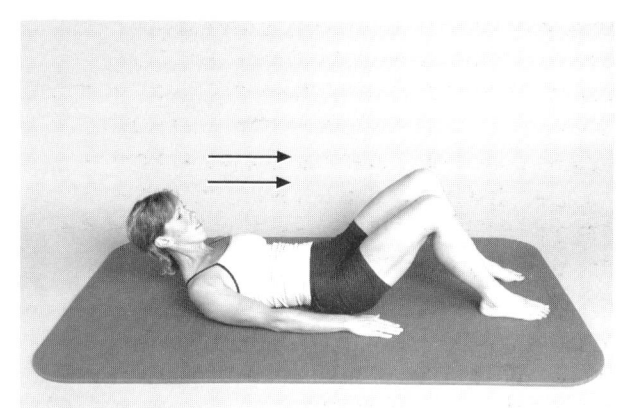

2. The eyes are a valuable tool to use with training as they help facilitate movement with exercises that require spinal articulation sequentially from the cervical to the lumbar spine as well as maintain cervical alignment throughout the exercise. Use visual imagery to cue your patient to look to or over the knees. Proper eye positioning can help alleviate neck tension. "Imagine your eyes as flashlights shining light over the knees."

3. If your patient has a short neck, cueing him/her to focus on the knees may result in compensatory cervical extension. Modify the cue to focus on the mid-thigh to support cervical neutral throughout the exercise.

Motor Coordination

Pilates coined the word *Contrology* and used it to describe the intentional, mindful attention of the mind to movement. His writings referenced the smooth, controlled, rhythmic movement of wild and domestic animals alike and encouraged humans to move in similar fashion. With practice, this controlled, intentional movement would become natural, seemingly innate, and unconscious (1).

Clinically, one of the benefits of the Pilates practice of Contrology is that it challenges *purposeful* motor coordination and, in some cases, can help facilitate neuromuscular reeducation when one's attention is focused on a particular muscle or movement. For this reason, we include motor coordination as a Pilates-based principle.

Each principle, from breathing to rib cage positioning, may be performed in isolation or layered on top of each other, until all are successfully coordinated together. This, coupled with stability before mobility, is at the heart of motor learning and skill coordination.

Teaching tips:

1. *When working with patients, initially teach the principles in isolation. We typically begin with breathing or pelvic position, depending on the patient's health condition, goals, and our objective assessment findings.*

2. *As each principle is mastered, another is added; the two are then coordinated, and so on. Which principle we decide to focus on next is dependent on our patient's desired outcome.*

3. *Once principles are coordinated together, stationary and/or stable movement patterns are coordinated with the principles. Generally, these patterns are performed in prone or supine positions. This process is repeated over and over as your patient progresses to more advanced movement patterns that challenge through coordination, endurance, strength, and balance. Our ultimate goal is movement efficiency and muscular control in sitting, standing, ADLs, and/or safe return to sport.*

Integrative Isolation

"It is very interesting to note the indisputable fact that no one modern activity employs all our muscles. But it is also quite obvious . . . each muscle should cooperatively and loyally aid in the uniform development of all muscles. . . . developing minor muscles helps to strengthen major muscles. . . . When all your muscles are properly developed, as a matter of course you will perform your work with minimum effort and maximum pleasure (1)."

Our interpretation? At the core of this Pilates-based principle is the thought that our body is one big kinetic chain: What occurs at the feet affects the knees, hips, pelvis, ribs, shoulders, and head. And vice versa: What happens at the core affects the rest of the chain, upper extremity to lower. Quality of movement demands that the entire body work together: the upper and lower body—torso and extremities—supporting each other's work in both an integrated and isolative manner. Case in point: Perform a standing biceps curl with no attempt to stabilize the body at the shoulder girdle, torso, or legs. Repeat the effort, applying the Pilates-based principle of integrative isolation. Can you tell the difference?

Use this drill with your patients to enhance their understanding of core stabilization and how it affects the quality of the work effort, whether it is in performing a therapeutic exercise or walking up a flight of stairs.

Relative to Pilates, each exercise has a purpose—for example, to strengthen the abdominals or stretch the erector spinae. Does that mean that other muscles are not working to support the movement? No. And that is the beauty of Pilates.

Mind-Body Principles

How often do you drive to a destination without remembering how you got there? Ever experience a muscle ache and wonder what you did the day before? These questions bring to light tenets important to Pilates practice—concentration and centering—that serve us well today in a technology-driven lifestyle.

Concentration

It strikes us that concentration and Pilates' Contrology work hand-in-hand to achieve desired motor control and coordination. Perhaps better termed mindfulness, concentration is one of the foundational principles identified in the original Pilates Method. From Pilates' perspective, concentration is a method of focusing the mind on what the body is doing at all times, from gross, simple motor movement patterns to the smallest, most complex patterns.

Moreover, concentration is a method of better connecting mind and body, fostering mental clarity, creativity, and the ability to leave occurrences of the day behind. According to Pilates, concentration allows one to gain the most benefit from an exercise by performing it correctly, with precision and good technique.

From a movement education perspective, concentration can help improve kinesthetic awareness, muscle reeducation, neuromuscular coordination, and movement quality throughout the kinetic chain. Of these, the latter require control through intentional, mindful movement.

Centering

Centering refers to the practice of initiating all movement from the body's center or the "girdle of strength." Today this girdle of strength is more commonly referred to as the core, the powerhouse of torso stabilization.

Our understanding of centering is simply the ability to control the muscles that comprise the powerhouse or trunk. The trunk is our functional platform: the ability to control it in the face of a misstep down the stairs or lunging for a tennis ball can translate to reduced injury risk or dysfunction.

Chapter References

1. Gallagher, S.P., Kryzanowska, R. 2000. *The Complete Writings of Joseph H. Pilates*. Philadelphia, PA: Bain Bridge Books.

2. STOTT *Pilates Comprehensive Matwork Manual*. 2001. Toronto, Canada: Merrithew Corporation.

3. Lee, D. 2003. *The Pelvis—Bridging the Gap Between Science and the Clinic*. Course notes. Edina, MN: Fairview Education Center, October 4-5.

4. Kendall, F.P., McCreary, E.K., Provance, P.G. 1993. *Muscles, Testing and Function, Posture and Pain*, Fourth Edition. Baltimore, MD: Williams and Wilkins.

chapter 5

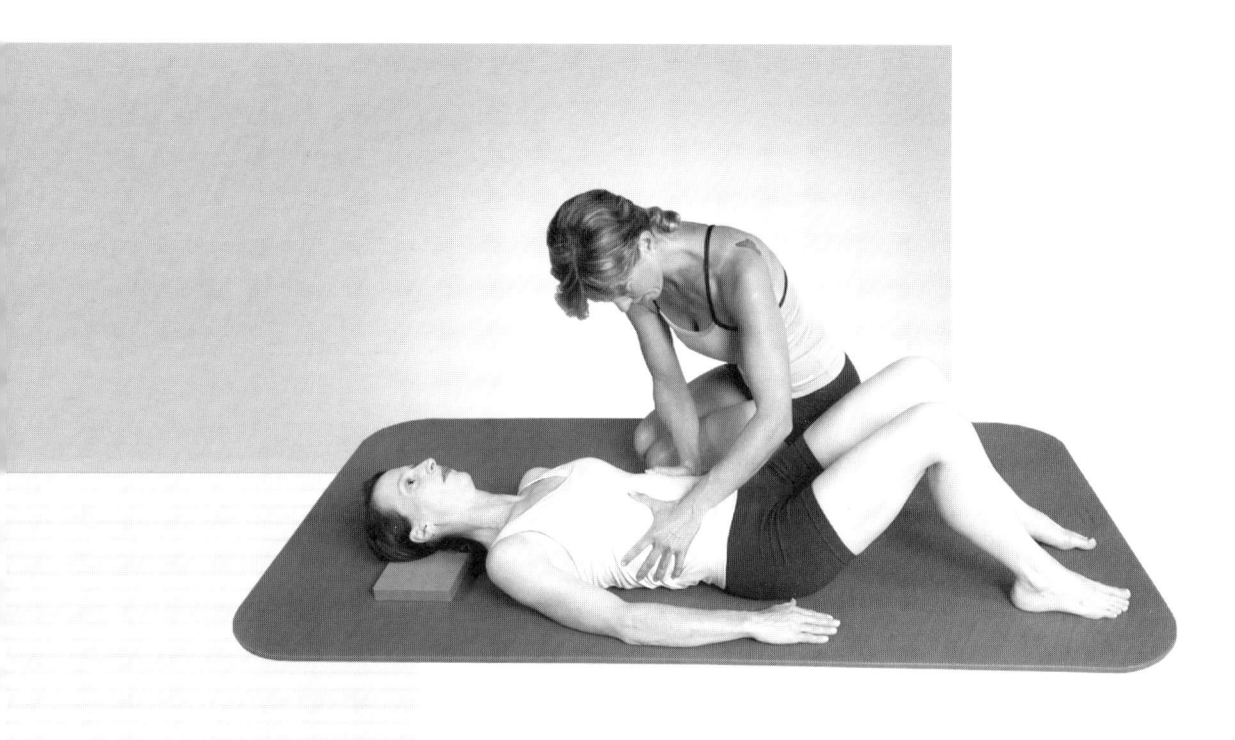

CORE
STABILIZATION
STRATEGIES:
BREATHING,
TRANSVERSUS
ABDOMINIS,
NEUTRAL PELVIS,
ABDOMINAL
BRACING

Body alignment and awareness are essential components in developing core stabilization or volitional control of our trunk. As we all know, some people have good body alignment and movement awareness and some do not. For patients who have poor alignment or movement awareness, core stabilization training can be challenging for the rehabilitation or fitness practitioner. You can try all the tricks in the book and it won't matter; the results are the same. There are no changes in faulty muscle recruitment or movement patterns.

How does one approach this challenge? This chapter provides you with additional assessment tools and teaching strategies to identify and correct faulty muscle recruitment patterns, assist with neuromuscular reeducation, and enhance core stabilization training for the challenging patient.

Assessing Breathing

It isn't a secret that breathing is essential for life as well as exercise. It is also a crucial element to assess during the musculoskeletal examination. Indeed, breathing affects core stabilization and movement. Surprised? Read on.

Clinically, the breathing assessment is composed of two parts (1). The first part evaluates the quality of the breath pattern at rest and its relationship to the torso. The second part examines abdominal muscle recruitment patterns.

Breathing Assessment at Rest, Part One

The first breathing assessment looks at the breath pattern at rest. The assessment can be performed in a hooklying position, in sitting or standing, or a combination thereof.

1. Ask your patient to breathe naturally and observe the normal resting breath pattern. Refer to our helpful hints. Proper breathing requires diaphramatic breathing.

2. Questions to ponder as you observe the breathing patterns: Is there more expansion in the abdominal or chest regions? Are the ribs moving laterally or posteriorly with breathing? Is there increased muscle definition (shadowing) indicative of overactive muscles (1)? Can your patient relax overactive muscles with verbal or hands-on cueing? Is there symmetrical or asymmetrical tone of torso muscles and rib movement? Can you feel unilateral or bilateral restriction in the rib cage with the breathing cycle?

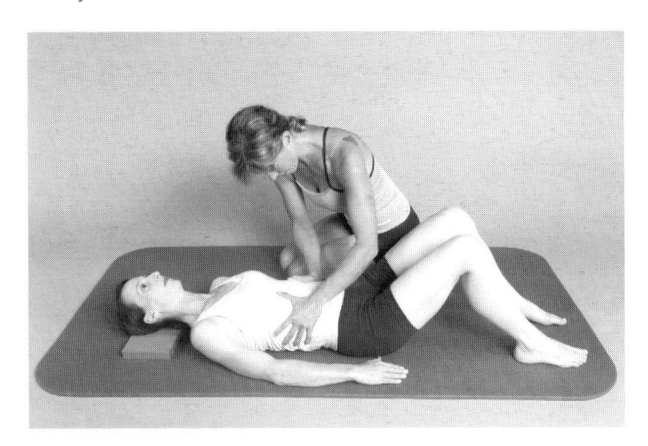

Helpful tip: After observing the breathing cycle, it is helpful to use your hands to sense any restriction in rib movement from all aspects: anterior, posterior, and lateral. This can be done with your patient in sitting, standing, or supine positions.

Hodges et al. identified common compensatory strategies with breathing:

- Restricted lateral and/or posterior rib cage expansion
- Shadowing present with tonic activity of the superficial abdominal muscles such as the external obliques (EO) and rectus abdominis (RA)
- Tonic obliques with the breathing cycle secondary to chronic low back pain (Upper chest breathing and accessory inspiratory muscle activation can accompany this faulty firing pattern. Normal activation pattern of the obliques occurs with forced expiration (2).
- Breathing into the upper chest
- Overdeveloped or tonic thoracolumbar erector spinae
- Decreased thoracolumbar segmental mobility

Breathing Assessment with Abdominal Contraction, Part Two

The second part of the breathing assessment suggested by Hodges examines general abdominal muscle activity with breathing and sets the stage for transversus abdominis assessment, which is addressed later in this chapter.

1. The test is performed in hooklying, sitting, or standing. Ask your patient or client to breathe naturally and recruit the abdominals slowly and gently with exhalation. Ideally, abdominal muscle recruitment should occur below the level of the umbilicus (1). The umbilicus draws in slightly and the lower abdominal region flattens, indicating the ability to contract the TrA independently and voluntarily.
2. Observe the contraction pattern and look for faulty muscle recruitment and movement patterns. Observations include: a) whether shadowing occurs across the anterior and posterior regions of the torso, which might indicate tonic muscle activity; b) whether the contour of the lower abdominal region changes; c) whether the upper abdominal muscles such as the external obliques or rectus abdominis are dominant; d) whether there is coordination of breath with abdominal contraction; and/or whether spinal alignment is maintained (1).

Helpful tip: Even the movement of the belly button can reveal something about your patient's breathing patterns. Does the umbilicus draw in or move to the right or left? This observation may tell you more about muscles that are dominant or inhibited.

Richardson, Jull, Hodges, and Hides demonstrated common compensatory strategies on exhalation with abdominal contraction (3):

Abnormal Movement

- Lumbar flexion, a result of increased external oblique and rectus abdominis activity
- Thoracolumbar flexion, a result of increased external oblique and rectus abdominis activity
- Depressed rib cage secondary to increased firing of the anteromedial external oblique

Observing the Abdominal Wall

- No observable contraction
- Bulging of the lower abdominal wall, indicating compensatory internal oblique (IO) firing
- Increased lateral abdominal wall excursion, external oblique muscle contraction with increased activity at the origin
- Inability to relax the abdominals

Compensatory Breathing Patterns

- Compensatory recruitment of the external and internal obliques with breathing
- Inability to breathe diaphragmatically
- Compensatory recruitment of the scalene and sternocleidomastoid muscles, which causes the abdominal wall to move inward

Compensatory Recruitment of Thoracic Erector Spinae

- Co-activation

Retraining Breathing

Breathing is innate. That said, learning how to breathe correctly is a skill and requires that the patient use the Pilates principles of concentration and centering. Moreover, you might be surprised at the positive patient outcomes that ensue with increased breathing capacity.

If you identify, for example; muscle hypertonicity and/or faulty diaphragmatic breathing pattern in your assessment, relaxation training and/or manual therapy techniques should be initiated first to normalize diaphragmatic breathing pattern before you progress your patient to the Pilates breath principle.

Once normal diaphramatic breathing is restored, initiate retraining of the breath pattern as described under the Pilates breathing principle. Remember, we advocate a *gentle, passive exhalation*, not the typical active exhalation endorsed by many Pilates practitioners.

If your patient lacks posterior or lateral rib expansion with inhalation, see the additional training techniques listed below for options.

Helpful tips:

1. *Every effort should be made to retrain breathing in neutral pelvis and spine. Some clinicians find success by retraining breathing in different positions or by incorporating equipment, such as in sidelying on a stability ball, which can facilitate a stretch similar to manual techniques or can provide greater sensory feedback.*

2. *Use relaxation training to foster concentration with controlled breathing. Select the training position that is comfortable for the patient. This might be in hooklying if the external oblique muscles are hyperactive or in a yoga-style "child's pose" position if the thoracolumbar erector spinae are hypertonic (4).*

3. *With normal diaphragmatic breathing pattern excursion of the diaphragm will occur just distal to the base of the sternum with inhalation. If you do not observe this excursion normal breathing mechanics are not present.*

4. *Use imagery to increase rib cage expansion laterally, posteriorly, or in combination.*

Imagery Examples:

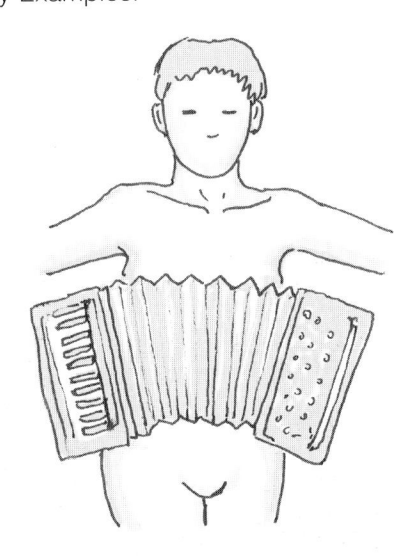

- To increase lateral excursion of the ribs, imagine that the ribs are expanding toward the elbows like an accordion
- To increase posterior excursion of the ribs while supine, imagine that the ribs are expanding into the floor like melting butter
- To increase lateral and posterior mobility of the ribs, imagine that the ribs are a room with a ceiling and floor. As you inhale, breath into the sides and floor of the room, keeping the ceiling still.

  Relaxation Training Example: Inhalation is gentle and expiration is passive. Cue your patient: "Gently deepen your breath to increase your feeling of relaxation, but do not force your breath." Training can last anywhere from a minute to several minutes and can be enhanced with visual imagery and touch. If tonic activity is not reduced, use equipment such as biofeedback or additional manual therapy techniques to relax overactive muscles.

5. Use tactile cueing to facilitate increased rib cage expansion posteriorly, laterally, or a combination of both, and to decrease compensatory external oblique firing prior to TrA recruitment.

Tactile Cueing Example:

- Clinician places his/her hands bilaterally on the patient's lateral rib cage and cues the patient to expand the ribs into the clinician's hands with inhalation, feeling the ribs pull away from the hands with exhalation. Follow with the patient placing his/her own hands on the rib cage to experience the same.
- Clinician spreads his/her hands along the patient's lateral rib cage and facilitates lateral rib cage expansion with inhalation by applying pressure down and across the ribs diagonally and giving a quick stretch at the end of the exhalation phase. Follow the quick stretch with resisting lateral rib cage expansion to facilitate the external intercostal muscles.

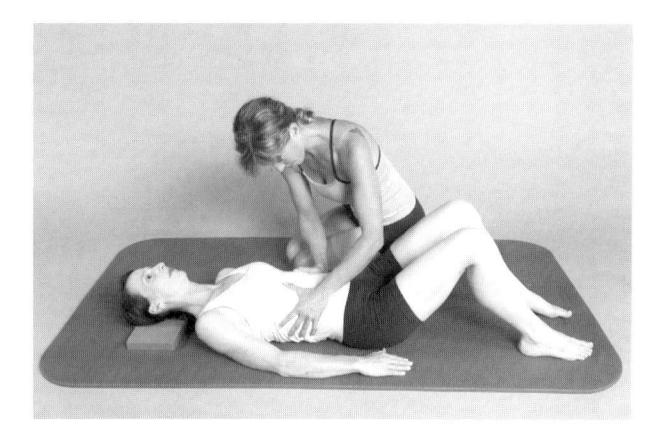

6. Use equipment such as a mirror to help your patient self-monitor rib cage mobility and to provide sensory feedback.

Equipment Example:

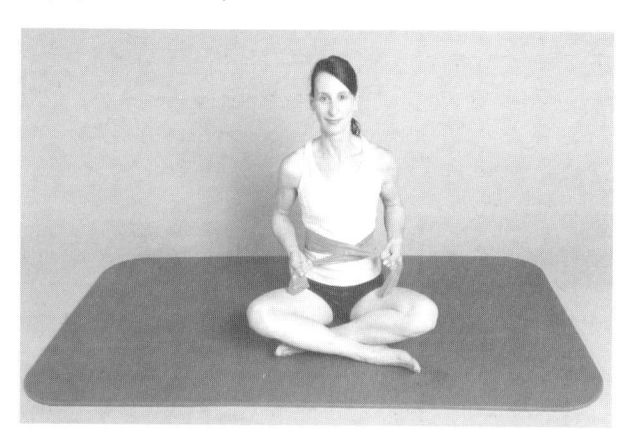

Place an exercise band, belt, towel, or bedsheet around the patient's lower posterior and lateral ribs and cross it in front of body. Ask the patient to gently pull the ends of the equipment away from the body to create slight tension along the rib cage and expand the ribs laterally, posteriorly, or in combination into the equipment with inhalation. Adding more resistance by gently tightening the band can encourage a deeper range of motion on inhalation and is helpful for patients who have a difficult time correcting faulty breathing patterns.

7. Use kinesthetic cueing. Patients who have poor body awareness and alignment (i.e., thoracic kyphosis) with breathing may benefit from this simple exercise.

Kinesthetic Example:

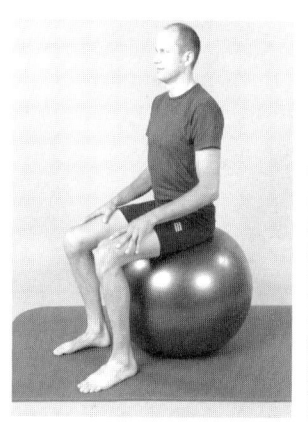

Ask your patient to sit tall and inhale, breathing into the back and sides of the ribs.

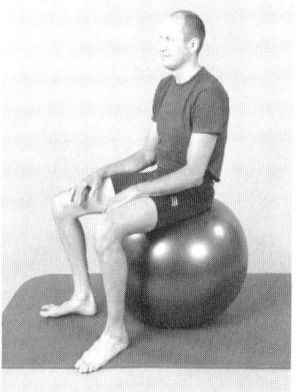

Next, ask him or her to collapse and breathe. With each exercise, ask your patient to observe the changes in breath and rib cage expansion when the spine is aligned and not aligned. The patient should note an increase in breathing capacity with good alignment.

Transversus Abdominis

The transversus abdominis plays a crucial role in core stabilization. Although it isn't the only muscle to contribute to stability, it has been shown to contribute to lumbo-pelvic stabilization through lumbar stiffness, sacroiliac stability (3,5,6), tightening of the thoracolumbar fascia, and an increase in intra-abdominal pressure, each important for quality movement (2,3,6).

Core stabilization is affected by a delayed or absent TrA contraction, and rehabilitation is essential to restore a normal TrA recruitment pattern. It is important to note that we don't advocate TrA training if a normal recruitment pattern is present. Moreover, we do not emphasize its isolative recruitment in Pilates exercise as some methods currently encourage. As large muscle groups, the abdominals, the lower back muscles, and other important torso stabilizers must be trained in an integrated manner.

Assessing the Transversus Abdominis for Dysfunction

Rehabilitation of the TrA starts with assessment. The focus of the evaluation is not on measuring strength, but on the precision and pattern of muscle fiber recruitment. Clinically, Richardson, Hodges, and others have suggested two primary methods to assess your patient's ability to contract the TrA independently from other abdominal muscles: the indirect and the direct methods (2,3).

These methods are great for educating your patients about the relationship of the abdominals to the back muscles and the role of the torso muscles as stabilizers in movement. Ideally, this education will carry over to ADLs and other functional movement activities.

The first method uses a pressure biofeedback unit to monitor pressure changes with volitional TrA contraction (2,3). The second method requires the clinician to palpate and observe TrA contraction as well as the activity of other abdominal muscles (2,3).

Method One: Pressure Biofeedback Unit

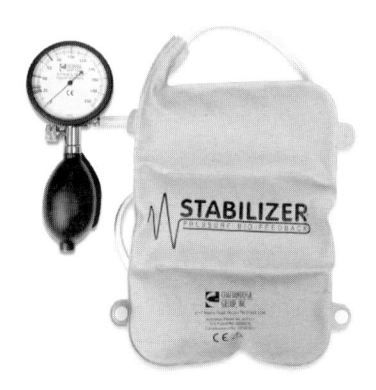

Developed by Hodges, the indirect method of testing TrA is performed in the prone position with the arms relaxed at the sides and using the anatomical landmarks of the umbilicus and ASIS for inflatable pad placement. Align the center of the pad with the umbilicus and the bottom border of the pad with both anterior superior iliac spines (2,3). Increase the pressure to 70 mmHg and note any small pressure changes that are occurring secondary to normal abdominal activity with breathing for a resting baseline (2,3).

Cue your patient to lift the navel slowly up and away from the pad with natural exhalation while keeping the lumbo-pelvic region still, and observe the pressure changes (2,3). Once a normal recruitment pattern is demonstrated, test TrA endurance by having the patient hold the contraction for 10 seconds and performing the test up to 10 repetitions (2,3). An abnormal test occurs when there is either no change, an increase in pressure, or less than a 2 mmHg change in pressure. If abnormal, repeat the test (1,3).

Other compensatory strategies using the pressure unit method include (2,3):

- Posterior pelvic tilt/lumbar flexion
- Contraction of the external obliques, characterized by rib cage depression
- Inability of the TrA to fire or overactivity of other abdominals such as the EO and RA muscles

Method Two: Palpation

The palpation method of TrA testing is performed in hooklying.

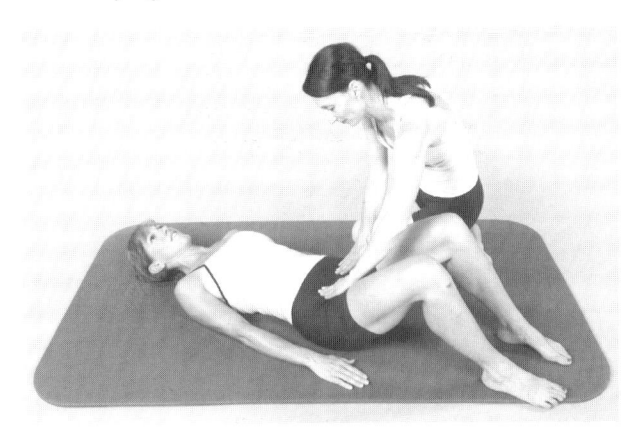

1. Ask your patient to relax the abdominals. Then place both thumbs or the middle three fingers 2 centimeters medial and inferior to the ASIS and gently burrow the fingers deeply into the abdominal area. In this position, you will be able to monitor the TrA and internal oblique muscle recruitment patterns with breathing and attempts at a voluntary contraction (1).

2. Ask your patient to slowly pull his/her navel in gently with normal exhalation while you observe and palpate the TrA contraction. With correct contraction of the TrA, you should feel a slowly developing, deep tension in the abdominal wall beneath the fingers. You also may feel your fingers move toward the midline, much like a corset tightening around the hips, indicating TrA fiber recruitment (1).

Helpful tip: Observe the TrA contraction pattern, looking for faulty muscle recruitment and movement patterns as noted in the second part of the breathing assessment test, and palpate contraction. If a TrA contraction is absent or there is IO substitution characterized by a bulging into your fingers, assess the TrA recruitment pattern with a submaximal pelvic floor (PF) contraction. A co-activation pattern exists between the TrA and the pelvic floor and can be used as a training tool as described later (2,3,6).

Common compensatory strategies using the palpation method include (2,3):

- A dominance of, or substitution by, the internal oblique muscles may be palpated via a rapid development of tension in the abdominal wall, a superficial muscle contraction, such as from the EO, or when the palpating fingers are pushed out of the abdominal wall
- An altered or absent TrA contraction; the contraction may be phasic and/or there is asymmetrical firing of the right and left sides
- Inability to maintain neutral pelvis
- Altered diaphragmatic breathing pattern: upper chest or abdominal breathing

Practitioner's tip: A bilateral TrA contraction is necessary for contributing to lumbo-pelvic stabilization (1). Mechanical dysfunction of the lumbar spine and/or pelvis can affect the TrA muscle recruitment patterns. Restore faulty lumbar and pelvis mechanics first and then retest TrA contraction.

Retraining the Transversus Abdominis

The focus of TrA retraining is facilitation of a normal recruitment pattern independent of other abdominal muscles. If superficial abdominal overactivity is noted with assessment, the initial training focus is to decrease overactivity with relaxation training as previously described. Following that, work toward a correct neuromuscular TrA contraction.

The recommended TrA training positions are (2,3):

Sidelying

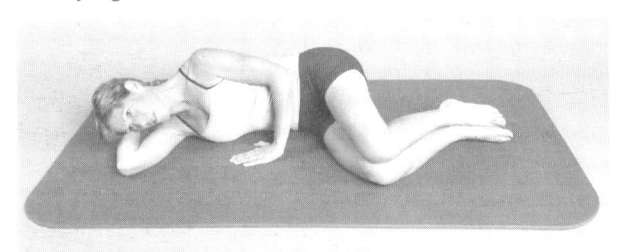

Four-point

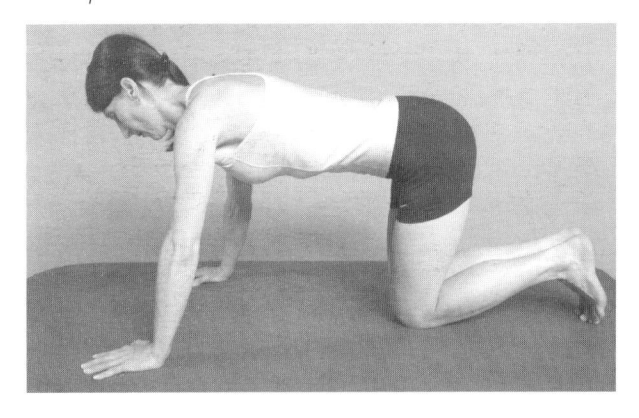

Prone

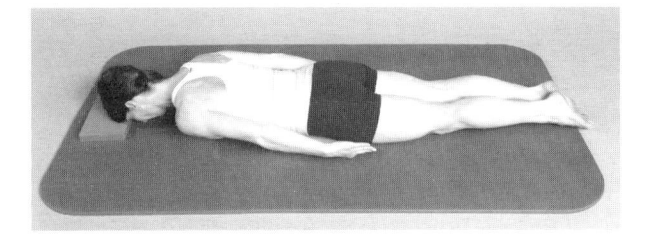

Hooklying

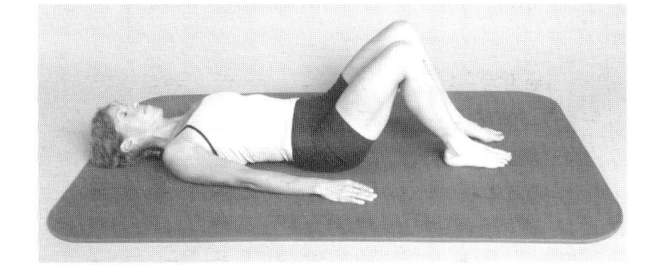

Helpful tip: As you begin neuromuscular reeducation of the TrA, remember that research has demonstrated that TrA recruitment can be affected by low back pain (3,7-10). Choose your training position based on the required recruitment intensity and your patient's comfort by selecting a pain-free position that might include sidelying or four-point (2,3). Such training positions may help reduce hypertonic abdominal muscles such as the external obliques or an overactive rectus abdominal muscle.

Successful training of the TrA focuses on the precision of muscle contraction and requires the practitioner to use various skill sets that include:

- Technical instruction that might include description of the TrA's anatomical location, muscle action, and role in lumbo-pelvic stabilization
- Patient observation: Let your patient visualize and/or palpate a correct recruitment pattern by using yourself as a model. Help your patient to see you contract your TrA. If appropriate, allow your patient to palpate your muscle contraction.
- Provide clear and concise directions. For example, "Draw your navel toward the spine slowly and gently (submaximal contraction); breathe out and feel your lower abdomen slowly flatten beneath your navel."
- Palpate the TrA contraction while cueing and provide feedback on the recruitment pattern to enhance TrA isolation

Practitioner's tip: Encourage self-palpation of the contraction to provide valuable sensory feedback, improve the quality of the contraction, and enhance your patient's kinesthetic awareness. As with breathing, it is a learned skill and begins with teaching your patient about the function of the TrA, how to anatomically locate the TrA and IO muscles, and where to place his or her hands to monitor the contraction. Ask your patient what he or she feels when contracting the TrA. Flattening? Bulging? Nothing? Unilateral or bilateral contraction?

Troubleshooting

If your patient indicates he or she feels nothing or has no idea what the contraction should feel like, choose another technique from your toolbox, such as a submaximal pelvic floor contraction, visual imagery, or equipment, to achieve the desired motor response. Recommended repetitions for a TrA home training program are three to five times daily to avoid fatiguing the TrA until a normal recruitment pattern is restored. The focus should be on precision and bilateral symmetry of the contraction (1).

Additional Training Techniques for the Transversus Abdominis: The Pelvic Floor and Abdominal Bracing

1. Research shows that a co-activation pattern exists between the pelvic floor and TrA muscles (2,3,6,11,12). Because these muscles are in the same neurological loop, use a pelvic floor contraction to co-activate the TrA when a patient has (2,3):

- Abnormal function of the TrA
- Problems relaxing the external obliques
- Difficulty in performing an isolated TrA contraction
- Ipsilateral or asymmetrical TrA contraction by cueing a unilateral pelvic floor contraction or when cueing techniques have been exhausted (2,4)

Helpful tip: Once patients are able to contract their TrA via pelvic floor contraction, coach them to contract their TrA coinciding with a PF contraction with progression to an independent TrA contraction.

2. You do not have to be an expert in physical therapy–women's health to use the pelvic floor as a method of co-activating the TrA. Keep it simple and within your scope of practice. An isolated pelvic floor contraction is necessary to train the TrA contraction efficiently when a normal TrA recruitment pattern is disrupted.

3. Avoid assuming that your patient knows how to contract the pelvic floor correctly if he or she is performing Kegel exercises, or that the pelvic floor and Kegels are associated with one another. Training begins with educating the patient about the basic pelvic floor anatomy, muscle action, and its role in lumbo-pelvic stabilization. Discuss the interrelationship between the two muscles: contracting the pelvic floor tightens the TrA to contribute to spinal stability, and vice versa. Contracting the TrA facilitates tightening of the pelvic floor, which is beneficial in keeping the pelvic floor muscles strong and preventing incontinence.

4. When instructing a patient to tighten the pelvic floor, keep the following things in mind:

- Perform a submaximal contraction of the PF to facilitate the transversus abdominis muscle (2)
- Watch for faulty recruitment patterns that include gluteal and hip adductor activation
- Hone your verbal cueing, which is definitely an art with pelvic floor instruction. This is a foreign and private area for many patients, and cues need to be selected carefully. Use simple cues. Cue your patient to pull the pelvic floor up and in and ask what he/she feels. If a patient has poor awareness with PF contraction, cue him/her to tighten the muscles as if trying to stop urinating. If the patient has difficulty performing this, have him/her try the same exercise as a test at home by contracting the pelvic floor muscles and stopping urination in midstream to increase self-awareness.
- Remember, this is only a test and not an exercise. Performing repeated pelvic floor contractions while urinating has been shown to lead to urinary tract infections. For further information, see below and Chapter 11 (Imagery) for further training options for the pelvic floor.

Train the TrA with the use of pelvic floor contraction with the following options:

- Begin TrA/pelvic floor training with an isolated submaximal pelvic floor contraction to co-activate the TrA (2)
- Progress to a combination of submaximal pelvic floor contraction and conscious TrA contraction
- Contract the pelvic floor unilaterally to enhance unilateral TrA contraction (4)

5. Use Imagery:

- To cue the TrA: "Feel as if your hipbones are sliding together like an elevator door closing
- To cue the pelvic floor: "Imagine sitting on a diamond composed of the following landmarks: ischial tuberosities, pubic bone, and tailbone. Pull all four points together and up with natural exhalation (13)."

6. Use kinesthetic cueing: This exercise will increase your patient's awareness of abdominal/extensor co-activation and general core stabilization. It's best implemented with kinesthetic direction, followed in two phases of training.

Abdominal Bracing in Practice

Begin abdominal bracing training by asking your patient to feel what it's like to have the abdominals contract incorrectly. Direct him or her to suck the abdominal area in, followed by abdominal bulging without abdominal tightening (abdominals are slack).

Next, have the patient begin to feel abdominal bracing in the following ways:

1. Cue the patient to slide the ribs gently toward the hips and feel the tension of the obliques with or without palpation.

2. Cue the patient to slide the two ASIS bilaterally together as if they are shutting an elevator door to facilitate TrA contraction.

3. Cue the patient to put the first two steps together. If an abdominal brace contraction is performed correctly, there will be a tensing of the abdominal area with co-activation of the spinal extensors.

Phase one: Ask your patient to sit on a chair with good posture. Stand behind the patient with your hands on his/her mid-back. Cue the patient to resist moving and to avoid using his/her hands or feet when you try to push him/her forward.

Phase two: Use the same exercise, but now ask the patient to exhale prior to resisting the movement. Ask the patient to identify the differences between phases one and two. The normal response is a deep tightening of the abdominals, indicating use of the abdominals and a stronger torso with breath than without. This same exercise can progress to standing.

7. Use equipment: Use a mirror, ultrasound, or pressure biofeedback to provide visual feedback of TrA contraction. Remember to advance the skill by discontinuing the use of equipment once your patient has successfully learned (and felt) what proper use of the abdominals should feel like.

Additional Training Techniques for the Transversus Abdominis: The Hip Adductors

Like the pelvic floor, the hip adductors have a neurological connection to the TrA. Use hip adductor contractions as a tool to facilitate the pelvic floor to co-activate the TrA (14,15). Use the hip adductors as a means of indirect strengthening of the TrA when the patient has:

- Abnormal function of the TrA and the training methods above have failed
- A lack of sensation of the abdominal wall secondary to surgery
- Progressed to a combination of hip adductor contraction and conscious pelvic floor contraction

1. Use Imagery:

- To cue the hip adductors: "Imagine you are holding an orange between your thighs. Squeeze the orange to create juice"

2. Use Equipment:

- Place a small ball or rolled-up towel between the thighs to enhance sensory feedback of the hip adductors

Teaching tip: Watch for femoral internal rotation as a compensatory strategy with hip adductor training.

Teaching Neutral Pelvis

Teaching the concept of neutral pelvis and spine is the foundation for efficient functional movement. What is neutral? Why move in neutral? How do you teach the concept of neutral and find it? These are questions common to both rehabilitation and fitness professionals.

Whether your focus is on improving cardiovascular fitness, strength, flexibility, or Pilates-based training, a neutral pelvis is essential to developing core stabilization and to enhancing posture and maximal use of the upper and lower extremities with activities of daily living, work, and sports.

Neutral Spine

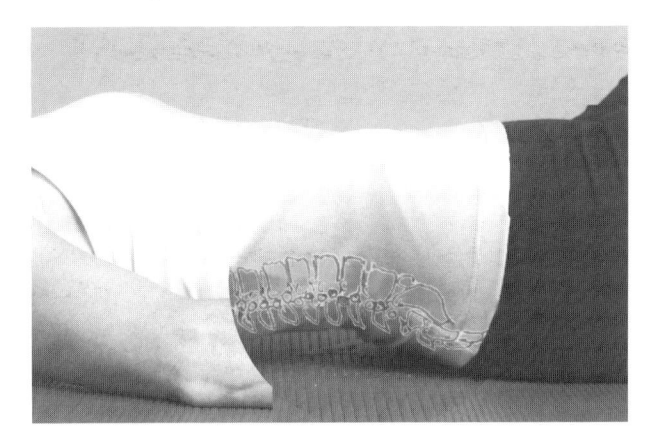

When the pelvis is in neutral alignment, the natural lordosis of the lumbar spine is supported and creates a sense of balance for the vertebrae, muscles, joints, myofascial tissue, and ligaments (16). The body is in balance and in its strongest position; the body's efficiency is maximized and stress is minimized. Remember, the body is a machine. If neutral pelvis is not maintained, the body will take the path of least resistance. Overuse injuries, hypermobility, and degenerative changes may occur secondary to changes in normal lumbo-pelvic mechanics and compensatory strategies elsewhere in the body.

Pelvic Clock

If your patient has a hard time finding neutral pelvis alignment or stabilizing the pelvis in the transverse plane, use the Pelvic Clock exercise to enhance kinesthetic awareness and control.

Based on the work of Moshe Feldenkrais, the Pelvic Clock exercise can be used to assess weak areas of the abdominal muscles, restrictions in lumbar segments, lumbo-pelvic control, and stabilization in all planes of movement: sagittal, frontal, and transverse (17). Once faulty movement patterns are identified, you can begin neuromuscular reeducation of the lumbo-pelvic region.

The starting position for the Pelvic Clock is in hooklying with the knees bent and the feet flat.

Imagine that a clock has been placed on top of the abdomen between the pubic bone and sternum: 12 o'clock is at the base of sternum (xiphoid process), 3 o'clock is at the right anterior superior iliac spine, 6 o'clock is at the pubic bone, and 9 o'clock is at the left ASIS.

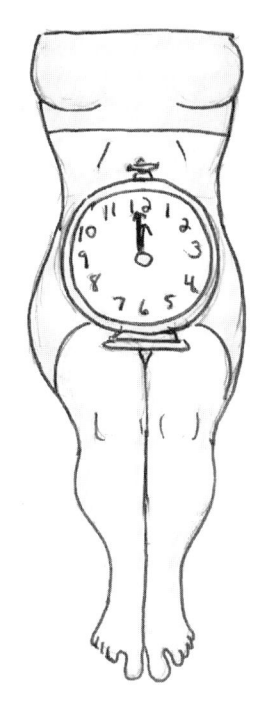

Assess movement patterns from 12 to 6 (lumbar extension), 6 to 12 (lumbar flexion), 9 to 3 (left pelvic/right lumbar spine rotation), and 3 to 9 (right pelvic/left lumbar rotation), both clockwise and counterclockwise.

Place your thumbs on the slope of either the superior or inferior ASIS and note any asymmetry. Or, if asymmetry is present from the start, observe when the asymmetry changes as your patient moves toward 12 o'clock, becoming either more symmetrical or more asymmetrical (17). Repeat this process, observing pelvic movement toward 6 o'clock.

Next, assess pelvis symmetry or asymmetry in the transverse plane. The movement should be one of relatively pure pelvic rotation toward 3 and 9 o'clock without the ASIS moving cephally or caudally (17). Finally, assess the quality of lumbo-pelvic control in both clockwise and counterclockwise movements.

Common compensatory strategies using the Pelvic Clock include (17):

- Moving to 6 o'clock: right ASIS lower than left
- Moving to 12 o'clock: left ASIS higher than right, overactive gluteals, or sequential articulation of the lumbar spine does not occur
- Moving from 9 to 3 o'clock: right anterior innominate rotation
- Moving from 3 to 9 o'clock: hip hiking left or excessive right lumbar extension

Once your assessment is complete, teach your patient to perform the Pelvic Clock and self-monitor his/her movement. Teach your patient to locate his/her ASIS with the thumbs and place them on the slope of either the superior or inferior ASIS to monitor pelvic movement.

Teaching tip: Begin by teaching your patient pelvic movement awareness first in the sagittal and transverse planes with progression to a combination of movements in clockwise and counterclockwise directions. Once pelvic awareness is mastered, have the patient find neutral pelvis by giving him/her the following cues: "Move your pelvis between 6 o'clock and 12 o'clock while maintaining pelvic stability side to side. Next, find the midpoint between these ranges to determine your neutral pelvic position."

Additional Training Techniques

1. Use imagery: For example, cue: "Roll a marble from your pubic bone to your navel."

2. Use tactile cueing: Hands-on training by the clinician or self-guided pelvic movement.

3. Equipment: Ask your patient to sit on a chair or ball in neutral alignment so that he/she can feel the entire spine. Ask the patient to feel changes in the body when not aligned. Mirrors and pressure biofeedback are also helpful.

Chapter References

1. Hodges, P.W. 2002. Science of Stability: Clinical Application to Assessment and Treatment of Segmental Spinal Stabilization for Low Back Pain. Course notes, Bloomington, MN.

2. Hodges, P.W. 2002. *Science of Stability: Clinical Application to Assessment and Treatment of Segmental Spinal Stabilization for Low Back Pain.* Course Manual, Bloomington, MN.

3. Richardson, C., Jull, G., Hodges, P., Hides, J. 1999. *Therapeutic Exercise for Spinal Segmental Stabilization in Low Back Pain: Scientific Basis and Clinical Approach.* Edinburgh, U.K.: Churchill Livingstone.

4. Lee, D. 2003. The Pelvis—Bridging the Gap Between the Science and the Clinic. Course notes, Fairview Education Center, Edina, MN, October 4-5.

5. Richardson, C.A., Snijders, C.J., Hides, J.A., Damen, L., Pas, M.S., Storm, J. 2002. The relation between the transversus abdominis muscles, sacroiliac joint mechanics, and low back pain. *Spine* 27(4): 399-405.

6. Lee, D. 1999. *The Pelvic Girdle: An Approach to the Examination and Treatment of the Lumbo-Pelvic-Hip Region.* Edinburgh, U.K.: Churchill Livingstone.

7. Hodges, P.W., Richardson, C.A. 1998. Delayed contraction of transversus abdominis in low back pain associated with movement of the lower limb. *J Spinal Disord* 11(1): 46-56.

8. Hodges, P.W., Richardson, C. 1996. Inefficient muscular stabilization of the lumbar spine associated with low back pain: A motor control evaluation of transversus abdominis. *Spine* 21(22): 2640-2650.

9. Ferreira, P.H., Ferreira, M.L., Hodges, P.W. 2004. Changes in recruitment of the abdominal muscles in people with low back pain: Ultrasound measurement of muscle activity. *Spine* 29(22): 2560-2566.

10. Hodges, P.W., Richardson, C.A. 1999. Altered trunk muscle recruitment in people with low back pain with upper limb movement at different speeds. *Arch Phys Med Rehabil* 80: 1005-1012.

11. Sapsford, R.R., et al. 2001. Co-activation of the abdominal and pelvic floor muscles during voluntary exercises. *Neurourology and Urodynamics* 20: 31-42.

12. Sapsford, R.R., Hodges, P.W. 2001. Contraction of the pelvic floor muscles during abdominal maneuvers. *Arch Phys Med Rehabil* 82:1081-1088.

13. DiGiulio-DuBeau, L. 2003. STOTT Pilates Mat-Based Stability Ball Workout. Course notes, Idea Fact Fest, Rosemont, IL, April 25-27.

14. Hulme, J.A. 1999. Beyond Kegels: Assessment and Treatment of Incontinence. Course notes, Minneapolis, MN, February 19-20.

15. Hulme, J.A. 2000. Research in geriatric urinary incontinence: Pelvic muscle force field. *Top Geriatr Rehabil* 16(1): 10-21.

16. Vogel, A. 2001. Helping clients find neutral spine. *ACE Certified News* 7(2): 6-7.

17. Bookhout, M.R. 2002. Exercise as an Adjunct to Manual Medicine. Course notes, Minnesota American Physical Therapy Association Spring Conference, Brooklyn Park, MN, April 19-21.

chapter 6

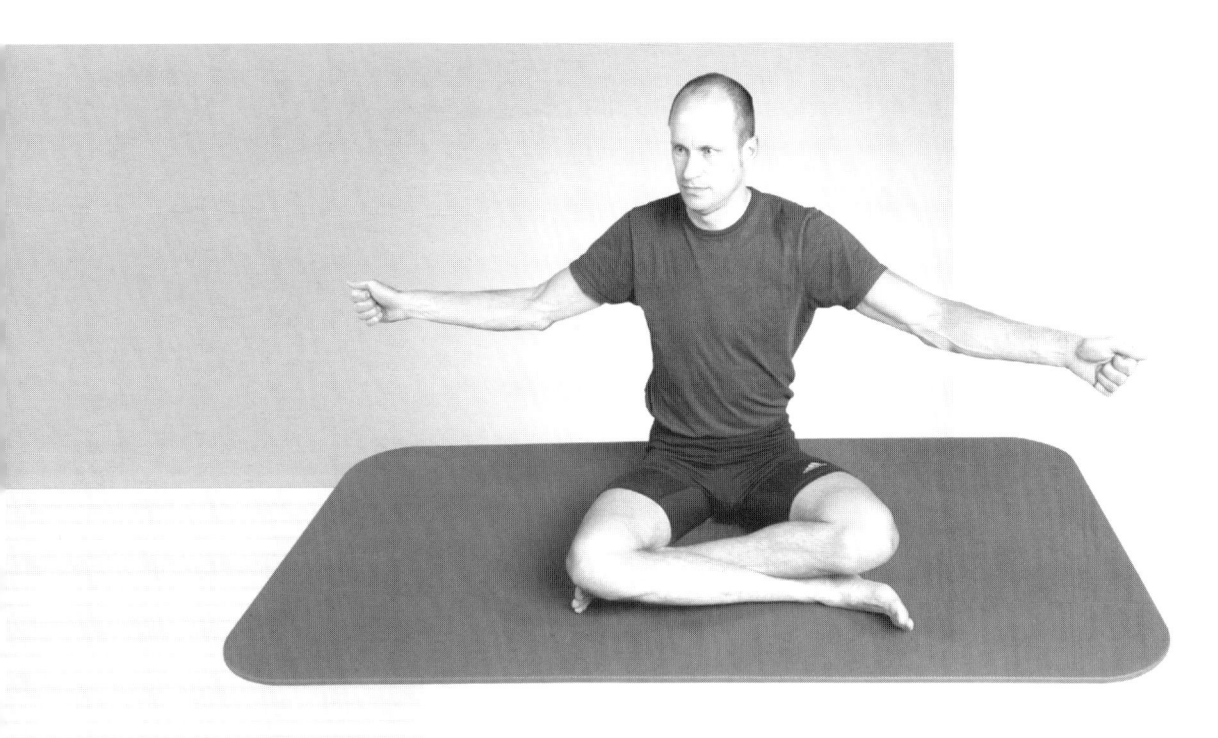

FUNDAMENTAL
EXERCISES:
THE PRINCIPLES IN
ACTION

The original Pilates Matworks regimen consists of about 35 exercises. For the average person, not to mention the athlete or the patient, most exercises are quite challenging and require significant abdominal, lower back, and upper body strength, as well as good kinesthetic awareness and body control.

As the science of movement has improved over the years, many knowledgeable practitioners have updated the regimen. Today, it is not uncommon to see modifications and variations of the same exercises or new exercises based on the original ones. These updates help the average, albeit less fit, person perform the exercises safely and successfully and prepare to work toward the original exercises.

From a rehabilitation perspective, many of the original Pilates exercises are inappropriate in a clinical setting. That said, the intent and purpose of the original exercises and the focus on centering or working from the girdle of strength, now termed core stabilization, have direct applicability.

This chapter reviews what we consider to be the Pilates fundamentals and applies and coordinates the principles to basic movement of the lower and upper extremities. As mentioned in earlier chapters, our focus is stability before mobility. Patients must master the foundational movement patterns before advancing to more difficult exercises.

Stability Before Mobility

An essential component in advancing a patient is his or her understanding and demonstration of the Pilates-based principles identified in Chapter 4. Ask your patient what muscles he or she feels with movement. Examine the movement. Are faulty movement patterns present? Rib cage popping? Abdominal breathing?

If compensatory strategies are present, avoid progressing your patient until core stabilization is mastered. Break down the movement pattern into smaller components.

Once your patient has mastered the principles of core stabilization, introduce Pilates-based mat exercises that first emphasize single-joint and uniplanar movements. Fundamental exercises that emphasize stability are generally those where the body has the most contact with the mat (supine/prone) and/or where the movement is uniplanar.

Once the patient has mastered the fundamental mat exercises without faulty movement patterns, choose exercise patterns that challenge stability, coordination, and mobility. Progress to less stable positions, such as sidelying, sitting, or four-point, or consider using equipment to challenge stability. You can also introduce multiplanar movement patterns of the upper and lower extremities to challenge coordination, stamina, and mobility.

Lower Extremity Patterns with Neutral Pelvis: Sagittal Plane

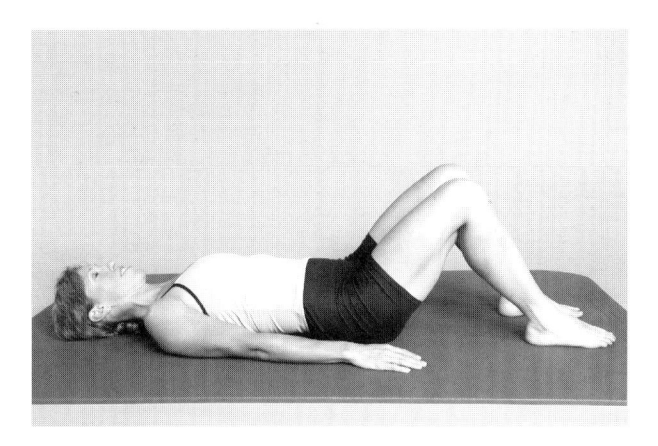

Starting Position for All Exercises*: Hooklying with neutral pelvis, head, and neck alignment, arms alongside the body, elbows slightly bent, with the palms facing down on the mat. (*Exception: Movement Pattern 8.)

Practitioner's tip: The goals of the following exercises are to maintain neutral, with weight distributed equally on low back and pelvis. Avoid weight shifting from side to side and reduce upper body tension. Breath helps facilitate the motion and recruitment of the deep stabilizing muscles.

Movement Patterns 1-8
Purpose:

- To isolate hip movement independent of the pelvis and spine in the sagittal plane. Perform initially in supine and progress to weight-bearing positions, such as sitting and standing.
- Challenge dissociation of the femur from the pelvis with advanced lower extremity movement patterns, stabilizing with the muscles of the hip and pelvis

Clinical Application:

- Use initial movement patterns when dissociation of the hip from the pelvis and spine is not occurring. These patterns create the foundation for gait, running mechanics, lifting, and transitional movements such as sit to stand. Advanced patterns challenge torso stabilization against various lower extremity lever lengths and gravity (in standing) with asymmetrical/symmetrical lower extremity patterns.

- Suggested patient populations: Total hip replacement rehabilitation; patellofemoral pain syndrome; introductory/intermediate lumbar stabilization exercises; excessive lumbar lordosis; hip bursitis

Repetitions: 5, depending on patient goals

Faulty Movement Patterns: Increased lumbar lordosis with leg extension; pelvis imprinting with hip flexion; lateral pelvic tilt; rib cage popping; upper body tension

Movement Pattern 1: Heel Slide

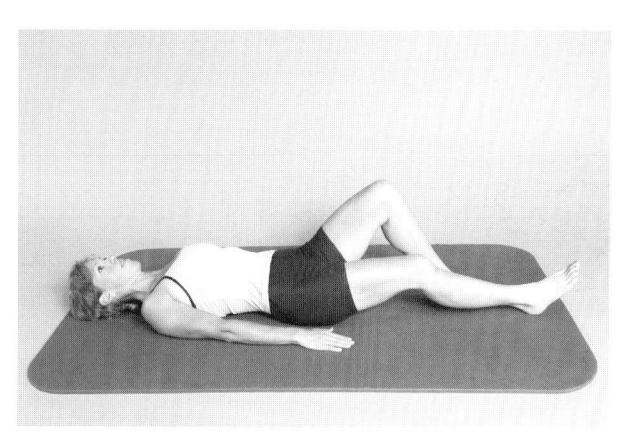

Inhale through the nose, engage the abdominals, and slide the heel on the mat as the hip/knee extend in a straight line from the sitz bone, maintaining neutral. Exhale and slide the heel back to the starting position. Repeat on the opposite side.

Movement Pattern 2: Bilateral Heel Slides

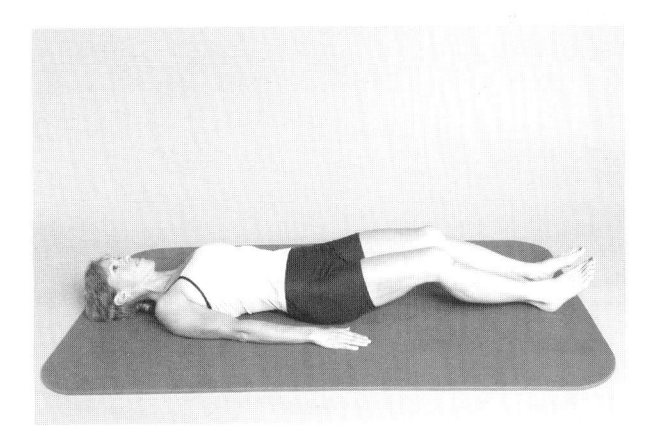

Inhale, engage the abdominals, and slide both heels on the mat as the hips/knees extend from the sitz bones, maintaining neutral. Exhale through pursed lips and slide the heels back to the starting position.

Movement Pattern 3: Single Tabletop (knee and hip flexed to 90 degrees)

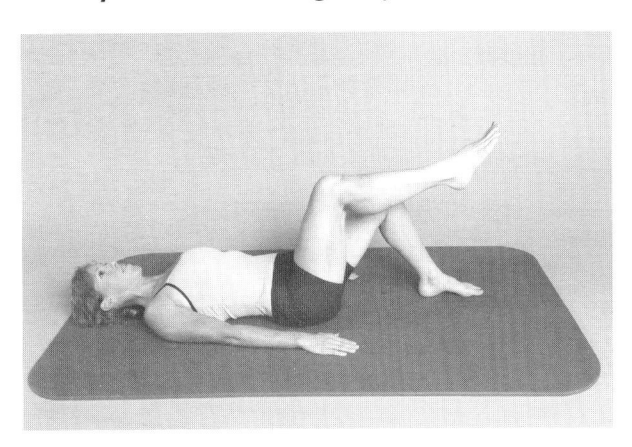

Inhale to prepare, breathing into the back and sides of the ribs. Exhale, maintaining neutral pelvis, and flex the hip to 90 degrees to bring one leg up into tabletop position. Inhale and lower the foot back to the mat. Repeat on the other side. To advance: Add Single Tabletop with arm patterns of your choice.

Movement Pattern 4: Heel Slide with Single Tabletop

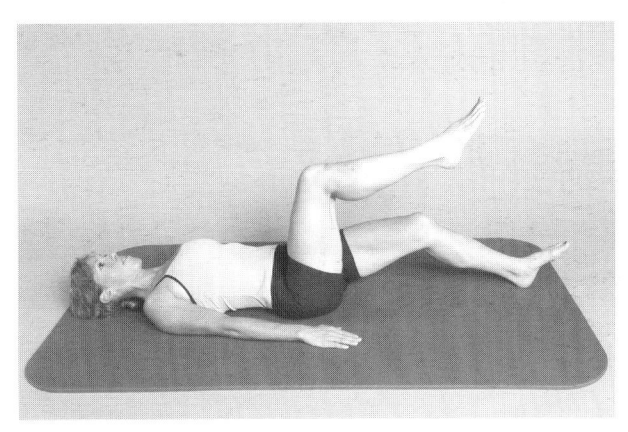

Keep one leg in tabletop position as above. Inhale to prepare, breathing into the back and sides of the ribs. Maintain neutral pelvis and slide the heel on the mat as the hip/knee extend in a straight line from the sitz bone. Exhale and slide the heel back to the starting position. Repeat on the other side.

Movement Pattern 5: Single Tabletop with Knee Extension

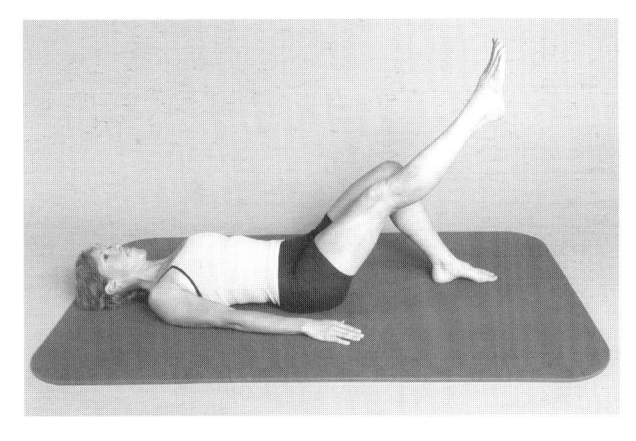

Keep one leg in tabletop position as above. Inhale to prepare, breathing into the back and sides of the ribs. Exhale, maintaining neutral pelvis, and extend the leg in tabletop at the knee. The hip remains flexed at about 90 degrees. Inhale to flex the knee, returning to the initial position. Repeat on the other side.

Movement Pattern 6: Single-Leg Bicycle

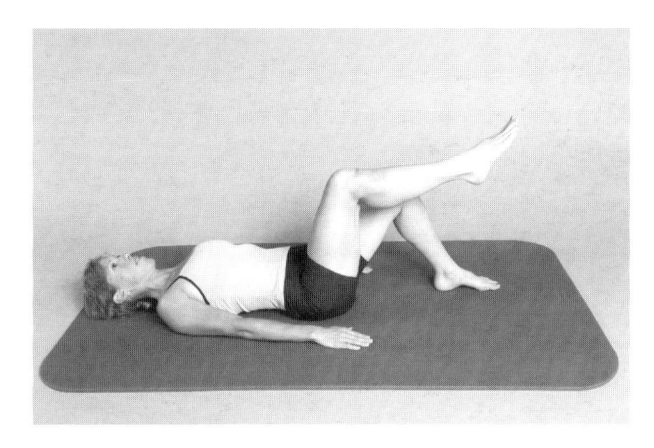

Keep one leg in tabletop position as above. Inhale to prepare, breathing into the back and sides of the ribs.

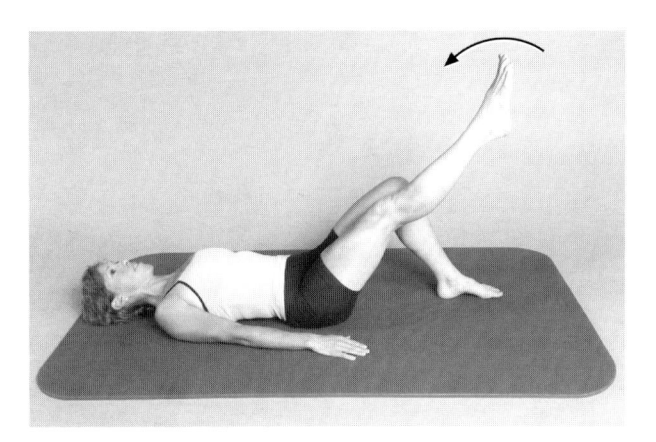

Exhale, maintaining neutral pelvis, and extend the knee and hip to a 45-degree diagonal, not allowing weight to shift to that side. Inhale to draw the hip/knee back to the initial position. Repeat the pattern. The weight and rhythm of the leg will challenge torso stability.

Movement Pattern 7: Single-Leg Developé with Foot Variations

Keep one leg in a bent knee position. Inhale to prepare, breathing into the back and sides of the ribs. Exhale, maintaining neutral pelvis, and extend the hip to a 45-degree diagonal, not allowing weight to shift to that side.

Inhale through the nose and lower the extended leg toward the floor, maintaining neutral pelvis against the weight of the leg. The ankle is dorsiflexed. Exhale to lift the extended leg up to a 45-degree diagonal. The ankle is plantar flexed. Inhale and draw the hip/knee back to the initial position. Repeat the pattern.

Movement Pattern 8: Single Tabletop in Unilateral Standing (knee and hip flexed to 90 degrees)

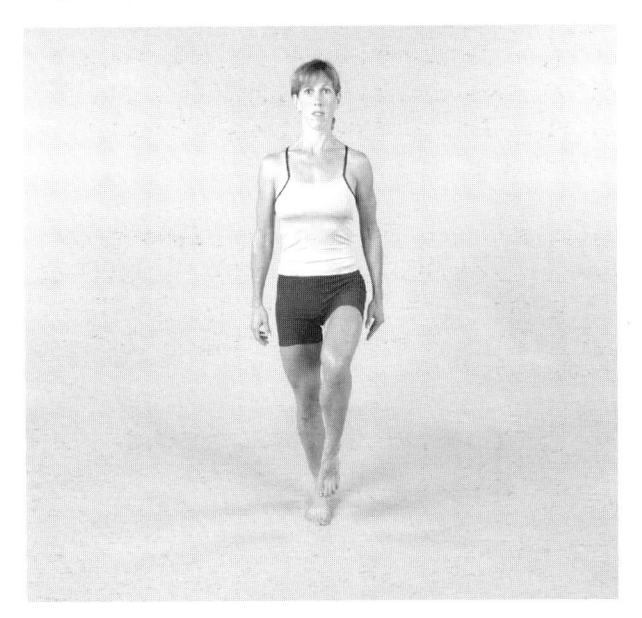

Start in standing with neutral pelvis/spine. Inhale, breathing into the back and sides of the ribs. Exhale, maintaining neutral pelvis, and flex the left hip to tabletop position while maintaining a stable base of support on the right (stance) leg. Inhale and return to the starting position. Repeat on the other side.

Helpful tips: Strive to maintain body weight centered and the spine elongated, despite removing a stability point. Patients should not lean back or to the side, and the anterior super iliac spines (ASIS) should remain level bilaterally. Avoid hyperextending the right knee and flexing the toes by applying even pressure to all four borders of the foot.

Lower Extremity Patterns with Neutral Pelvis: Multiple Planes

Movement Pattern 1: Single-Leg Knee Stirs

Start in hooklying with neutral pelvis, head, and neck alignment, one leg in a bent knee position and the other aligned with the ASIS, arms alongside the body, elbows slightly bent, with the palms facing down on the mat.

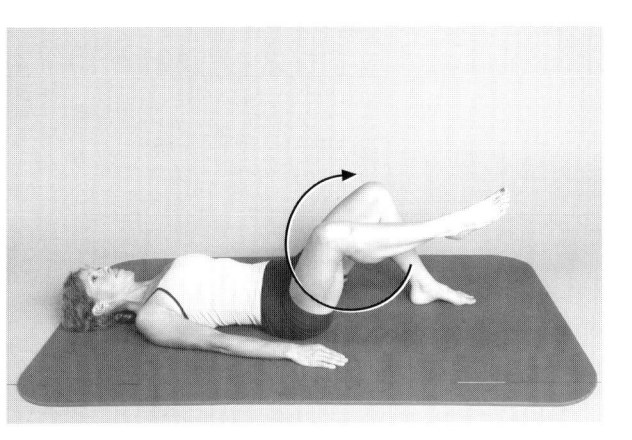

Inhale through the nose, breathing into the back and sides of the ribs, maintaining neutral pelvis. "Draw" a half circle (hip circumduction) with the patella, adducting the hip across the midline and then extending it. Exhale to complete the circle, abducting the hip away from the midline and flexing it to the starting position. Maintain neutral with the movement. Repeat five times in one direction. Inhale and pause to change directions. Repeat on the other leg.

Purpose:

- To isolate movement independent of the pelvis and spine. Knee Stirs also lay the groundwork for advanced Pilates exercises in later chapters
- To challenge torso stability with hip circumduction

Clinical Application:

- Use this movement pattern when dissociation of the hip from the pelvis and spine is not occurring and neuromuscular reeducation of the hip is needed in the frontal and sagittal planes
- Suggested patient populations: Hip osteoarthritis; hip adductor strain; sport-specific training: soccer, dancing, gymnastics
- Use to enhance approximation for the unstable hip with specific cueing: "Sink the femur into the hip socket" or "Imagine using your leg bone to stir a pot of chili"

Repetitions: 5 each direction, depending on patient goals

Faulty Movement Patterns: Not maintaining neutral; inability to stabilize the pelvis, resulting in weight shift side to side or pelvic rotation; inability to isolate the hip from the pelvis; upper body tension; Valsalva

Movement Pattern 2: Bent-Knee Fallout (1)

Start in hooklying with neutral pelvis, neutral head and cervical alignment, the arms alongside the body, elbows slightly bent with the palms facing down on the mat.

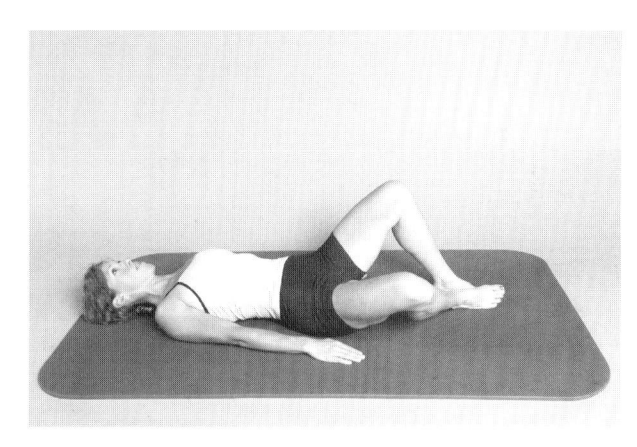

Inhale through the nose and slowly drop the knee out to the side (hip external rotation) while maintaining neutral pelvis. Contact of the opposite foot with the floor supports movement through stabilization. Exhale to draw the leg in toward the midline (hip internal rotation) to the initial position.

Variation: Inhale and drop both knees out to the side (hip external rotation). Exhale to draw the legs in toward the midline (hip internal rotation) to the initial position.

Purpose:

- To isolate hip movement independent of the pelvis and spine and to introduce movement in the transverse plane, stabilizing with the muscles of the hip and pelvis

Clinical Application:

- Use this movement pattern when dissociation of the hip from the pelvis and spine is not occurring
- Suggested patient populations: Essential lumbar stabilization exercise; hip adductor strain; hip bursitis; total hip replacement with posterior approach (contraindicated for anterior approach during the first six weeks postoperative or per physician protocol). Use as an adjunct to manual therapy for a tight anterior hip capsule.

Repetitions: 5, depending on patient goals

Faulty Movement Patterns: Increased lumbar lordosis with hip external rotation; pelvis imprinting with hip internal rotation; lateral pelvic tilt occurring with Bent-Knee Fallout; rib cage and/or abdominal popping; upper body tension

Movement Pattern 3: Hip External Rotation with Knee Extension (Bent-Knee Fallout/Heel Slide Progression)
Start in hooklying with neutral pelvis, neutral head and neck alignment, the arms alongside the body, the elbows slightly bent, with the palms facing down on the mat.

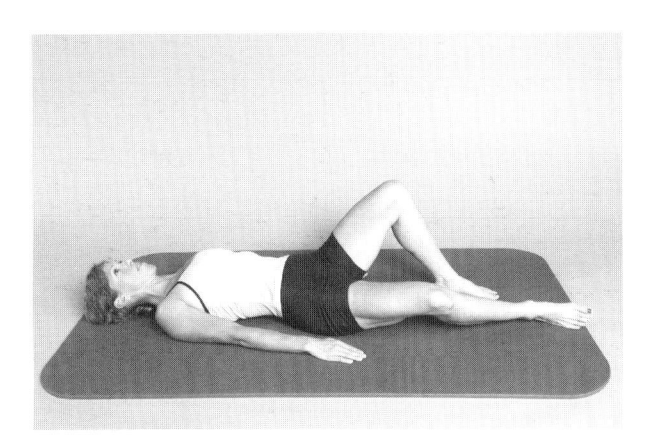

Inhale through the nose and drop the knee out to the side (hip external rotation) while maintaining neutral pelvis and extend the hip/knee out with the heel sliding away from the sitz bones. Exhale to draw the leg in toward the midline (hip internal rotation) and flex the knee and hip (with the heel maintaining contact with the mat) to the initial position.

Purpose:

- To isolate hip movement independent of pelvis and spine movement in the transverse and sagittal planes, stabilizing with the muscles of the hip and pelvis

Clinical Application:

- Use this advanced movement pattern to challenge dissociation of the hip from the pelvis in the sagittal and transverse planes
- Essential lumbar stabilization exercise
- Suggested patient population: Tight anterior hip capsule; one-joint hip flexor tightness; hip adductor strain; sport-specific training—kicking fundamentals (soccer), dancing

Repetitions: 5, depending on patient goals

Faulty Movement Patterns: Increased lumbar lordosis with hip external rotation; pelvis imprinting with hip internal rotation; lateral pelvic tilt occurring with Bent-Knee Fallout; rib cage and/or abdominal popping; upper body tension

Lower Extremity Patterns with a Posterior Tilt (Imprinted)

Movement Pattern 1: Double Tabletop

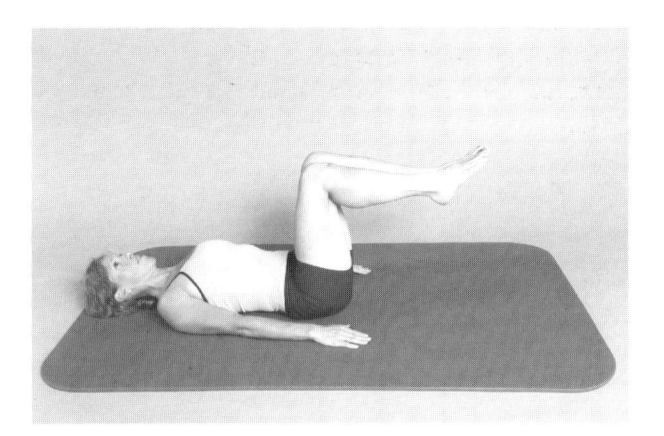

Inhale through the nose. Exhale, imprint the pelvis, and lift one leg up into the tabletop position, followed by the other. Inhale to lower one foot to the mat. Exhale to lower the other foot.

Movement Pattern 2: Heel and Toe Taps

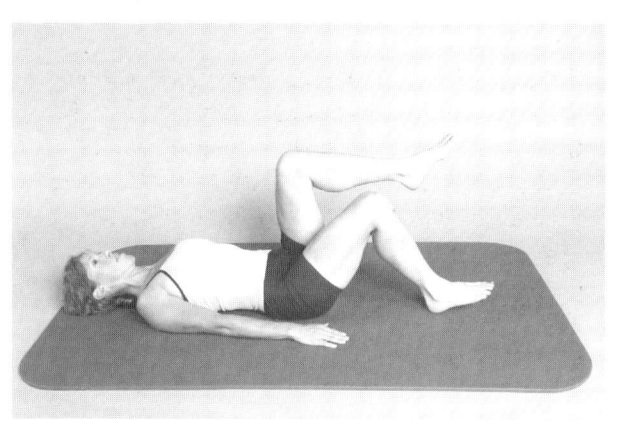

Start supine with the legs in double tabletop and the pelvis in a posterior tilt. Inhale to prepare.

Exhale and lower one heel to the floor without changing pelvic position. The movement should initiate at the femur/pelvis, not the tibia. Inhale and lift the heel and return the leg to the initial position. Exhale and lower the other heel to repeat. Variation: Tap the toes instead of the heels.

Movement Pattern 3: Heel and Toe Taps with Arm Lift

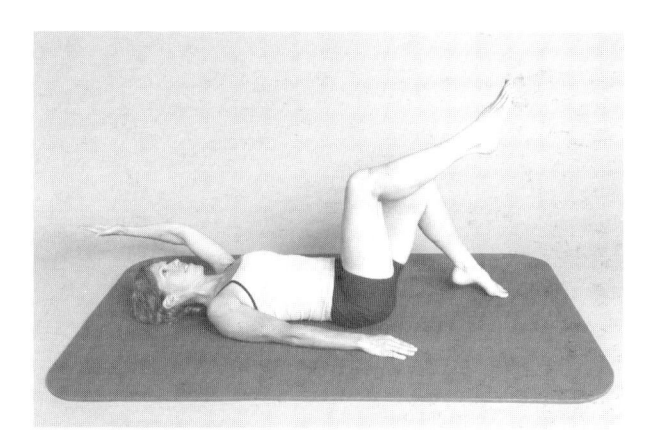

Start supine with the legs in double tabletop and the pelvis in a posterior tilt. Inhale to prepare.

Exhale and lower one heel to the floor without changing pelvic position. The movement should initiate at the femur/pelvis, not the tibia. Simultaneously lift the opposite arm over the head. Inhale and lift the heel and return the leg and arm to the initial position. Exhale and lower the other heel to repeat. Variation: Tap the toes instead of the heels.

Movement Pattern 4: Double Tabletop Heel and Toe Taps with Spine Flexion

Start supine with the legs in double tabletop, the pelvis in a posterior tilt, and the spine flexed. Inhale to prepare.

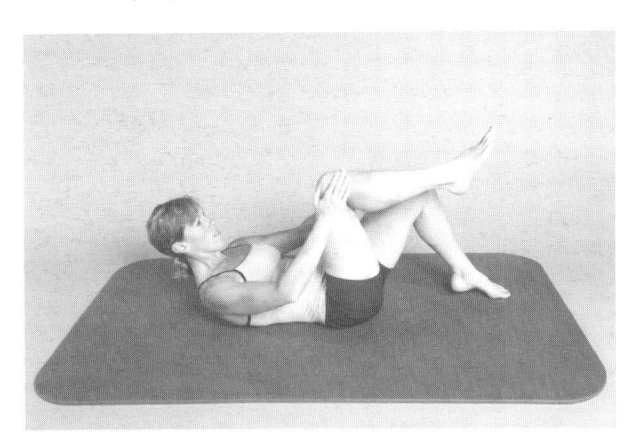

Exhale and lower one heel to the floor without changing pelvic position. The movement should initiate at the femur/pelvis, not the tibia. Inhale and lift the heel and return the leg to the initial position. Exhale and lower the other heel to repeat. Variation shown: Tap the toes instead of the heel.

Movement Pattern 5: Tabletop with Bent-Knee Fallout

Start supine with the legs in double tabletop and the pelvis in a posterior tilt.

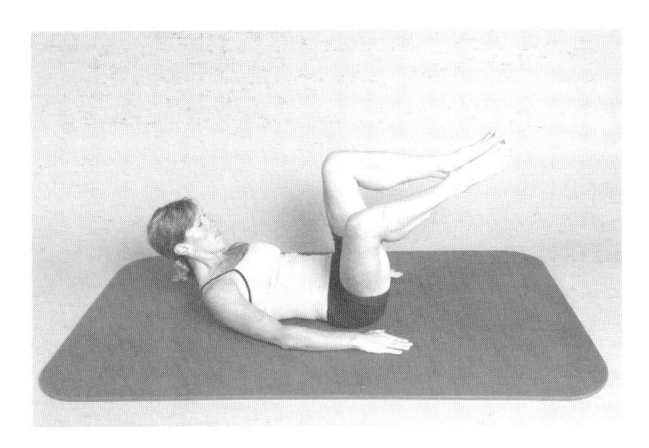

Inhale to connect with the abdominals and externally rotate both hips, maintaining an imprinted pelvis and keeping the heels together. Exhale and internally rotate the hips back to neutral (2).

Movement Pattern 6: Bend and Stretch (Bilateral external rotation at hip)

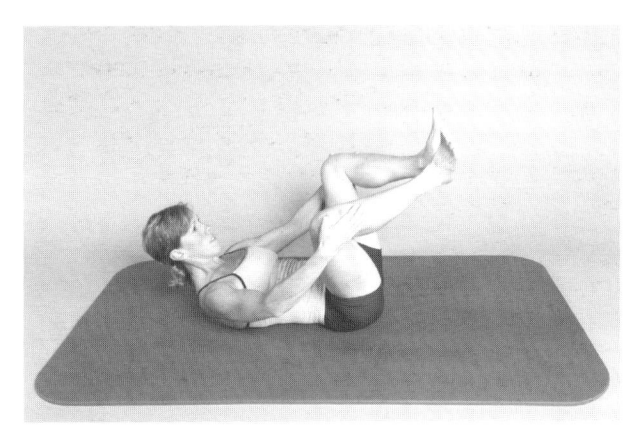

Start supine with the pelvis in a posterior tilt, the knees and hips flexed, and the hips externally rotated past the shoulders. The heels are together and the toes apart, with the ankles dorsiflexed. Inhale to connect with the abdominals.

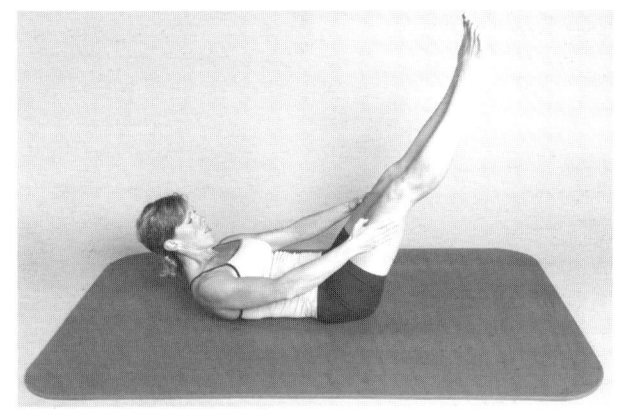

Exhale and press the heels together as the knees/hips extend and the hips adduct to extend the legs on a diagonal. Maintain hip external rotation. The ankles are plantar flexed. Inhale and return to the initial position. Flex the knees/hips/ankles, drawing the heels into the sitz bones.

Faulty Movement Patterns: Exaggerated posterior pelvic tilt (sacrum lifting); inability to maintain pelvic position; inability to stabilize the pelvis from the femurs; rib cage and/or abdominal popping; upper body tension; weight shifting; overactive gluteals; legs deviating from midline; Valsalva; inability to coordinate breath with movement

Upper Extremity Patterns in Neutral Pelvis

Start in hooklying with neutral pelvis, head, and neck alignment, the heels hip-width apart, arms alongside the body, elbows slightly bent, with the palms facing down on the mat. The distal ribs should be in contact with the mat for the normal resting position.

Movement Pattern 1: Arm Scissors

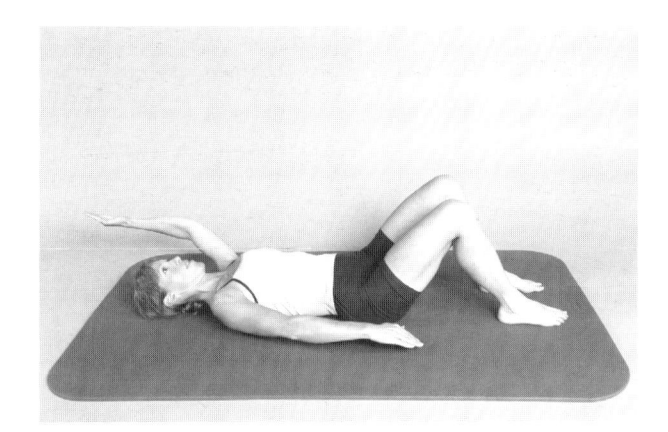

Exhale and flex one shoulder to 180 degrees overhead and extend the other shoulder to the mat simultaneously while maintaining abdominal connection and contact of the lower ribs against the mat. Inhale and change arm positions.

Movement Pattern 2: Snow Angels

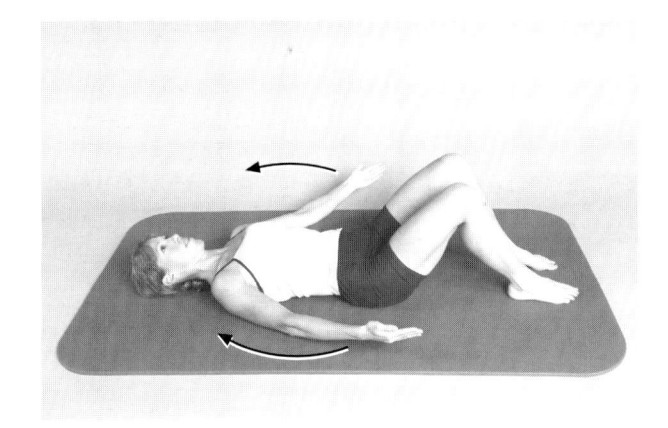

Inhale to prepare. Exhale and externally rotate the shoulders and abduct to 180 degrees, maintaining abdominal connection and contact of the lower ribs against the mat. Inhale and internally rotate the shoulders and extend the shoulders to the initial position.

Movement Pattern 3: Arm Circles

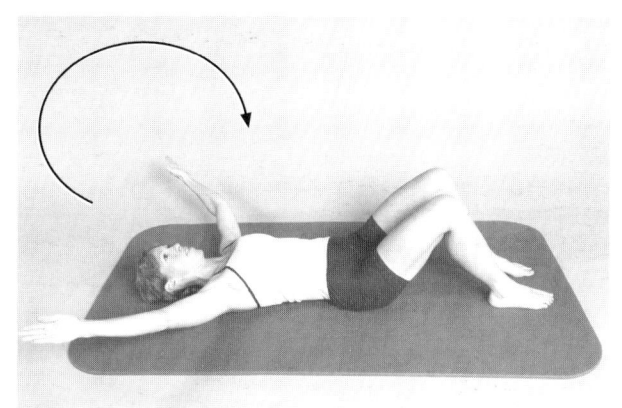

Inhale to prepare. Exhale and flex the shoulders to 180 degrees overhead, maintaining abdominal connection and contact of the lower ribs against the mat. Inhale and medially rotate the shoulders to 90 degrees, adducting the shoulders to the initial position.

Movement Pattern 4: Windmill Arms

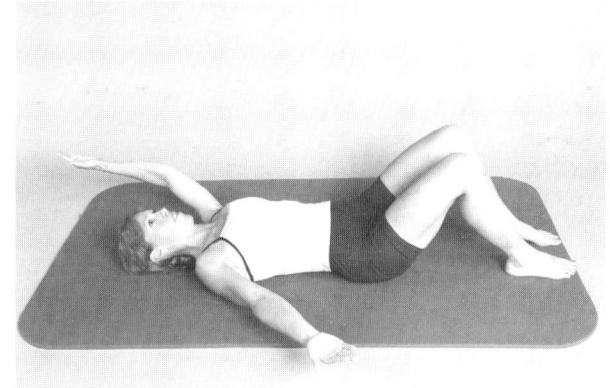

Exhale to flex the left shoulder to 180 degrees. Inhale and medially rotate the right shoulder, adducting it to the initial position while simultaneously externally rotating the left shoulder and abducting it to 180 degrees. Extend the left shoulder to the initial position and flex right shoulder 180 degrees while maintaining abdominal connection and contact of the lower ribs against the mat. Repeat the pattern in the other direction.

Movement Patterns 1-4
Purpose:

- To challenge torso/pelvic stabilization against movement of the shoulder with progression from uniplanar to multiplanar upper extremity movement patterns

Clinical Application:

- Movement patterns are a fundamental exercise for ADLs, such as dressing and reaching into a cupboard above shoulder level or preparing a basketball player for retraining basketball mechanics—throwing, shooting, and rebounding—with rehabilitation of the shoulder
- Suggested patient populations: Use as an adjunct to shoulder mobilization and/or shoulder dysfunctions that include bursitis/rotator cuff tendonitis or frozen shoulder

Repetitions: 5-10, depending on patient goals

Practitioner's tip: Once your patient has mastered these arm patterns, add challenge by adding leg patterns of your choice.

Faulty Movement Patterns: Rib cage popping secondary to decreased shoulder/thoracic mobility and/or latissimus dorsi tightness; lumbar lordosis; tension in chest, upper back, and neck; Valsalva; inability to coordinate breath with movement; hyperextended elbows

Purpose:

- To develop kinesthetic awareness of the posterior pelvic position with open kinetic chain training of the lower extremities

Clinical Application:

- Advanced lumbar stabilization training in open kinetic chain positions
- Suggested patient populations include those who require sport-specific training: divers, swimmers, gymnasts, dancer, ice skaters

Repetitions: 5-10, depending on patient goals

Fundamental Movement Patterns

Spine Rolls in Supine

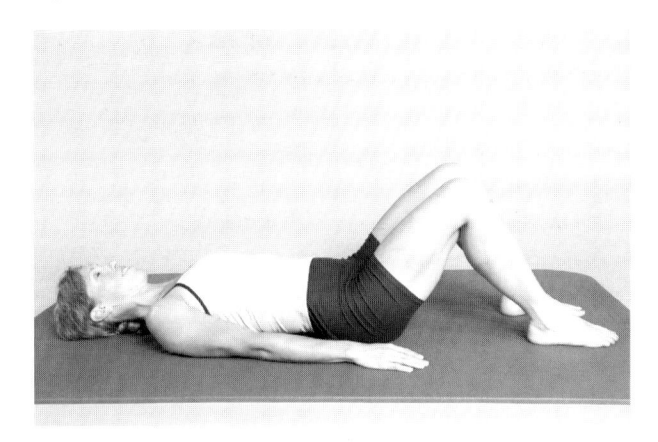

Start supine with neutral spine, head, and cervical alignment, the heels hip-width apart, the arms alongside the body, the elbows slightly bent, with the palms facing down on the mat.

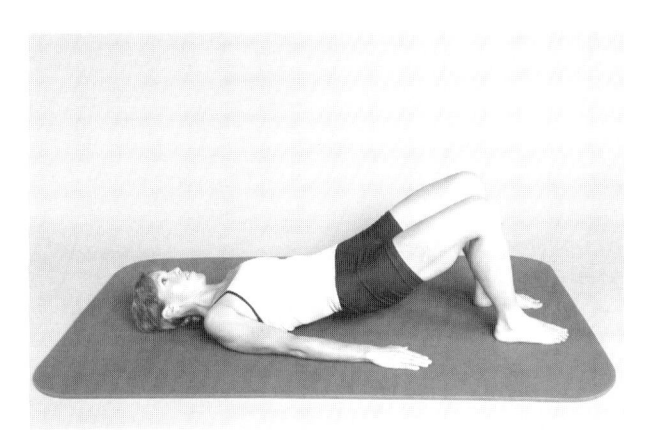

Inhale and breathe into the back and sides of the ribs. Exhale and imprint the pelvis, sequentially rolling the spine off the mat, leading with the tailbone and continuing to the upper thoracic region. Avoid putting pressure on the cervical spine. Inhale to hold. Exhale and sequentially roll the spine back onto the mat, leading with the upper thoracic spine.

Purpose:

- Spine Rolls focus on simultaneous mobilization of the hips into flexion/extension and spinal articulation. The rectus abdominis and obliques facilitate rolling through the spine.

Clinical Application:

- Spinal articulation
- Abdominal, gluteal, and hamstring strengthening
- Lengthening the one-joint hip flexors
- As an adjunct to manual therapy to reinforce sequential and segmental articulation of hypomobile segments
- Neuromuscular reeducation of hypomobile segments

Repetitions: 5-10, depending on patient goals

Variation: Place a towel or small ball between the knees.

Faulty Movement Patterns: Not rolling through the spine sequentially; not leading with the tailbone; missing segments of the spine; abdominal bracing (EO); overactive gluteals; abdominal popping; Valsalva; upper body tension; inability to coordinate breath with movement

Teaching tips:

1. *With hypomobile thoracic segment(s), focus on relaxing the thoracic spine back to the mat versus trying to force the spine to the mat to reduce compensatory gluteal firing and external oblique activity (3).*

2. *Avoid using a pillow beneath the head, which increases pressure on the cervical spine.*

3. *To decrease hamstring cramping and enhance gluteal firing, apply more pressure at the heels while maintaining stability through the rest of the foot. It may be helpful to introduce this exercise with small ranges of motion, such as beginning articulation only at the lumbar spine, progressing to low thoracic, mid-thoracic, and so on.*

Bridge Prep

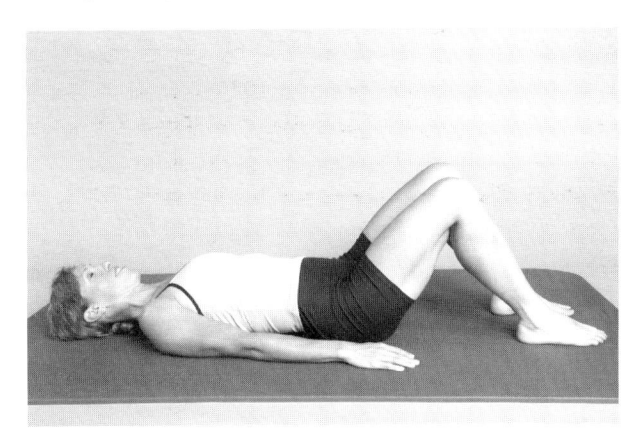

Start in hooklying with neutral pelvis, head, and cervical alignment, the legs parallel, the heels hip-distance apart, the arms alongside the body, the elbows slightly bent, with the palms down.

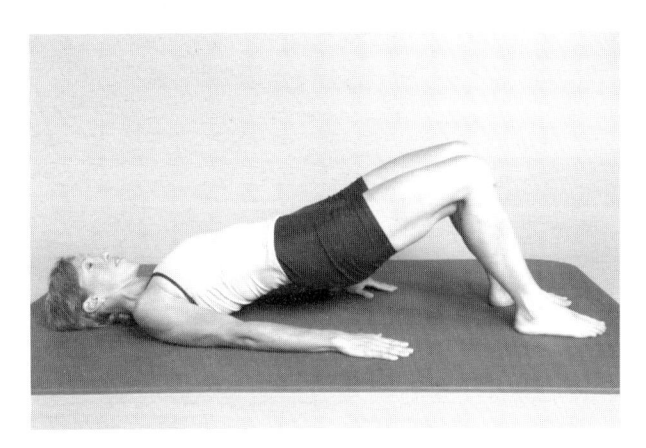

Inhale to refocus breathing. Exhale and lift the torso off the floor as one unit, keeping the pelvis and spine neutral, extending the hips to create a bridge position with pressure on the upper thoracic spine. Be sure to push the feet evenly into the floor to increase hip extensor involvement. Inhale and maintain neutral pelvis and spine. Exhale to return the torso back to the mat.

Purpose:

- To maintain neutral spine and pelvis with mobilization of the hip and spine
- Mobilize the hip joint through flexion and extension
- Coordination of the primary and secondary stabilizers (TrA, obliques, multifidus, hip adductors/abductors/hip extensors).

Clinical Application:

- Useful in teaching patients to isolate hip movement from the pelvis and stabilize the torso in the closed kinetic chain position
- Essential lumbar stabilization exercise
- Excellent exercise to strengthen the hip extensors, hip abductors/adductors, abdominals, and lumbar stabilizers and lengthen the one-joint hip flexors
- Suggested patient populations: Hamstring strain; sacroiliac joint (SIJ)/anterior innominate dysfunction; patellofemoral syndrome; hip bursitis; hip adductor strain
- Foundational pattern for sport-specific training for runners, cross-country skiers

Repetitions: 5-10, depending on patient goals

Practitioner's tips:

1. To lengthen the one-joint hip flexors, cue the individual to push the knees forward simultaneously with the bridge while maintaining neutral pelvis and keeping the upper torso still.

2. A patient with long femurs may have difficulty maintaining neutral pelvis as they lift up into the bridge secondary to limited room between the pelvis and femur. Modify the starting position by moving the heels farther away from the ischial tuberosities, but realize that the gluteals will be more challenged in this position.

3. *This exercise can be used to reeducate the gluteus maximus muscle when there is compensatory firing of the hamstrings and back extensors with a squat. Stimulate the quadriceps muscles slightly to decrease hamstring activity and enhance gluteus maximus firing (4). Once the gluteus maximus firing pattern has been normalized with the bridge, progress to the squat.*

4. *Avoid using a pillow, which will increase pressure on the cervical spine.*

Faulty Movement Patterns: Inability to stabilize the pelvis, resulting in anterior or posterior tilting and/or unilateral pelvic rotation; hip rotation; Valsalva; abdominal popping; pressure on the cervical spine; upper body tension; the torso moving forward or backward; hyperextended elbows; inability to coordinate breath with movement

Hip Extension Preps

Start prone on the mat, hands beneath the forehead, the spine and pelvis in neutral, the legs extended long, hip-distance apart, the ankles dorsiflexed, and the toes extended.

Practitioner's tip: Use a pad under the ASIS to support neutral pelvis with excessive lumbar lordosis when the patient is not able to maintain neutral with use of the abdominals. Progress to no pad.

Movement Pattern 1 (5):

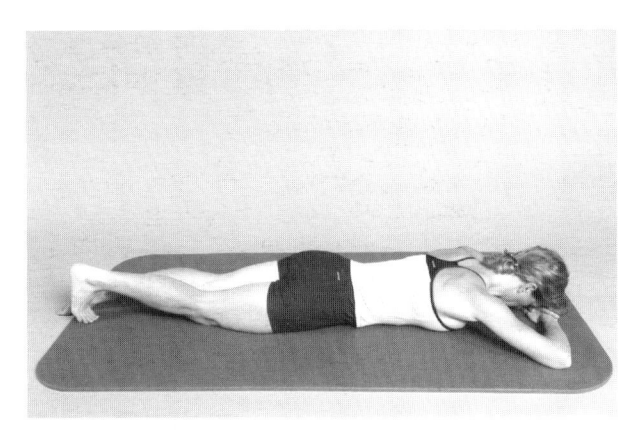

Inhale to stabilize the spine and pelvis. Exhale, contract the abdominals, then the gluteals, and extend one knee while keeping the ankle dorsiflexed. Inhale to flex the knee and return it to the floor. Exhale and repeat on the opposite side.

Movement Pattern 2 (5):

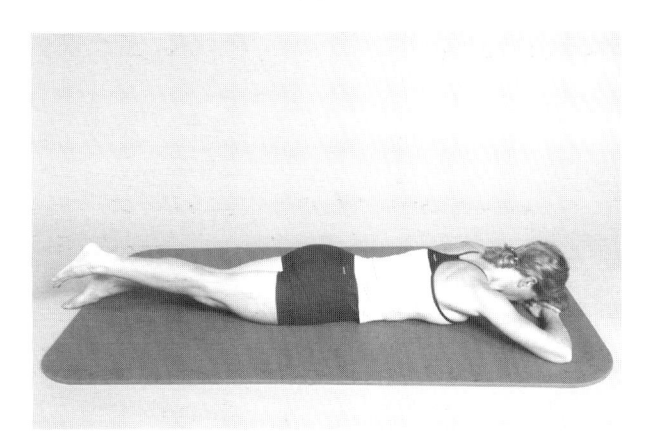

Inhale to stabilize the spine and pelvis. Exhale, contract the abdominals, then the gluteals, and extend one knee. Inhale and maintain lumbo-pelvic stabilization while plantar flexing the ankle and lifting the leg. Exhale to dorsiflex the ankle. Inhale and flex the knee, returning to the floor. Exhale and repeat on the opposite side.

Purpose:

- To challenge pelvic and spinal stability
- To mobilize the hip joint to extension and normalize the hip extensor firing pattern via gluteus maximus neuromuscular reeducation

Clinical Application:

- Coordinating pelvic stability with hip mobility
- Hip extensor strengthening
- Beginning lumbar stabilization exercise
- Reeducation of the gluteus maximus recruitment pattern
- Challenging unilateral movement
- Suggested patient populations: Use with rehabilitation of post-hamstring strains; SIJ/anterior innominate dysfunction; gait training; retraining running mechanics

Repetitions: 5-10, depending on patient goals

Variations: Prone on a stability ball; standing, with or without arm patterns

Equipment: Pad/towel beneath the ASIS

Faulty Movement Patterns: Anterior tilting of the pelvis as a result of decreased hip extension secondary to one-joint hip flexor/anterior hip capsule tightness and/or not stabilizing the spine/pelvis with the abdominals; pelvic rotation as a result of not stabilizing with the TrA and/or multifidus/obliques, resulting in body weight shifting unilaterally; hinging at the lumbar spine (T-L junction); hyperextended knee; upper body tension; thoracic flexion as a result of excessive external oblique muscle contraction; Valsalva; inability to coordinate breath with movement

Trunk Extension with Arm Patterns
Trunk Extension 1:

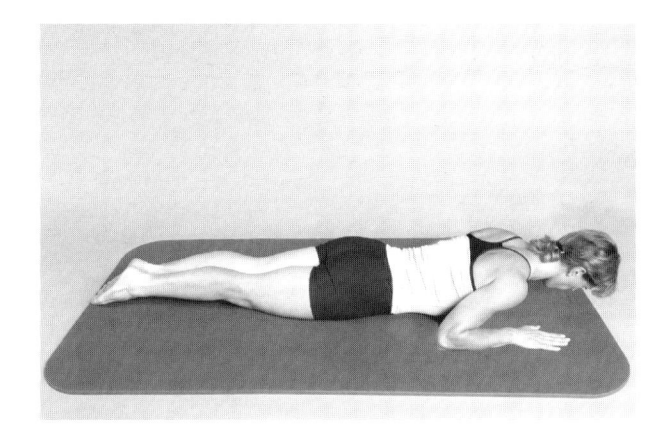

Start prone with neutral pelvis, head, and neck alignment, the elbows bent, hands aligned just outside the shoulders on the mat, the legs extended and the hips adducted, and the ankles plantar flexed.

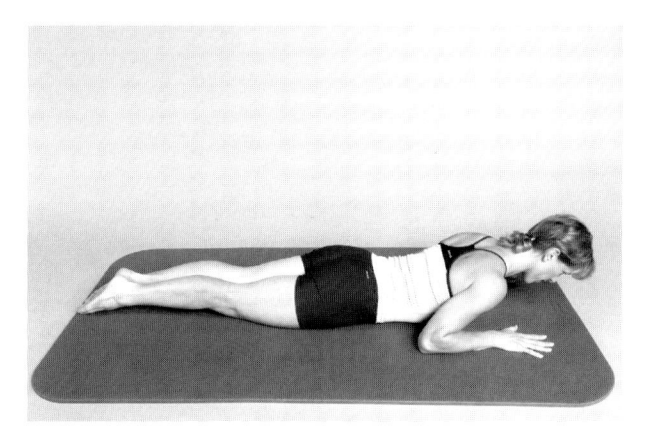

Inhale to prepare. Exhale, gently depress and retract the scapulae, and extend the cervical and thoracic spine slightly off the mat, keeping the lower ribs on the mat and minimal pressure on the forearms and hands. Inhale and hold the extended position. Exhale to the initial position.

Helpful tips:

1. Patients with excessive thoracic kyphosis should position the hands wider to open up the chest or use a pillow to support the chest. Your decision will be based on the severity of the kyphosis.

2. Place a towel or pad beneath the ASIS if your patient has difficulty maintaining neutral. Be sure to check gluteal stabilization.

Trunk Extension 2:

Start prone with neutral pelvis, head, and neck alignment, the arms long on the mat and the palms facing the thighs, the legs extended and the hips adducted, and the ankles plantar flexed.

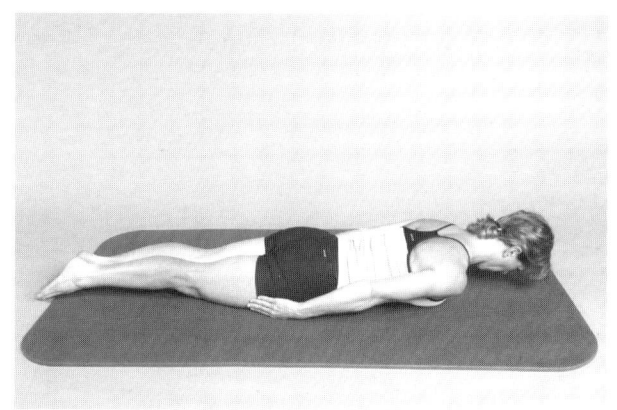

Inhale to prepare. Exhale, gently depress and retract the scapulae, and extend the thoracic spine and shoulders slightly off the mat, reaching the shoulders toward the toes. Inhale to stay, breathing without losing abdominal/gluteal connection. Exhale to the initial position.

Teaching tip: Remember that the cervical spine should align with the thoracic spine and not go into excessive extension. Cue the patient to use eye position as a guideline in finding the cervical position for this exercise. Most of the emphasis in this exercise is on thoracic extension.

Purpose:

- Spinal extension with lumbo-pelvic stabilization

Clinical Application:

- Use this exercise to increase upper/mid-back erector spinae strength while maintaining neutral pelvis, scapular/rib cage stabilization
- Use as an adjunct to mobilization or muscle energy techniques for FRS dysfunction of the thoracic spine (flexion, rotation, sidebend)
- This is an excellent exercise for an individual who has an increase in kyphosis or osteoporosis. Challenge the individual by changing the position of the arms.

Repetitions: 5-10, depending on patient goals

Variations: Two breaths; arm positioning; equipment

Faulty Movement Patterns: Anterior pelvic tilt; ribs popping into the mat; legs lifting off the floor; neck hyperextension/hyperflexion; scapular elevation; inability to fire the gluteals as stabilizers; flexion at the thoracolumbar junction, a result of increased external oblique and rectus abdominis activity; upper body tension; Valsalva; inability to coordinate breath with movement

Torso Rotation: Supine Knee Sways

Start in hooklying with neutral pelvis/spine, head, and neck alignment, the heels hip-width apart, the hips adducted. The arms are alongside the body, elbows slightly bent, with the palms facing down.

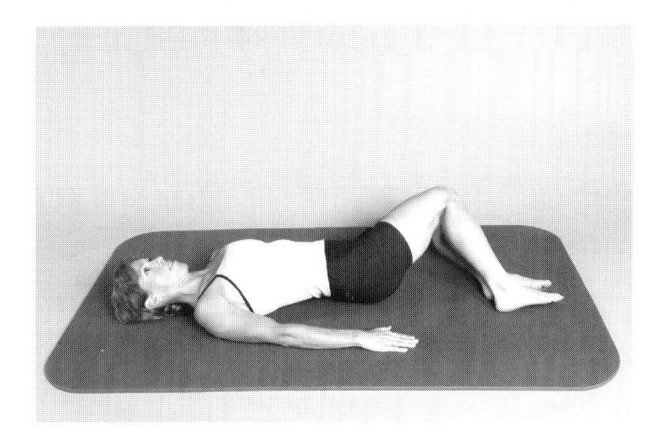

Inhale, maintain neutral pelvis, and sway the knees together away from the midline. Maintain foot contact with the mat. Exhale to draw the legs in toward the midline. Repeat in other the direction.

Purpose:

- To mobilize the mid- to low-thoracic spine sequentially
- To maintain hip and lumbo-pelvic stabilization
- Oblique stretching and multifidus strengthening
- To increase proprioception of movement via feedback from the mat

Clinical Application:

- Use this movement pattern when sequential articulation of the mid- to low-thoracic spine is not occurring
- Use for neuromuscular reeducation of the obliques. Use as an option for introductory oblique retraining

Repetitions: 5-10, depending on patient goals

Variations: Four-breath pattern; reverse breathing; the legs in tabletop, the pelvis imprinted with the knees flexed or extended

Faulty Movement Patterns: Inability to rotate sequentially; rib cage popping; hyperlordosis or posterior tilt; upper body tension; Valsalva; inability to coordinate breath with movement

Spine Twist Prep with Legs and Arms

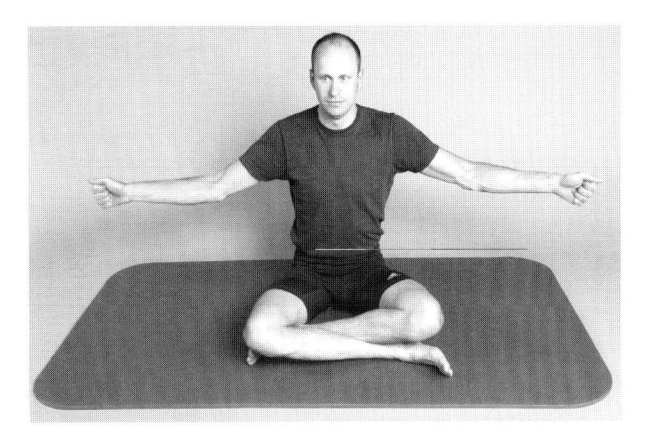

Start by sitting with neutral pelvis, spine, and neck, the shoulders aligned over the pelvis, the legs crossed in front of the body (tailor sit), the shoulders abducted to 90°.

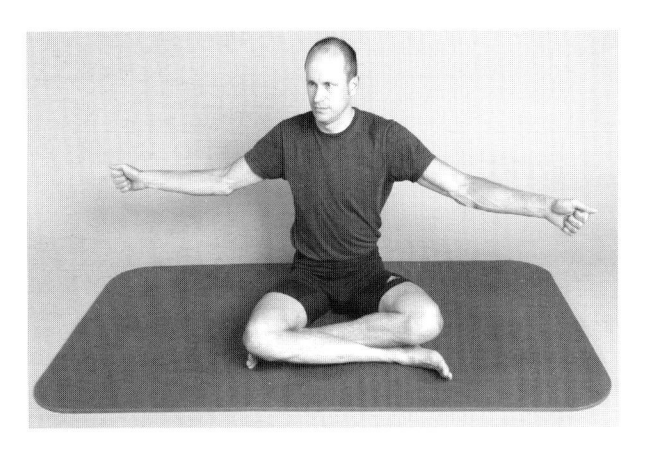

Inhale and reconnect with the abdominals. Exhale and rotate to the right three times, increasing rotational range with each exhale. Inhale to return to the center. Exhale to rotate to the left three times.

Variation: Arms crossed on chest

Purpose:

- Foundational Pilates exercise to introduce spinal rotation
- To stabilize the shoulders and pelvis with spinal rotation
- To strengthen the obliques, multifidus
- Pelvic stabilization through the TrA and the pelvic floor

Clinical Application:

- Provides the opportunity to observe/challenge spinal rotation and pelvic stabilization capabilities
- Strengthening of the internal obliques ipsilaterally and the external obliques and multifidus through concentric/eccentric contraction contralaterally
- Isometric strengthening of the scapular stabilizers and shoulder abductors
- Suggested patient populations: Use with patients who have scoliosis, shoulder dysfunctions that include bursitis/rotator cuff tendonitis (baseball players/pitchers) (6). Use this exercise as an adjunct to mobilization or muscle energy techniques of the thoracic spine. Also use this exercise to challenge dynamic stabilization for athletes who play tennis, golf, basketball, or softball. This is a nice exercise for ergonomic and body mechanics training.

Repetitions: 3-6 times to each side, depending on patient goals

Faulty Movement Patterns: Pelvic rotation; spinal rotation occurring at the upper thoracic spine as opposed the mid- to lower thoracic spine; posterior or anterior pelvic tilt; rib cage popping; leading with the head and shoulders

Chapter References

1. Sahrmann, S.A. 1992. In: McDonnell K, *Diagnosis and Treatment of Muscle Imbalances and Associated Regional Pain Syndromes*. Course Manual, Minneapolis, MN, February 28, 29, and March 1.

2. Bender, L. 2004. The Pilates Coach: Mini Ball Mat Workshop. Workshop notes, Idea Fact Fest, Rosemont, IL, April 23.

3. Lee, D. 2003. *The Pelvis: Restoring Function, Relieving Pain*, Edition 2. Course Manual, Minneapolis, MN.

4. McGill, S. 2004. *Ultimate Back Fitness and Performance*. Waterloo, Ontario, Canada: Wabuno Publishers.

5. Franke, B., Bauman, S. 1992. *Treatment of Muscle Imbalances*. Course Manual, Health Forum, Institute for Athletic Medicine, Saint Paul, MN, November.

6. Bruce, S.L. 2000. Shouldering pain. *Advance for Directors in Rehabilitation*. November, pp. 25-28.

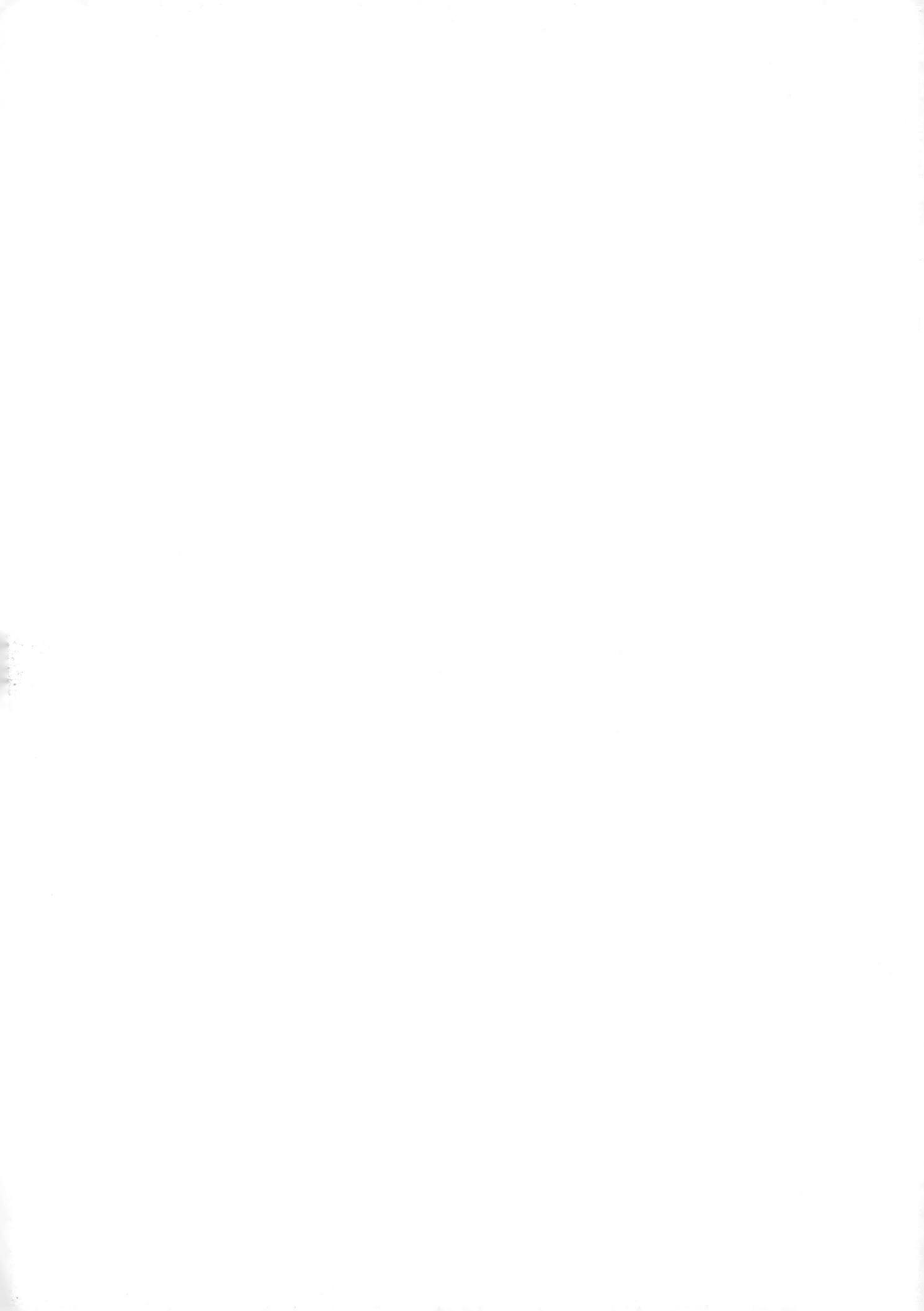

chapter 7

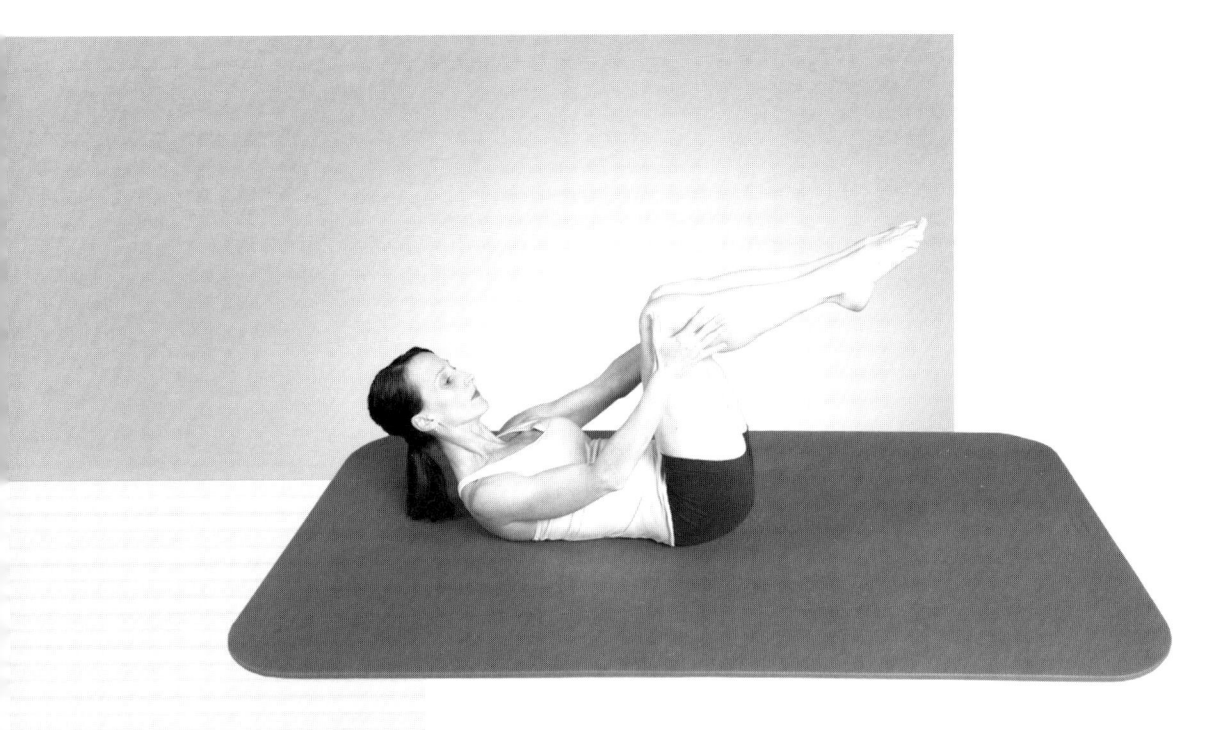

THE EXERCISES

In Pilates practice, the exercises generally follow a specific sequence. Pilates felt that the body responds best when exercises are performed consistently, in order. This format isn't conducive to rehabilitation specialists for many reasons, among them your patient goals and abilities.

For this reason, we've categorized the exercises by purpose and movement orientation so that you may pick and choose those that are best suited to your patient and his or her goals, maximizing the treatment outcome.

	Page
Spinal Flexion and Articulation	93
Spinal Extension, Mobility, and Stability	107
Torso: Stabilization, Rotation, and Lateral Flexion	111
Hips: Joint Mobilization and Muscle Strengthening	119
Upper Body Strengthening and Stabilization	132

Spinal Flexion and Articulation

"You're only as old as you feel" is a statement Pilates applied to the spine and his Contrology science. From his perspective, the spine is the lifeblood of movement and quality of life: the guide to your age is the degree of spinal flexibility. If your spine remains flexible into older adulthood, you are young. If it is inflexible as a young adult, you are old.

The following exercises focus on spinal flexion, mobility, and in one instance, rolling sequentially along the spine. Most of the exercises are progressions of the fundamentals and offer exercise ideas in all planes of motion, supine to sitting. Some are entirely new but are built on the foundation of the fundamentals and the principles.

Use your creativity and skill to add equipment or modify these exercises as appropriate for your patient.

Quarter Rollup with Neutral Pelvis

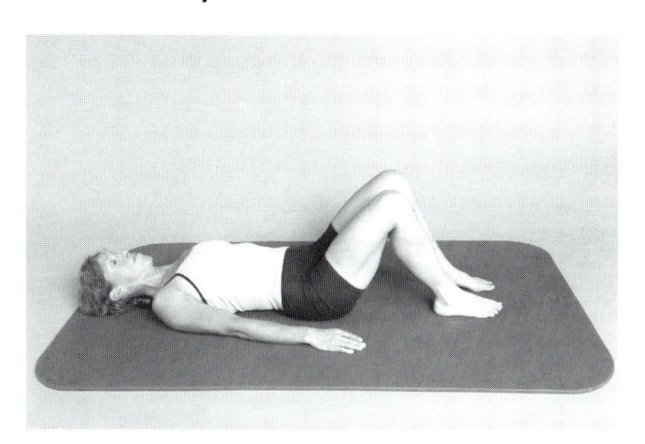

Start in hooklying with neutral pelvis, neutral head and neck alignment, heels hip-width apart, arms alongside the body, elbows slightly bent, with the palms facing down on the mat.

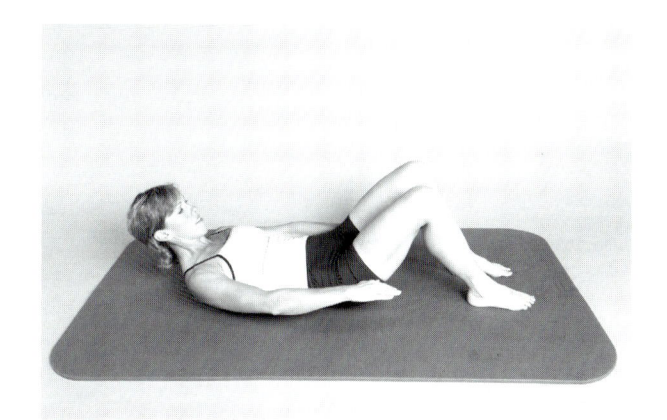

Inhale and breathe into the back and sides of the ribs. Maintaining neutral, exhale and sequentially flex the cervical to mid-thoracic spine, reaching the arms off the mat in line with the shoulders as the fingers reach for the toes. Inhale and hold the flexed position without losing abdominal connection. Exhale and sequentially roll the thoracic to cervical spine back to the mat, returning the arms to the initial position.

Purpose:

- Abdominal strengthening in neutral
- First exercise to coordinate several of the principles of stabilization
- To maintain neutral pelvis while mobilizing the thoracic spine into flexion
- To warm up the body

Clinical Application:

- Muscular emphasis includes isometric/concentric/eccentric contraction of the abdominals to stabilize the lumbo-pelvic region and flex the spine
- Suggested patient populations: Flat back posture, adjunct to muscle energy technique for thoracic spine such as ERS dysfunction (extension, rotation, sidebend)
- Essential lumbar stabilization exercise
- Contraindicated for osteoporosis

Repetitions: 5-10, depending on patient goals

Variations: Place one or two hands behind the head or vary arm positions to challenge lumbo-pelvic stabilization. Try this same exercise with the legs in tabletop.

Faulty Movement Patterns: Posterior tilt; gluteals firing; tailbone lifting off the mat; femoral rotation; abdominal popping; shoulder blade protraction; excessive neck flexion/extension; compensatory firing of the superficial neck flexors; inability to move segmentally; Valsalva; elbow hyperextension; upper body tension; inability to coordinate breath with movement

The Hundred

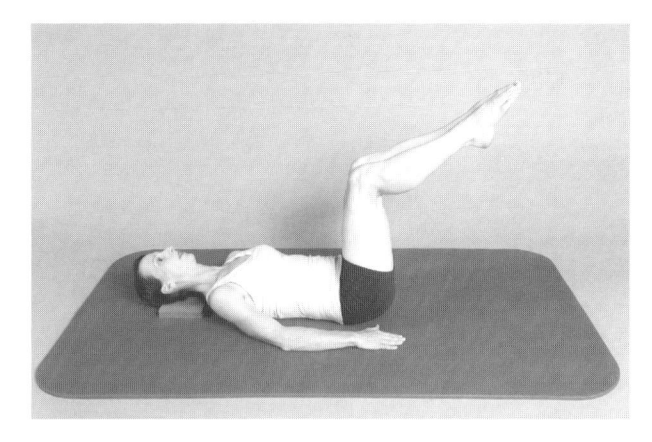

Start in tabletop with neutral pelvis, neutral head and neck alignment, the hips adducted, arms alongside the body, elbows slightly bent, with the palms facing down on the mat.

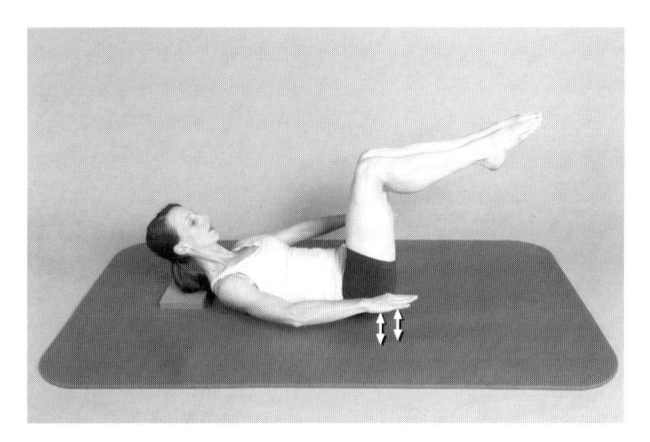

Inhale to prepare. Exhale and sequentially flex the cervical to mid-thoracic spine, reaching the arms off the mat in line with the shoulders as the fingers reach for the toes. Inhale and hold the flexed position without losing abdominal connection while the arms/shoulders gently "pulse" for a count of 5. Exhale to hold the flexed position and "pulse" the arms for a count of 5. Inhale to stay. Exhale and sequentially return the spine to the mat.

Variation: Keep feet on mat.

Practitioner's tips:

1. The original Hundred is performed as above for a total of 100 breaths (10 patterns of inhale/exhale) with the knees/hips extended on the diagonal. This is challenging even for the fit individual, much less a patient. Patients should be progressed to this end point or a variation of it, if appropriate. We often perform for 40 inhales/exhales and take a break.

2. Cue your patient to move through the shoulder with pulsing of the arms versus reaching through the hands to enhance the quality of movement and torso stabilization.

3. The patient needs to master the Quarter Rollup with Neutral Pelvis before progressing to the Hundred.

Purpose:

- Abdominal strengthening in the open and closed chain positions of the lower extremities while mobilizing the thoracic spine into flexion and the shoulders into slight extension/flexion
- Challenges coordination of upper extremity movement and the endurance of the primary and secondary torso stabilizers

Clinical Application:

- Challenges muscle endurance of the lumbo-pelvic and cervical/thoracic spine and shoulder regions. Muscular emphasis includes isometric/concentric/eccentric contraction of the abdominals to stabilize the lumbo-pelvic region and spinal articulation
- Open chain training of the lower extremities challenges lumbo-pelvic stabilization against the weight of the lower extremities and isometric hip flexor contraction
- Suggested patient populations: Use this movement pattern for neuromuscular reeducation of the scapular stabilizers with shoulder bursitis, rotator cuff tendonitis, and shoulder subluxation/dislocations with patients such as divers and cross-country skiers who perform a similar movement in sport

Repetitions: See Practitioner's tips; depending on patient goals

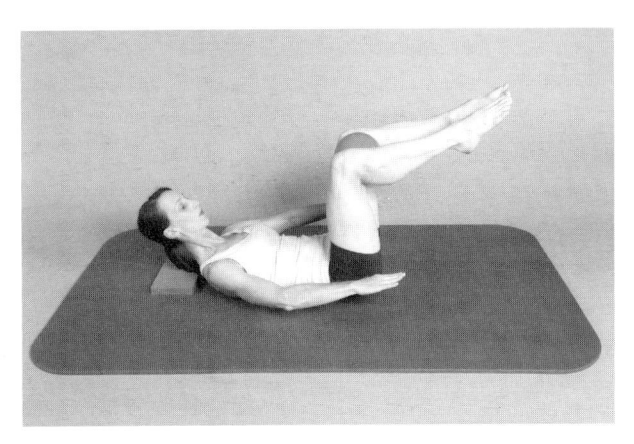

Increase the challenge by placing a small ball or stability ball between the ankles or knees.

Faulty Movement Patterns: Posterior tilt; gluteals firing; tailbone lifting off the mat; femoral rotation; abdominal popping; scapulae protraction; excessive neck flexion/extension; inability to move segmentally; hyperextended elbows; Valsalva; inability to coordinate breath with movement

Rollup

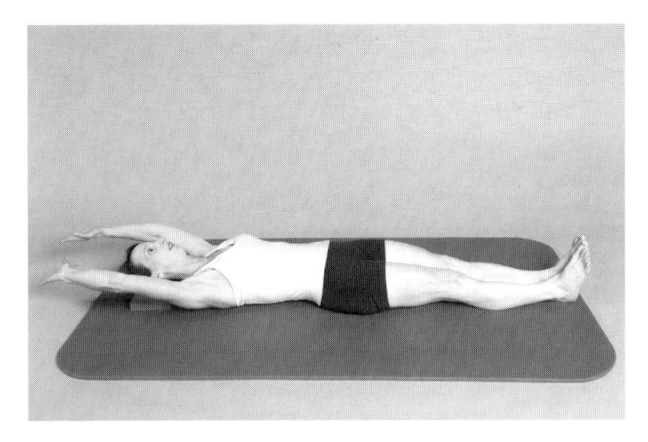

Start supine with neutral pelvis, the hips extended and adducted, the ankles dorsiflexed, the shoulders flexed to 180 degrees, and the lower ribs resting on the mat.

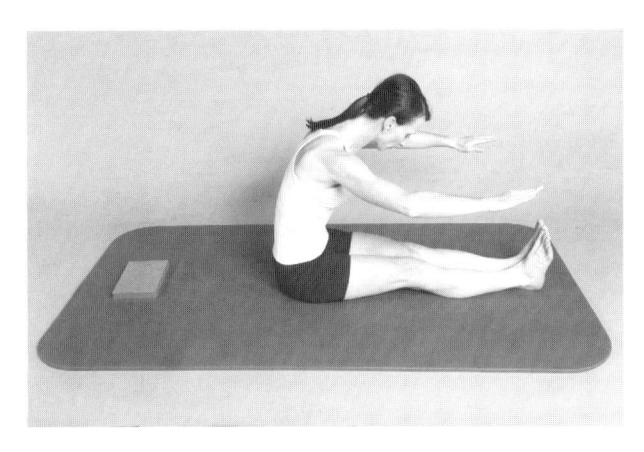

Inhale and flex the shoulders to 90 degrees. Exhale and begin to sequentially peel the spine off the mat from the cervical to the lumbar spine. Roll through imprint at lumbar spine.

The spine flexes, drawing the abdominals over the legs with the arms stretching parallel to the mat. Inhale and roll sequentially back to the mat, leading with the tailbone. The pelvis stays imprinted as the lumbar spine touches the mat. Exhale as the pelvis segues to neutral when the low thoracic vertebrae touch the mat. Continue rolling down and return the arms overhead to the starting position.

Practitioner's tip: Following our guideline of stability before mobility, the Quarter Rollup with Neutral Pelvis should be mastered before progressing to the full Rollup.

Purpose:

- Spinal mobility through sequential articulation
- Pelvic stability in varied positions
- Hamstring and erector spinae flexibility
- Abdominal strengthening
- Scapular stability

Clinical Application:

- IM/eccentric/concentric abdominal strengthening
- Spinal mobilization
- Elongation of the hamstrings and spinal extensors
- Challenges the abdominals secondary to greater range of motion
- Neuromuscular reeducation of the spine sequentially in the sagittal plane
- Suggested patient populations: Excellent exercise for individuals with flat back posture; Scheuermann's disease; supports pelvic mechanics with running. Use as an adjunct to spine mobilization techniques. Contraindicated for patients with a lumbar fusion or osteoporosis.

Repetitions: 5-10, depending on patient goals

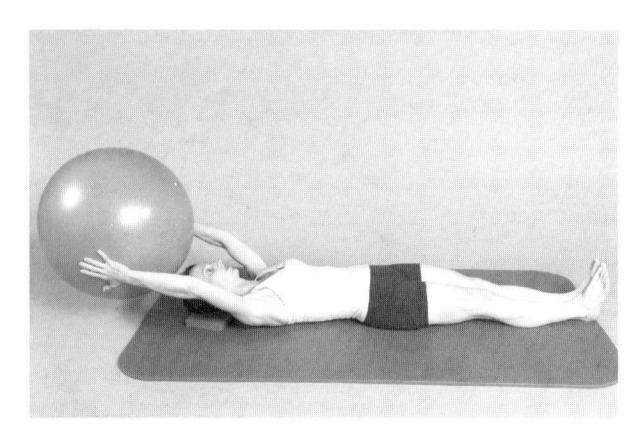

Place an exercise band, small ball, stability ball, or fitness circle in your patient's hands to help reinforce scapular stabilization and increase challenge.

Faulty Movement Patterns: Inability to mobilize segmentally; not articulating through portions of the spine; using momentum to roll up; scapular elevation/protraction; shoulder internal rotation; excessive cervical flexion; hip flexion; sliding on the mat; Valsalva; abdominal popping; upper body tension; compensatory trunk side bend as a result of rolling up or down unilaterally versus staying centered; inability to coordinate breath with movement

Rolling Like a Ball

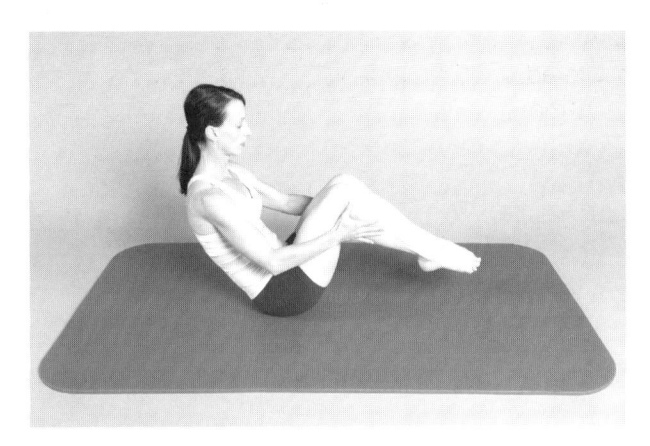

Start seated in spine flexion with a posterior tilt, balancing just behind the ischial tuberosities. The hips are adducted, the hips/knees flexed, the feet elevated off the mat and ankles plantar flexed. Spinal flexion creates a C-curve, with the scapulae stabilized. The hands are positioned at the outside of the calves or beneath the knees.

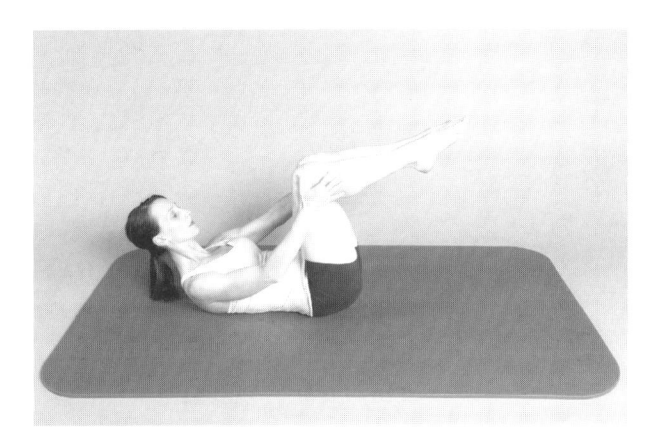

Inhale, maintaining the position of the spine, pelvis, hips, and knees, and gently roll back to the mid- to upper thoracic spine. Exhale; rock up to the initial position, maintaining the position of the spine, pelvis, hips, knees, and shoulders.

Purpose:

- To maintain spinal, hip, and knee flexion through stabilization
- Isometric abdominal strengthening
- Coordination of the primary and secondary stabilizers of the pelvis, spine, and shoulders
- To challenge balance
- Spinal massage

Clinical Application:

- Exercise focuses primarily on stability and challenges the abdominals/hip adductors/abductors/flexors/hamstrings isometrically to stabilize the spine and legs
- Prepatory exercises are helpful to teach stabilization of the pelvis from the femurs
- Sequential articulation of the lumbar and thoracic spine regions to achieve the starting position and rolling sequentially from the lumbar to the thoracic spine regions during the exercise (i.e., flat back posture)
- Suggested patient populations: Excellent training tool for patients such as athletes who lack stabilization of the lumbar spine secondary to lumbar hypermobility and muscle imbalances associated with sports such as diving, gymnastics, and dancing. Contraindicated for patients with osteoporosis.

Repetitions: 5-10, depending on patient goals

Variations:

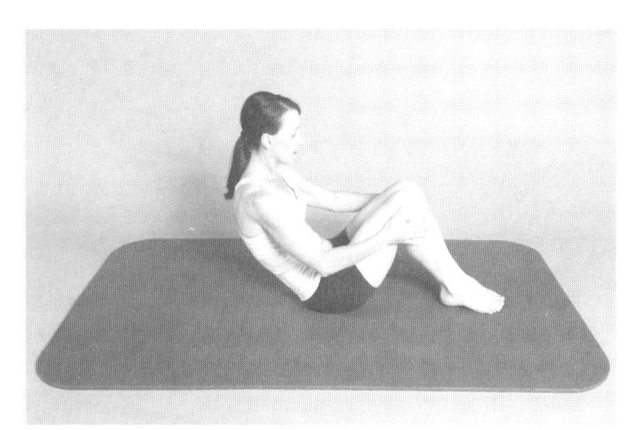

Prepatory exercise 1: With the feet on the mat, roll back halfway.

Prepatory exercise 2: With the feet off the mat, roll back halfway, balancing just off the sitz bones while maintaining the C-curve of the spine.

Faulty Movement Patterns: Anterior tilt; not maintaining the C-curve or posterior tilt, therefore missing the lumbar region (individual will fall heavily); scapular elevation or upper body tension; hyperextension or excessive flexion of the cervical spine; inability to stabilize the hips and knees, allowing the legs to extend or flex; inability to coordinate breath with movement; Valsalva; upper body tension

Single-Leg Stretch

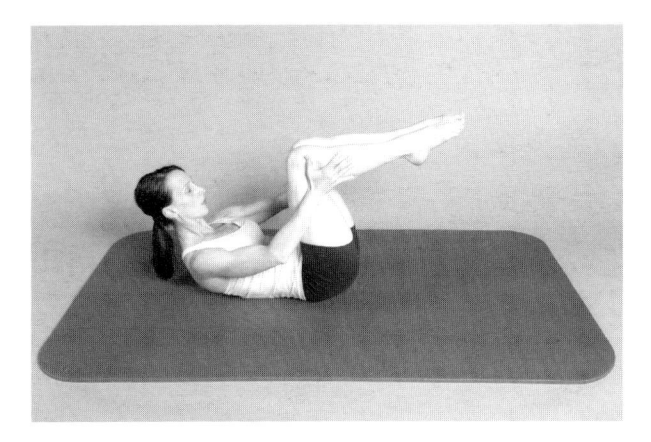

Start supine in cervical/thoracic flexion with the pelvis imprinted. The hips are adducted in tabletop, the ankles plantar flexed and elevated off the floor, and the hands on the outside of the calves.

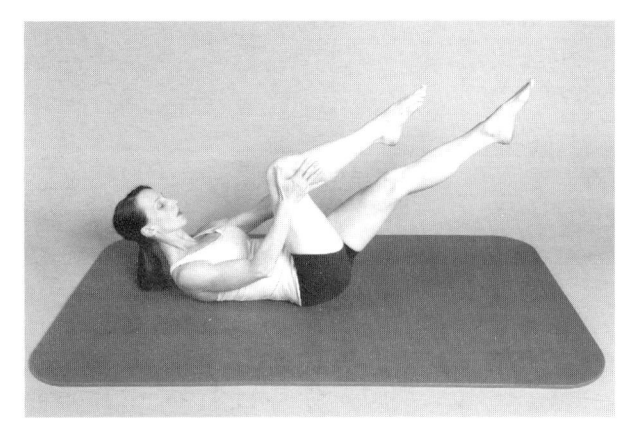

Inhale and connect with the abdominals. Exhale and extend at the hip, knee, and ankle, reaching one leg out on the diagonal. The opposite hand is positioned on the inside knee; the same-side hand is to the outside of the calf. Inhale to switch legs and hands. Exhale to extend the other leg at the hip, knee, and ankle.

Purpose:

- Lumbo-pelvic stability against asymmetrical rhythm of the lower extremities
- Pelvic stability via the TrA, multifidus, and obliques
- Abdominal strengthening
- Hip mobility through eccentric/concentric contraction of the hip flexors
- Stabilization of the shoulder, thoracic spine

Clinical Application:

- Coordinate the primary and secondary stabilizers of the spine and pelvis against the movement of the leg
- Suggested patient populations: Patients with lordotic posture, anterior innominate, hip bursitis, hamstring strain, patellofemoral dysfunction, and neuromuscular retraining of gait/running mechanics

Repetitions: 5-10, depending on patient goals

Variations

Variation 1: Alternate touching one heel to the floor or as low as possible while maintaining a posterior tilt.

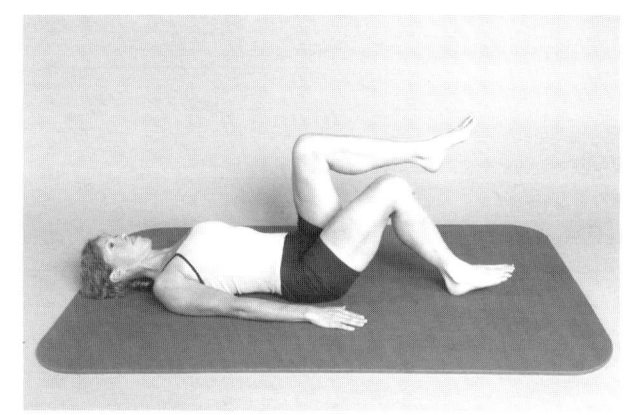

Variation 2: Perform as variation one. Keep the head on the mat during the heel taps (shown).

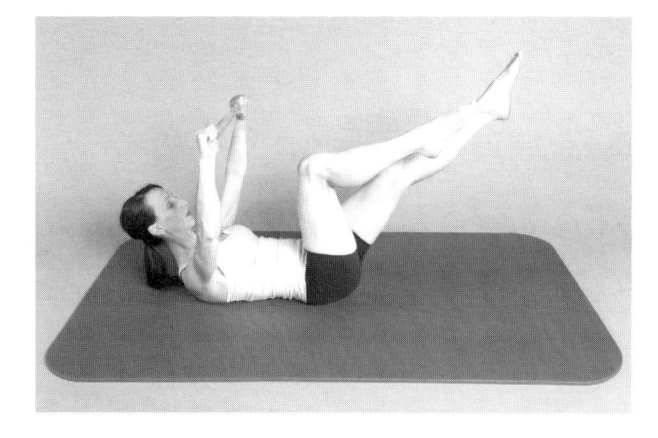

For more challenge, or to reinforce the principle of shoulder stabilization, place a stability ball or wooden doweling (shown) in your patient's hands and cue him/her to hold it stationary above the sternum.

Faulty Movement Patterns: Anterior pelvic tilt, or losing imprint; rocking back and forth on the mat, demonstrating an inability to stabilize; shifting weight from side to side with the leg pattern; the tibia drops as opposed to the femur moving away from the pelvis; excessive flexion/hyperextension of the cervical spine; abdominal popping; Valsalva; the torso collapsing; upper body tension; inability to coordinate breath with movement

Double-Leg Stretch

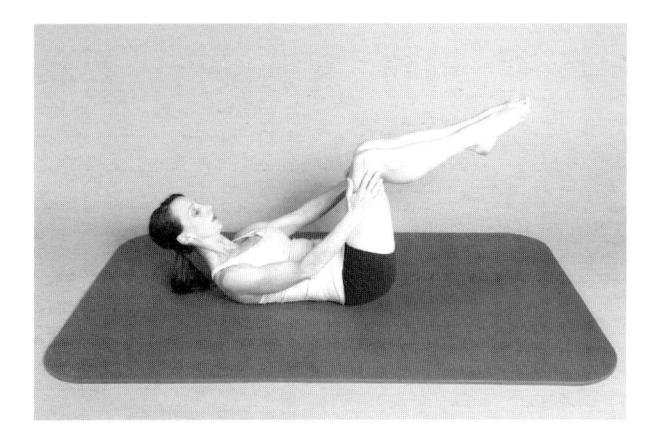

Start supine in cervical/thoracic flexion with the pelvis imprinted, the hips adducted in tabletop with the hips and knees flexed, the ankles plantar flexed and elevated off the floor, and the hands on the outside of the calves.

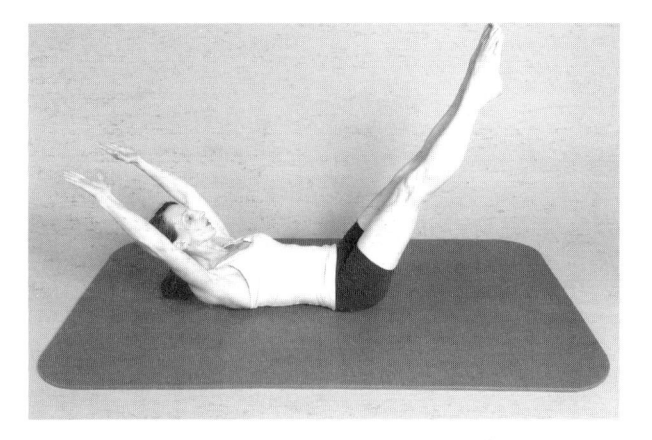

Inhale to prepare. Exhale, maintaining spinal flexion, and extend the hips/knees on the diagonal as low as possible while still maintaining a posterior tilt. The shoulders simultaneously flex overhead. Inhale to return the knees to tabletop while the arms reach out to the sides and down to return to the calves (creating a semicircle).

Purpose:

- Lumbo-pelvic stability with arm and leg patterns
- Hip and shoulder mobility
- Isometric/eccentric/concentric strengthening of the abdominals
- Scapular stability

Clinical Application:

- First exercise to challenge the abdominals in the long lever position
- Advanced lumbar stabilization exercise
- Focus is primarily on torso stability while creating patterns with the arms and legs
- Nice teaching tool to coordinate the primary and secondary stabilizers and to challenge the rib-to-hip connection with movement of the shoulders in multiple planes
- Suggested patient populations: Use with patients who experience shoulder dysfunctions, including glenohumeral instability and shoulder impingement. Advanced rehabilitation exercise for hip flexor tendonitis, patellofemoral syndrome, and pelvic dysfunction. This exercise simulates ADLs, such as reaching to a shelf, and can be used for sport-specific training for athletes whose sports require reaching, such as volleyball or gymnastics.

Repetitions: 5-10, depending on patient goals

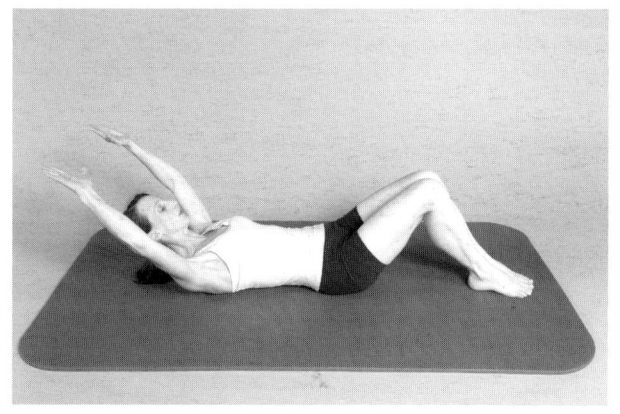

Variation: Start patients with their feet on the mat and using the arms only. Progress to legs in tabletop, arms only.

Faulty Movement Patterns: Inability to stabilize the lumbo/pelvic region; inability to maintain posterior tilt; inability to maintain spinal flexion with shoulders flexed; excessive neck flexion/extension; scapular protraction/elevation; rib cage or abdominal popping; inability to coordinate breath with movement, Valsalva

Criss Cross in Supine

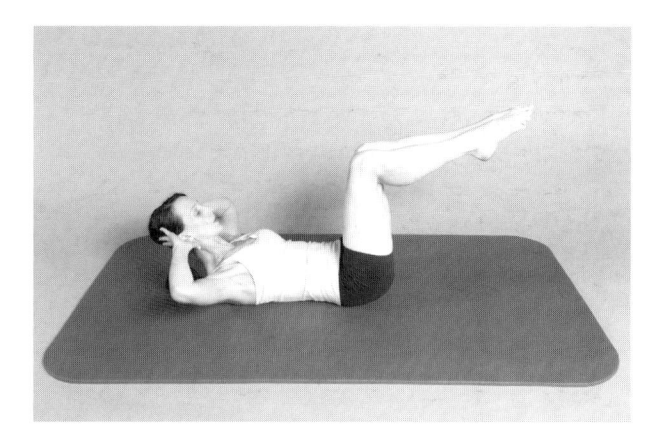

Start supine in cervical/thoracic spine flexion with the pelvis imprinted. The hips are adducted, with the hips/knees flexed, the feet elevated off the mat, the ankles plantar flexed, the hands cradling the head, and the scapulae stabilized.

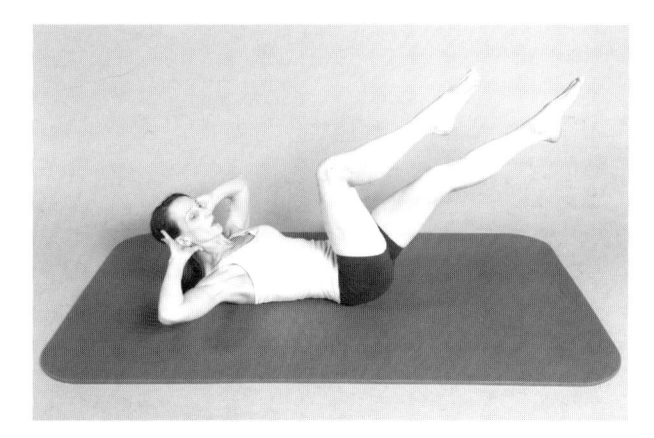

Inhale and deepen the connection with the TrA. Exhale to flex the thoracic spine and rotate the upper body as one unit toward the opposite hip, maintaining the pelvis imprint and thoracic flexion and keeping the elbows open. Simultaneously extend the other hip/knee to the diagonal. Inhale to rotate to the center. Exhale and repeat the pattern to the other side.

Purpose:

- Isometric/eccentric/concentric strengthening of the abdominals
- Contraction of the ipsilateral internal and contralateral external obliques and multifidus
- Coordination
- Eccentric/concentric contraction of the hip flexors
- Pelvic and spinal stabilization against rhythmic leg pattern

Clinical Application:

- Advanced torso stabilization exercise
- Coordination and stamina
- Suggested patient populations: Shoulder bursitis; rotator cuff tendonitis. Use this exercise for sport-specific training for tennis players, golfers, gymnasts, figure skaters, dancers, and baseball/softball players. This exercise is a nice adjunct to manual therapy for hypomobile thoracic vertebral segments.
- Ergonomic and lifting mechanics training
- See Single-Leg Stretch

Repetitions: 5-10, depending on patient goals

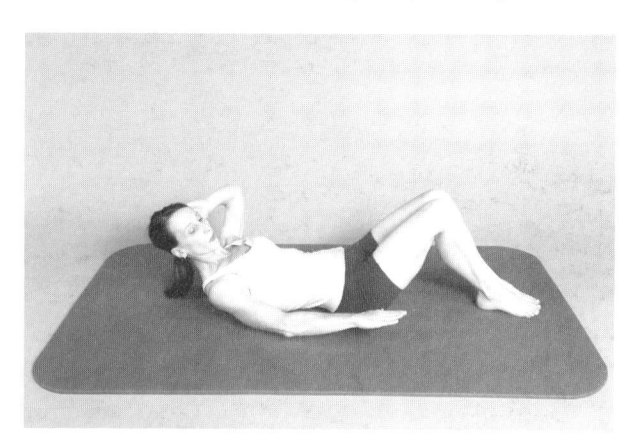

Variations: Begin the Criss Cross with the feet on the mat and one hand behind the head. Increase the challenge by placing both hands behind the head. Gradually progress your patient to legs in tabletop. Once mastered, add hip and knee extension; hands crossed on the chest to the opposite shoulders.

Faulty Movement Patterns: Inability to stabilize the lumbo-pelvic region, resulting in weight shifting from side to side or rocking back and forth on the mat; inability to maintain posterior tilt; rotation at the upper thoracic spine; neck hyperflexion/extension; scapulae elevation or protraction; elbows wrapping around the ears; abdominal popping; leading with the head and shoulders; inability to coordinate breath with movement; Valsalva

Criss Cross in Standing

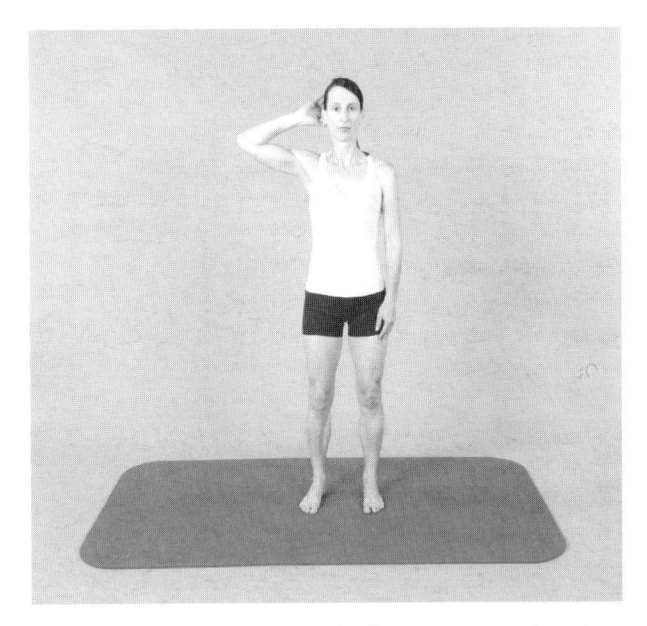

Start by standing in neutral alignment, one hand placed behind the head.

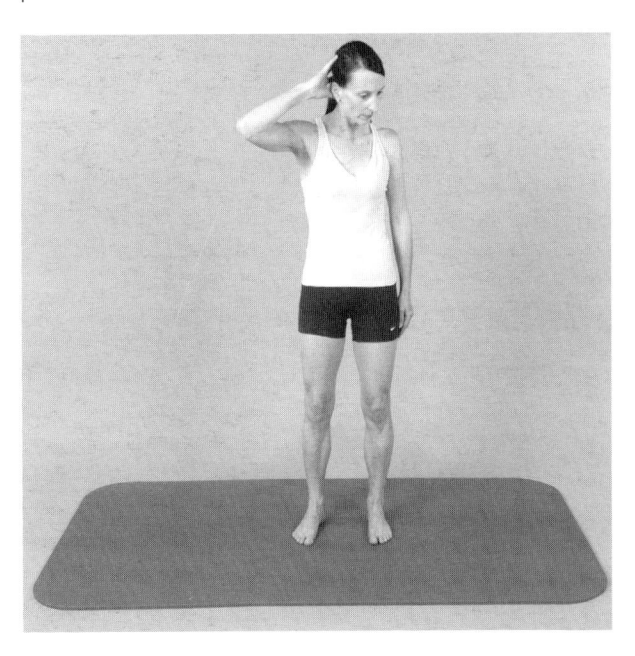

Inhale to prepare. Exhale to flex the thoracic spine and rotate the upper body as one unit toward the opposite hip, maintaining neutral and keeping the elbows open. Inhale to rotate back to the center, extending the spine.

To progress and challenge balance, flex the hip to tabletop as the spine flexes and rotates.

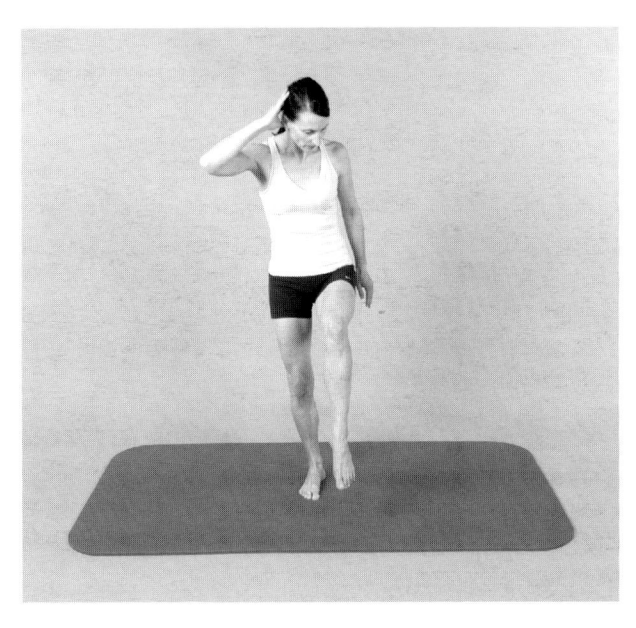

Purpose:

- Strengthening of the abdominals and other spinal rotators
- In progression: Eccentric/concentric contraction of hip flexors; pelvic and spinal stabilization against the leg pattern in standing

Clinical Application:

- Advanced lumbar stabilization strengthening for the spinal rotators in standing
- Contraction of the ipsilateral internal and contralateral external obliques and thoracic multifidus
- Coordination and endurance
- Suggested patient populations: Use this exercise for sport-specific training in athletes whose sports include cross-country skiing and tennis. This exercise can also be used for advanced ergonomic and lifting mechanics training.

Repetitions: 5-10, depending on patient goals

Faulty Movement Patterns: Inability to stabilize the lumbo-pelvic region, resulting in anterior or posterior tilt or lateral hip hiking; rotation at the upper thoracic spine; trunk side bend; lateral sway; inability to stabilize at the hip; scapulae elevation and protraction; elbows wrapping around the ears; abdominal popping; inability to coordinate breath with movement

Spine Stretch Forward

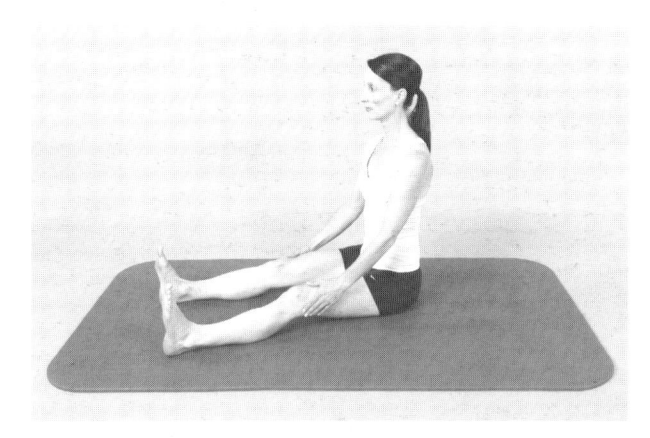

Start by sitting in neutral pelvis and spine, shoulders over the pelvis, with the hips flexed and abducted to about shoulder-width apart, the ankles dorsiflexed, and the hands on the outside of the hips.

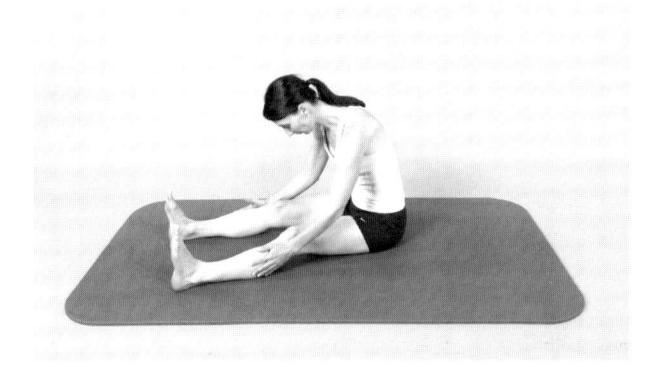

Inhale to lengthen the spine and connect with the abdominals. Exhale and sequentially flex the spine from the cervical to the lumbar segments. Keep the pelvis neutral while the hands move forward and past the knees as far as is comfortable. Inhale and breathe into the back and sides of the ribs. Exhale and sequentially restack the spine from the lumbar spine to the top of the head.

Purpose:

- Spinal mobility
- Segmental articulation
- Stretching of the erector spinae, hamstrings if tight
- Concentric/eccentric contractions of the abdominals and erector spinae
- Pelvic stability

Clinical Application:

- Spinal mobility in sitting; this exercise can serve as a progression of the Quarter Rollup.
- Suggested patient populations: Use as an adjunct to mobilization of the hypomobile thoracic and/or lumbar segments or to muscle energy techniques for thoracic ERS, lumbar paraspinal strain, flat back posture, and for sport-specific training for diving, long jumping.
- This exercise is contraindicated for patients with osteoporosis.

Repetition: 5, depending on patient goals

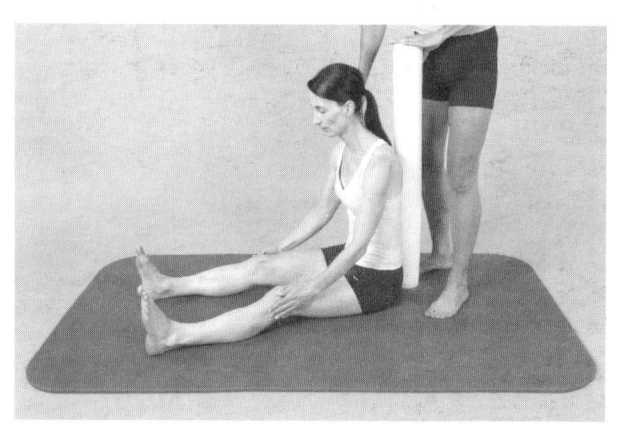

Variations: Sit or stand at the wall (or use perpendicular support at spine) in neutral alignment as a starting point for introducing this exercise. Follow the exercise steps as above.

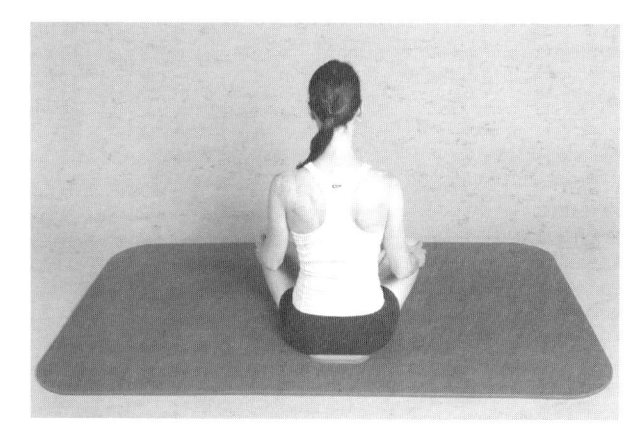

Helpful tip: Patients with tight hamstrings or a tight lower back will struggle with sequential articulation if they do not start with a neutral pelvis. To assist, place patients on a 2- to 3-inch pad to alleviate tightness and have them slightly flex the knees or cross the legs.

105

Faulty Movement Patterns: Hip rather than spinal flexion; posterior or anterior tilt at the start or end of the exercise; rib cage or abdominal popping; excessive neck flexion; scapular elevation/protraction; inability to articulate through the spine sequentially; hyperextended knees; Valsalva; femoral rotation; inability to coordinate breath with movement

Spinal Extension, Mobility, and Stability

Poor posture was a major concern for Pilates, so much so that he created his Matworks regimen, in part to stem what he saw as the cause of many health conditions and serious ailments. He even went so far as to invent a new type of sleeping mattress that was more conducive to the spine, good posture, and sleeping habits.

The following exercises focus on many postural muscles of the upper and mid-torso. As in other chapters, many exercises are progressions of the fundamentals and require stability before mobility. Most are performed prone and in the sagittal plane. The weight and movement of the arms challenge the core and the ability to maintain form.

Use your creativity and skill to add equipment or modify these exercises as appropriate for your patient.

Practitioner's tip: We often forget the pull of gravity on the center of the body. Be aware at all times that the abdominals, lower back, and gluteal muscles must work as partners for these exercises to be most effective.

Trunk Extension with Arm Patterns
Trunk Extension 1: Snow Angel

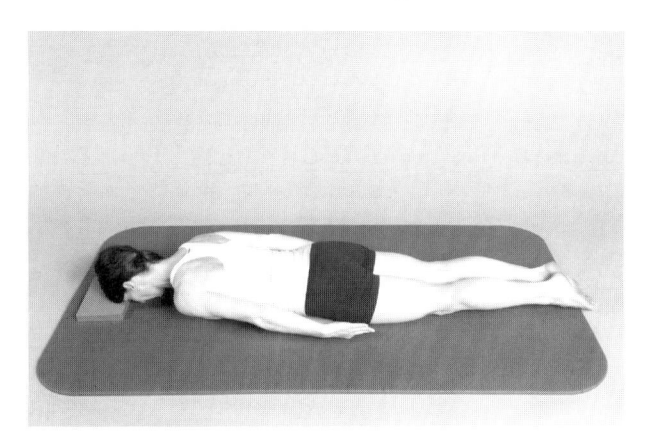

Start prone with neutral pelvis, head, and neck alignment, the shoulders relaxed in protraction, the arms long on the mat with the palms facing the thighs, the legs extended and the hips adducted, and the ankles plantar flexed.

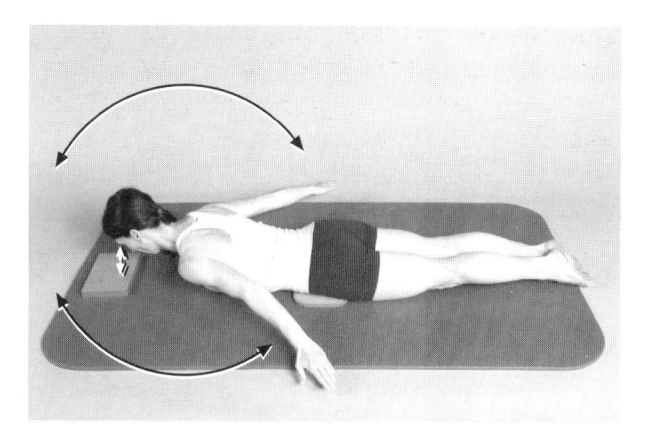

Inhale to prepare. Exhale, gently depress and retract the scapulae, and extend the cervical and thoracic spine slightly off the mat, reaching the fingers to the toes. Inhale and hold the extended position while abducting the shoulders to 90 degrees and then adduct to the starting position. Exhale to return to the mat with the shoulders relaxed.

Trunk Extension 2: Diamond Window

Start prone with neutral pelvis, head, and neck alignment, the elbows bent, with the hands beneath the forehead, the legs extended and the hips adducted, and the ankles plantar flexed.

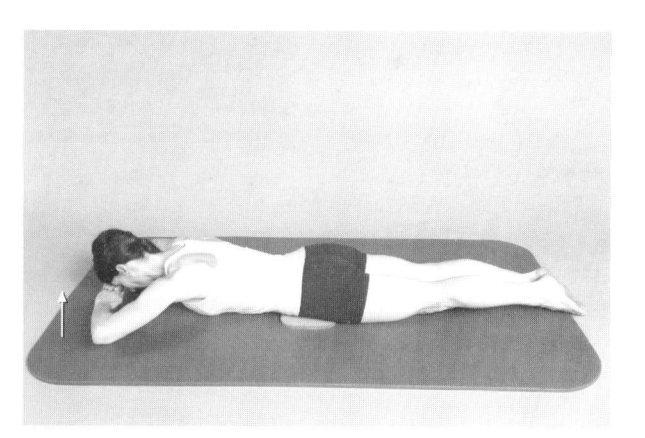

Inhale to prepare. Exhale, gently depress and retract the scapulae, and extend the cervical and thoracic spine off the mat, maintaining contact of the hands with the forehead. Inhale to stay; breathe without losing abdominal/gluteal connection. Exhale to the initial position.

Variation: Add rotation.

107

Trunk Extension 3: Arms Overhead

Start prone with neutral pelvis, head, and neck alignment, the arms overhead, the hips extended and adducted, the ankles plantar flexed.

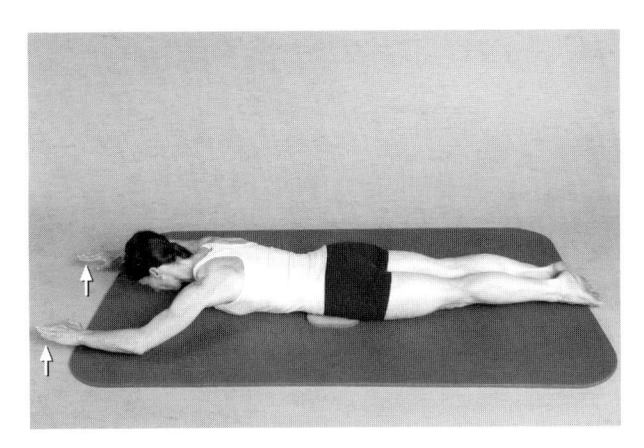

Inhale to prepare. Exhale, gently depress and retract the scapulae, and extend the cervical and thoracic spine off the mat and lift arms. Inhale to hold the slightly extended position. Exhale and return to the starting position (1). *Variation: Externally rotate the shoulders, thumbs facing the ceiling, to emphasize lower trapezius muscles.*

Teaching tips:

1. Patients who have excessive thoracic kyphosis will need to position the hands wider to open up the chest or use a pillow to support the chest. Your decision will be based on the severity of the kyphosis.

2. Place a towel or pad beneath the ASIS if your patient has difficulty maintaining neutral. Be sure to check gluteal stabilization.

3. Remember that the cervical spine should align with the thoracic spine and not go into excessive extension. Cue the patient to eye positioning as a guideline in finding the cervical position for this exercise. Emphasize thoracic extension.

Movement Patterns 1-3

Purpose:

- Spinal extension with lumbo-pelvic and scapular stabilization with varied lever lengths
- Maintain neutral pelvis with co-contraction of the gluteals and abdominals

Clinical Application:

- Use these advanced lumbar stabilization exercises to develop upper/mid-back erector spinae strength while maintaining neutral pelvis, scapular/rib cage stabilization
- This is an excellent exercise for individuals who have an increase in kyphosis, osteoporosis, or scapular weakness
- Challenge dynamic stabilization by changing the lever length via the arm position
- Other suggested patient populations: Use as an adjunct to mobilization of thoracic spine/muscle energy techniques for thoracic FRS dysfunction

Repetitions: 5-10, depending on patient goals

Variations: Changing breathing pattern; wooden dowel, body bar, or foam roller

Faulty Movement Patterns: Anterior pelvic tilt; rib cage or abdominal popping into the mat; legs lifting off the floor; flexion at the thoracolumbar junction, a result of increased external oblique and rectus abdominis activity; neck hyperextension/hyperflexion; scapular elevation; Valsalva; hyperextended elbows; upper body tension; inability to coordinate breath with movement; inability to fire gluteals as stabilizers

Swimming Progressions

Start prone with the arms overhead, the legs extended, hip-width apart and neutral, the ankles plantar flexed, and the spine and pelvis in neutral.

Movement Pattern 1: Opposite Arm and Leg

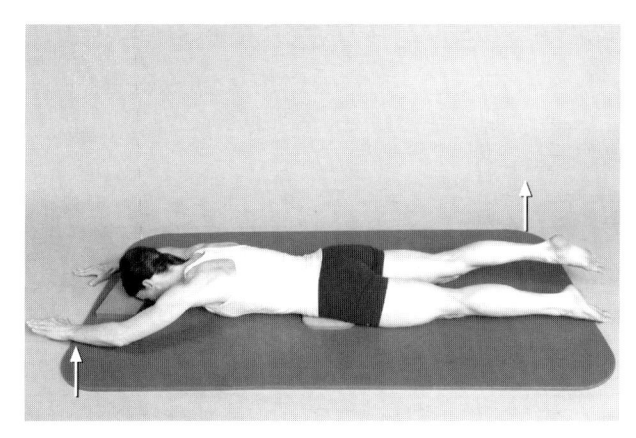

Inhale and breathe into the sides/back of the ribs. Exhale and extend the right hip/left arm off the floor (lift the opposite arm/leg), maintaining neutral spine and pelvis and scapular stabilization. Inhale to maintain the spinal position and connections with the abdominals and gluteals. Exhale to return the extremities to the mat at the same time. Repeat on the other side.

Movement Pattern 2: Upper Body Extension

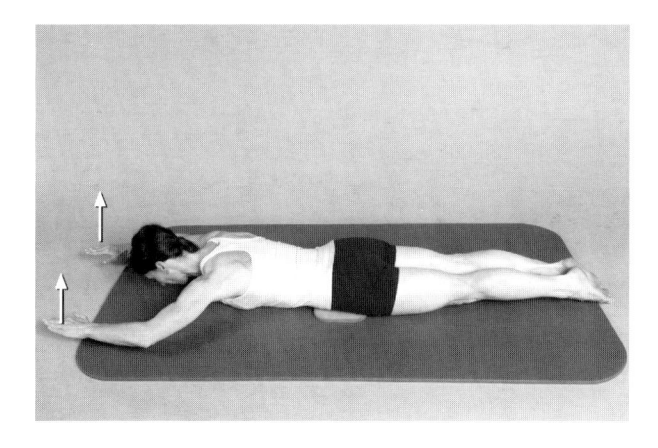

Inhale to connect with the abdominals. Exhale to extend the cervical and thoracic spine and lift the upper extremities off the floor, maintaining neutral spine and pelvis and scapular stabilization. Inhale to stay. Exhale to return the extremities/upper torso to the mat at the same time.

Movement Pattern 3: Lower Body Extension

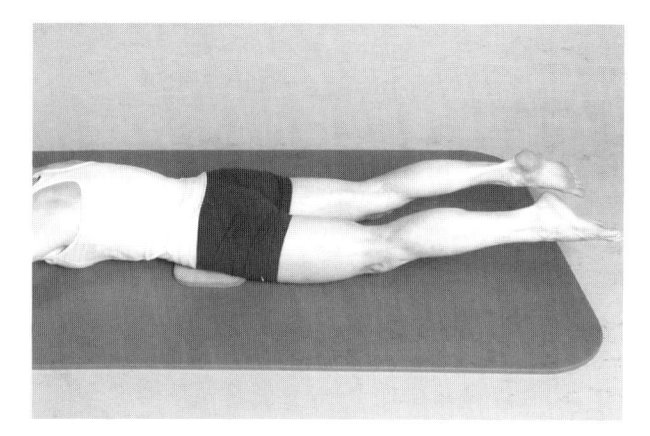

Inhale to connect with the abdominals. Exhale and lift the lower extremities off the floor, maintaining neutral spine and pelvis and scapular stabilization. Inhale to stay. Exhale to return the extremities to the mat at the same time.

Movement Pattern 4: Upper and Lower Body Extension

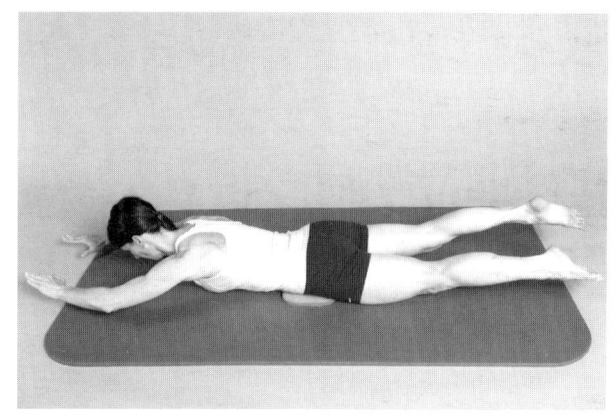

Inhale to connect with the abdominals. Exhale to extend the cervical and thoracic spine and lift the upper and lower extremities off the floor, maintaining neutral spine and pelvis and scapular stabilization. Inhale to stay. Exhale to return the extremities/upper torso to the mat at the same time.

109

Movement Pattern 5: Swimming Variation

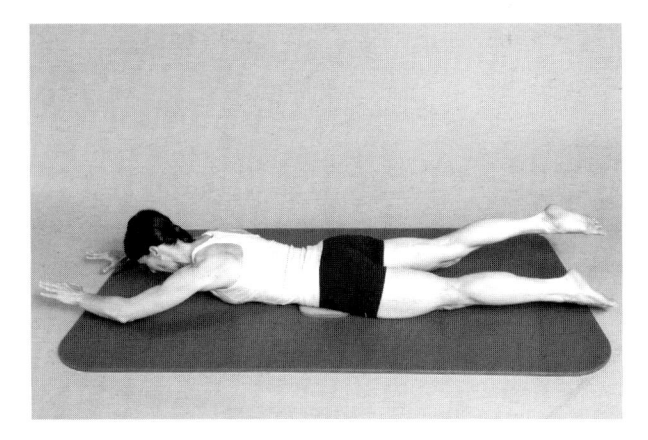

Inhale to connect with the abdominals. Exhale to extend the cervical and thoracic spine and lift the upper and lower extremities off the floor, maintaining neutral spine and pelvis and scapular stabilization. Inhale and lift the opposite arm and leg at a slow, controlled rate. Exhale to repeat on the other side.

Purpose:

- Abdominal/trunk and hip extensor strengthening
- Pelvic/spinal/scapular stability against movement of the arms and legs
- Coordination and balance

Clinical Application:

- Advanced lumbar stabilization exercise
- Strengthening of the abdominals, trunk, hip extensors, and shoulder flexors
- Coordination, endurance, and balance
- Hip and shoulder mobility
- Upper back strengthening for patients with kyphotic/lordotic posture
- Hip flexor stretch
- Suggested patient populations: Use with patients with SI joint dysfunction, hamstring strain, anterior innominate, rotator cuff tendonitis, hypermobility of the lumbar spine, anterior hip capsule/latissimus dorsi tightness, and lower trapezius weakness. This exercise can be used for sport-specific training for basketball, gymnastics, and swimming.

Variations: Quadruped or standing, with the options of lifting one arm, one leg, or a combination of both; hips externally rotated

Repetitions: 5-10, depending on patient goals

Helpful tips:

1. Place a towel or pad beneath the ASIS if your patient has difficulty maintaining neutral pelvis.

2. The patient must master Prone Hip Extension in Chapter 6 prior to performing Swimming Progressions.

Faulty Movement Patterns: Anterior pelvic tilt; scapular elevation, overusing the upper trapezius muscles; hyperextended elbows; Valsalva; rib cage and/or abdominal popping; weight shifting from side to side, indicating an inability to integrate stabilization principles; delayed or nonexistent firing of the gluteals; inability to coordinate breath with movement

Section References

1. *STOTT Pilates Comprehensive Matwork Manual.* 2001. Toronto, Canada: Merrithew Corporation.

Torso: Stabilization, Rotation, and Lateral Flexion

Many of the Pilates Matwork exercises focus on movement in the sagittal and frontal planes. There are a few that emphasize rotation, such as Spine Twist and Criss Cross, Side Bend and Saw, the latter two of which are not included in this handbook.

In our experience, rotation without compensatory strategies is one of the most difficult and challenging movements for our patients. Overrotation, lack of pelvic stability, compensatory upper thoracic rotation, and other faulty movement patterns can contribute to common musculoskeletal ailments that include chronic low back pain and neck pain.

The exercises in this section emphasize rotation and lateral flexion while maintaining pelvic and spinal stability. Remember to keep movements small, incremental, and if necessary, return to the fundamentals. Sometimes, we train the obliques isometrically with exercises such as the Side Plank before adding these concentric/eccentric contractions to give patients a sense of what oblique muscle activity feels like and as an initial neuromuscular reeducation and strengthening exercise.

Use your creativity and skill to add equipment or modify these exercises as appropriate for your patient.

Spine Twist in Sitting, Standing, and Lunge Positions
Movement Pattern 1: "Genie Arms"

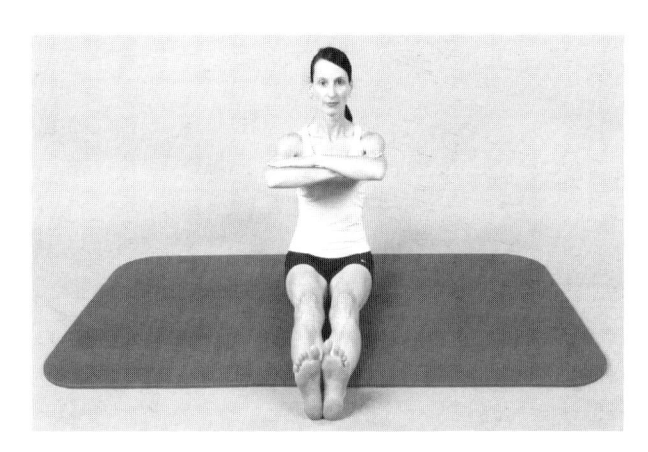

Start sitting with neutral pelvis, spine, and neck, the shoulders aligned over the pelvis and flexed/internally rotated to 90 degrees, with the hands on opposite elbows.

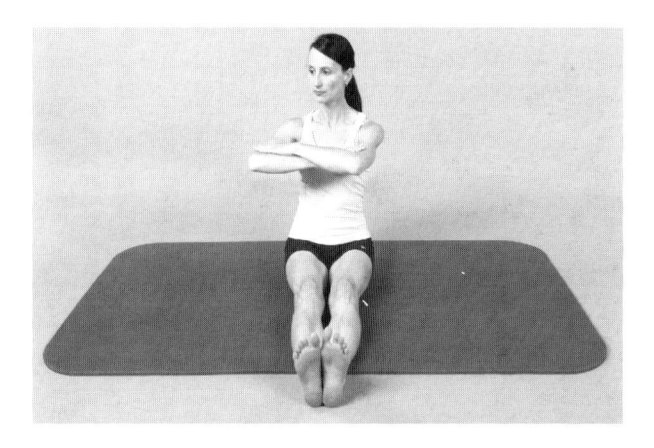

Inhale to reconnect with the abdominals. Exhale and rotate to the right once. Inhale and return to the center. Exhale and rotate to the left.

Variation: Sit in tailor position.

111

Movement Pattern 2: Arms Extended

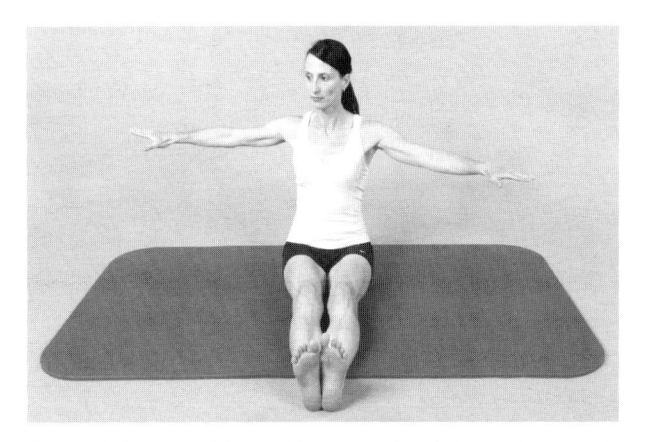

Start sitting position with neutral pelvis, spine, and neck, the shoulders aligned over the pelvis and abducted to 90 degrees, with the elbows slightly bent.

Variation: Sit in tailor position.

Inhale to reconnect with the abdominals. Exhale and rotate to the right once. Inhale and return to the center. Exhale and rotate to the left.

Variation 1: Tailor sit.

Variation 2: Rotate to each side three times, increasing the rotation with each pulse while maintaining lumbo-pelvic stability.

Movement Pattern 3: Standing with Arms Extended

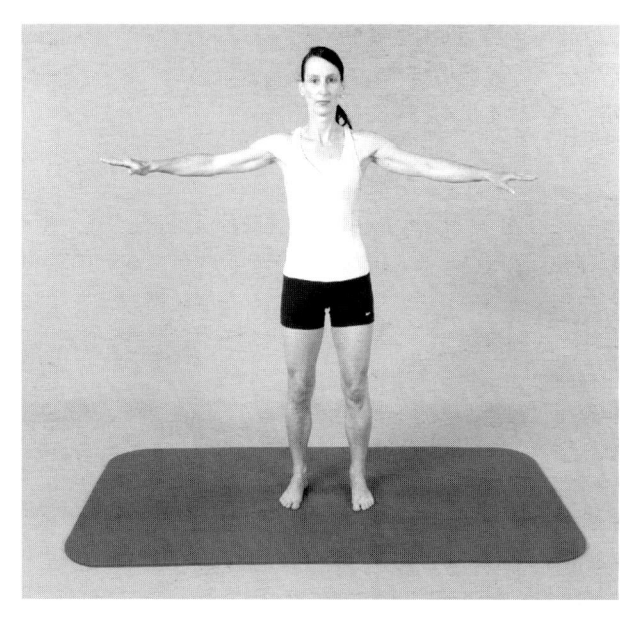

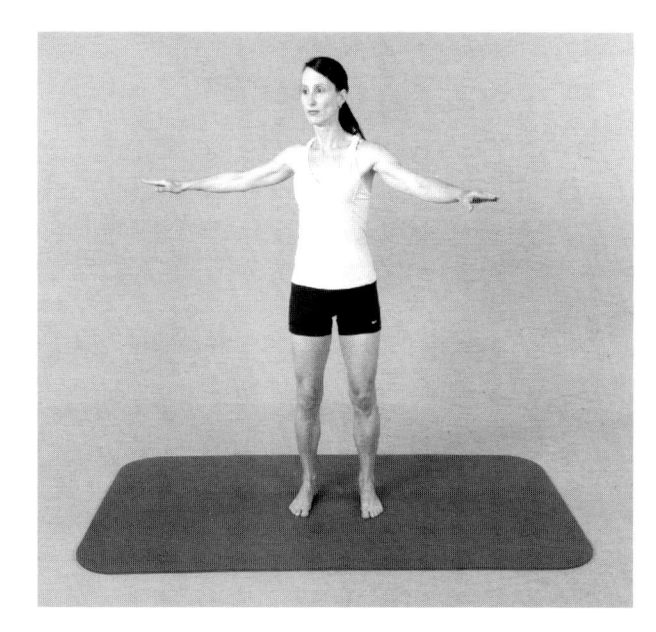

Start by standing with neutral pelvis, spine, and neck, the shoulders aligned over the pelvis and abducted to 90 degrees, with the elbows slightly bent.

Inhale to reconnect with the abdominals. Exhale and rotate to the right once. Inhale and return to the center. Exhale and rotate to the left.

Variation: Stand on one leg with the other leg in tabletop and rotate to the opposite side. Repeat the exercise with three pulses to the right and left as noted above.

Movement Pattern 4: Standing in Lunge Position with Arms Extended

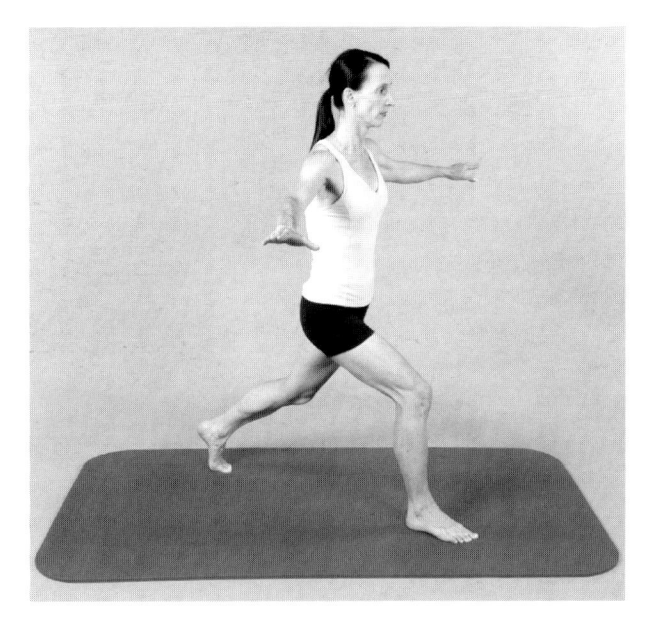

Start standing in a static lunge position with neutral pelvis, spine, and neck, the shoulders aligned over the pelvis and abducted to 90 degrees, with the elbows slightly bent.

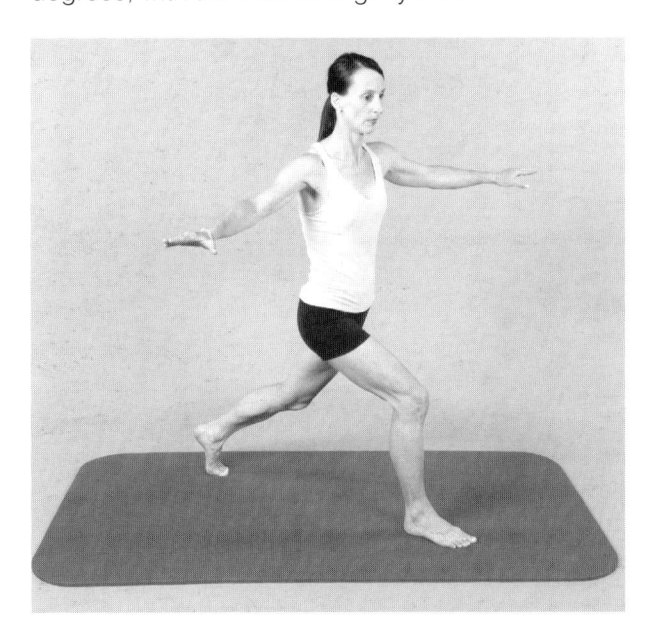

Inhale to reconnect with the abdominals. Exhale and rotate to the right once. Inhale and return to the center. Exhale and rotate to the left. Repeat the exercise with three pulses to the right and left as noted above.

Variation: Arms crossed at the chest.

Purpose:

- Beginner to intermediate Pilates exercises to introduce spinal rotation and progress the challenge by changing stability points
- To stabilize the shoulders and pelvis with spinal rotation
- To fire the internal obliques ipsilaterally and the external obliques and multifidus (thoracic) contralaterally
- Pelvic stabilization through the TrA and the pelvic floor

Clinical Application:

- Provides the opportunity to observe/challenge spinal rotation and pelvic stabilization capabilities in the sitting, standing, or lunging positions
- Strengthening of the obliques and other spinal rotators through concentric/eccentric contractions
- Isometric strengthening of the scapular stabilizers and shoulders abductors
- Suggested patient populations: Use this exercise as an adjunct to muscle energy techniques, joint mobilization of hypomobile thoracic segments, and/or to restore a normal oblique muscle recruitment pattern
- This exercise is beneficial for the athlete with shoulder dysfunction, such as bursitis/rotator cuff, tendonitis in golfers, and sport-specific movement patterns. You can also use the exercise for neuromuscular reeducation of the torso rotators for athletes such as ice skaters, runners, and cross-country skiers.
- Contraindicated for patients with osteoporosis

Practitioner's tips:

1. *Scapular stability is lost when the elbows are hyperextended with the shoulders held in an abducted position. Cue your patient to reach the shoulders away from the body toward the opposite walls versus the fingertips to decrease the potential for hyperextended elbows.*

2. *To decrease compensatory trunk side bend, cue your patient to imagine that the body is rotating around a rotisserie while keeping the spine elongated.*

113

3. Tactile cueing may help patients find the oblique muscles and feel them "fire" with movement.

Repetitions: 5, depending on patient goals. Start with one rotation and increase rotations to three on each side.

For more challenge in all positions, try holding a ball or exercise band with slight resistance in the hands.

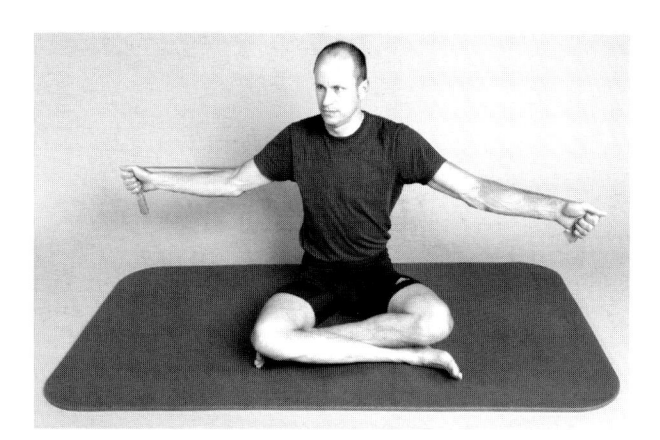

Faulty Movement Patterns: In sitting, pelvic rotation; functional leg length discrepancy with the legs extended/hips adducted; spinal rotation occurring at the upper thoracic spine as opposed to the mid- to lower thoracic spine; posterior or anterior pelvic tilt; rib cage popping; leading with the head and/or shoulders; hyperextended elbows; upper body tension; hyperextended knees in standing; hip or pelvic rotation in the lunge position; the knee coming anterior of the ankle on the forward leg in the lunge position; pelvic rotation secondary to tight hip flexors on the back leg in the lunge position

Reverse Curl with Rotation

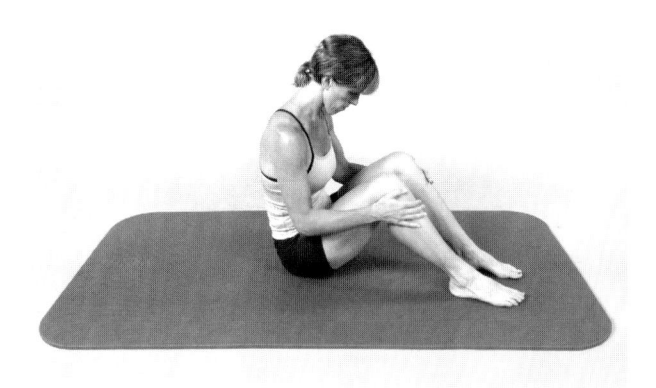

Start by sitting with the hips flexed, knees bent, and legs hip-width apart with the spine flexed over the lower extremities. The pelvis is in an imprinted position. The arms are flexed to rest naturally on the legs.

Movement Pattern 1: Arms Relaxed

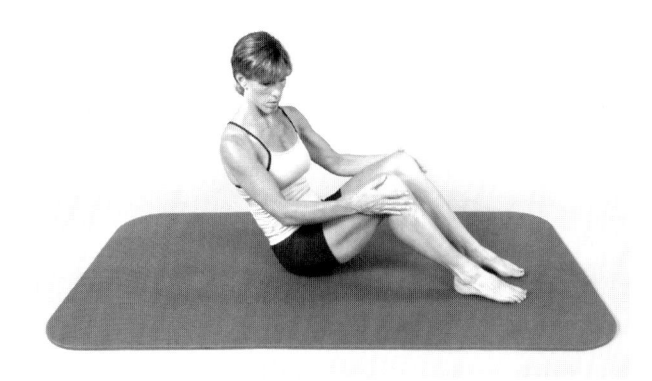

Exhale and sequentially articulate the pelvis/spine to roll the pelvis away from the femurs to extend the hips. Roll to the low thoracic spine, keeping the feet on the floor. Inhale to return to the initial position, reversing the sequence.

Movement Pattern 2: Long Lever Arm with Rotation

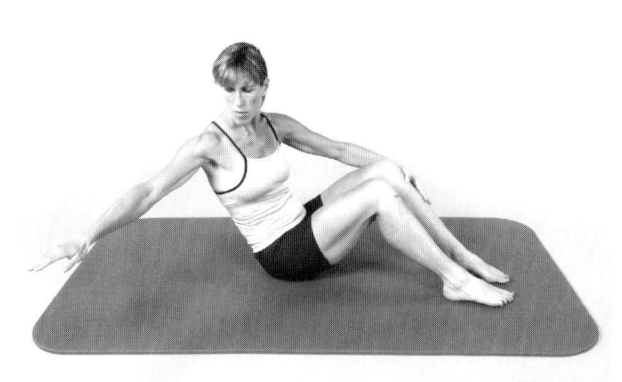

Exhale and sequentially articulate the pelvis/spine (imprint) to roll the pelvis away from the femurs as above. Simultaneously rotate the torso to the right while extending at the shoulder, palm down. Roll about halfway back, keeping the pelvis stable and the feet on the floor. Inhale to return to the initial position via hip flexion. Repeat on the other side.

Helpful tips:

1. *To maintain cervical stabilization throughout the exercise, cue the patient to follow the third finger with the eyes on rotation.*

2. *To guide arm movement, use imagery to cue the patient to imagine they are drawing a "smiley" face with the hand.*

Purpose:

- To strengthen the spinal flexors/extensors/rotators, shoulder and hip muscles
- To stabilize the shoulder girdle and the lower extremities in the sagittal plane of movement during spinal articulation, with or without rotation
- To fire the internal obliques ipsilaterally and the external obliques and multifidus contralaterally
- Lumbo-pelvic stabilization and spinal articulation

Clinical Application:

- Advanced torso stabilization exercises that challenge the spinal flexors/extensors with rotation, pelvic stabilization, and shoulder/hip strengthening
- Essential exercise for reteaching torso/lumbo-pelvic stabilization for activities such as mountain biking, gymnastics, and rowing
- Contraindicated for lumbar disc dysfunction, lumbar fusion, and osteoporosis
- Suggested exercise for shoulder/scapular dysfunction for the throwing athlete

Repetitions: 5-10, depending on patient goals

Variation: To add challenge, reverse the breathing pattern.

Faulty Movement Patterns: Pelvic rotation; hip rotation; spinal rotation occurring at the upper thoracic spine as opposed to the mid- to lower thoracic spine; anterior or lateral pelvic tilt; rib cage or abdominal popping; weight shifting to the unilateral sitz bone, which may result in trunk side bend or lateral pelvic tilt; leading with the head or shoulders; hyperextended elbows; Valsalva; inability to coordinate breath with movement

Trunk Side Bend

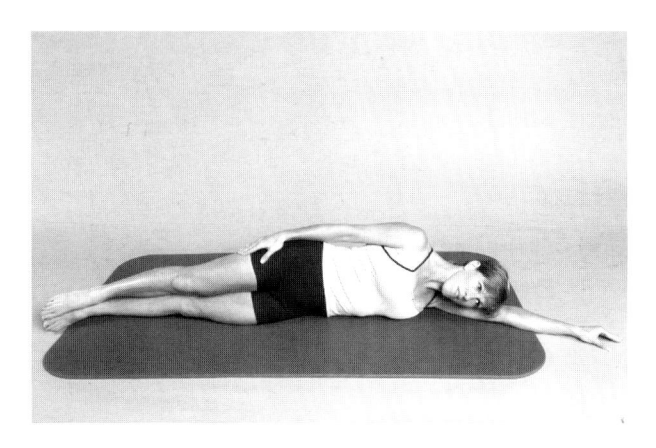

Start in sidelying with the pelvis and spine in neutral. The hips are adducted and in line with ankles and the shoulders and ASIS are aligned. The shoulder on the floor is flexed, providing support for the head; the arm on top is placed on top the thigh. The scalpulae are stabilized. Inhale to connect with the abdominals.

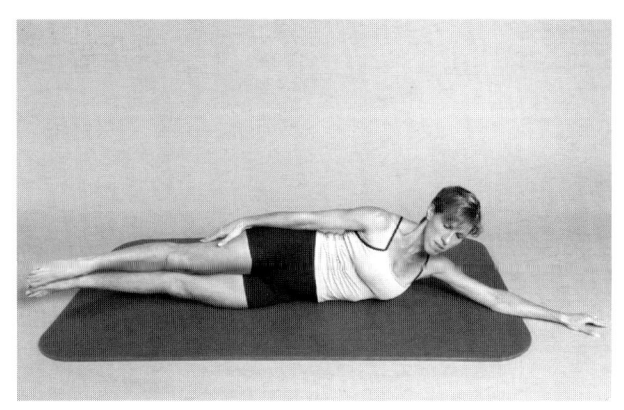

Exhale to lift the upper and lower extremities off the mat at the same time, moving sequentially from the top of the head to the toes. The arm reaches long down the thigh. The waistline will gently press into the mat. The head follows the line of the spine. Inhale to return to the starting position.

Purpose:

- Concentric/eccentric contraction of the hip adductors/abductors/lateral flexors
- Lateral spine flexion via ipsilateral contraction of the internal/external obliques, multifidus, and paraspinals
- Challenge pelvic/spinal stability in sagittal and transverse planes
- Hip mobility

Clinical Application:

- Lengthening and strengthening of the lateral spine flexors
- Strengthening of the hip abductors/adductors, lateral spinal flexors
- Scapular stabilization
- Balance and coordination
- Hip mobility
- A nice adjunct to conventional exercises for patients with scoliosis; sport-specific training for dancers and other sports that require lateral flexion, such as volleyball

Repetitions: 10, depending on patient goals

Variation: Follow the exercise description as above, this time holding the trunk in side flexion and adding two breaths; inhale while bringing the arm overhead and exhale while returning the arm to the hip.

Note: Also see Hip Abduction/Adduction Progressions.

Mermaid: Lateral Flexion in Sitting

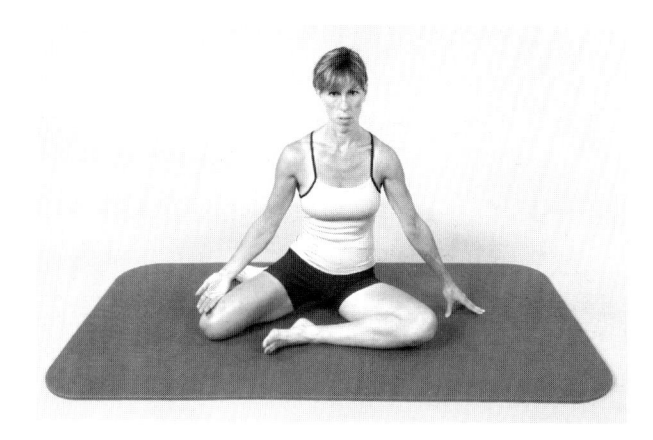

Sit on the floor with the right hip internally rotated and the left hip externally rotated with the foot in proximity to the right thigh, the right hand resting on the lower leg, and the left fingertips on the floor aligned with the shoulders.

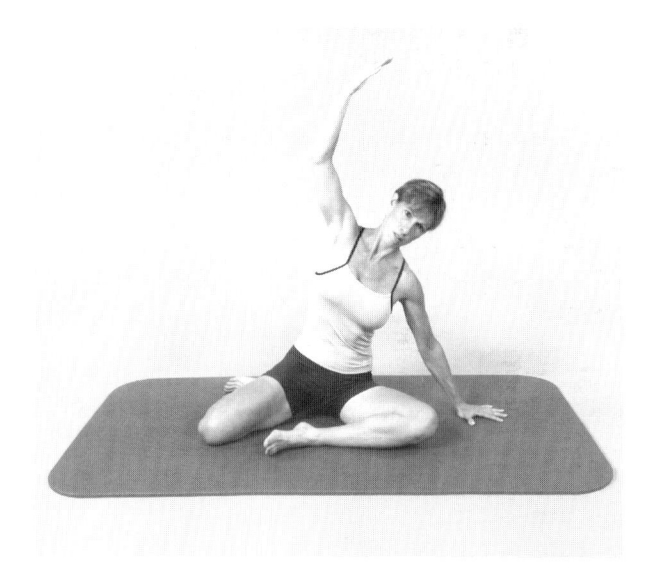

Inhale and abduct the right shoulder to 180 degrees. Exhale and perform a left trunk side bend while maintaining neutral pelvis. Inhale and breathe into the back and sides of the ribs. Exhale and return to neutral spine and then lower the shoulder to the initial position. Repeat on the opposite side.

Helpful tips:

1. Cue patients to elongate the spine as they perform a trunk side bend versus just side bending to enhance lengthening and strengthening of the lateral flexors.

2. Cue patients to reach the ischial tuberosity toward the floor with the trunk side bend to maintain neutral pelvic alignment.

Purpose:

- To mobilize the spine and lengthen/strengthen the lateral torso flexors and paraspinals in the frontal plane with neutral pelvis

Clinical Application:

- Lengthening and strengthening of the lateral torso flexors
- Concentric/eccentric contraction of the ipsilateral trunk side benders, including the quadratus lumborum, internal/external obliques, and paraspinals
- A nice adjunct to conventional exercises for individuals with scoliosis and myofascial release of the diaphragm

- Suggested patient populations: Use this exercise for neuromuscular reeducation of the breathing pattern with emphasis on ipsilateral breathing in the trunk side bend position. The exercise is also used in sport-specific training for dancers and others whose sports require lateral flexion (volleyball, etc.).

Repetitions: 5, depending on patient goals

Variations: Follow the exercise description above for the trunk side bend. Extend the hips, lifting the upper thighs off the floor; add a two-breath pattern; add torso rotation.

Faulty Movement Patterns: Inability to stabilize the pelvis, resulting in anterior, posterior, lateral pelvic tilting or rotation; rib cage or abdominal popping; scapular elevation/protraction; hyperextended elbows; inability to articulate through the spine; weight shifting

Hips: Joint Mobilization and Muscle Strengthening

This section is one of our favorites, focusing on the muscles around the hip, particularly the gluteus medius and maximus. These muscles must be strong for many reasons: hip stability, gait, balance, fall prevention, and sports performance.

Here you will find variations on many exercises already used in the clinical setting and some new exercises you have probably never seen before. Most are progressions of the fundamentals but increase challenge via ankle dorsi- and plantar flexion and less stable positioning, such as sidelying.

Use your creativity and skill to add equipment or modify these exercises as appropriate for your patient.

Practitioner's tip: As always, pelvic stability is key. Begin your focus at the pelvis and move to the extremities once your patient masters this fundamental.

One-Leg Circle

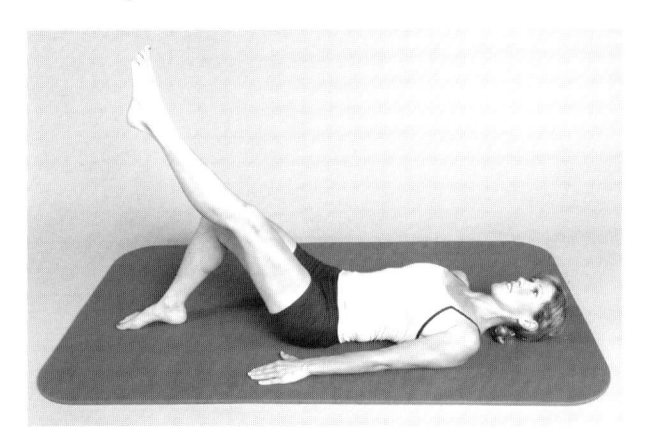

Start supine with neutral pelvis, one leg extended in the air with the hip flexed to 90 degrees, the other leg extended at the knee and hip, the arms alongside the body, the scapulae stabilized, the elbows slightly bent, palms down on the mat, and the ankles plantar flexed.

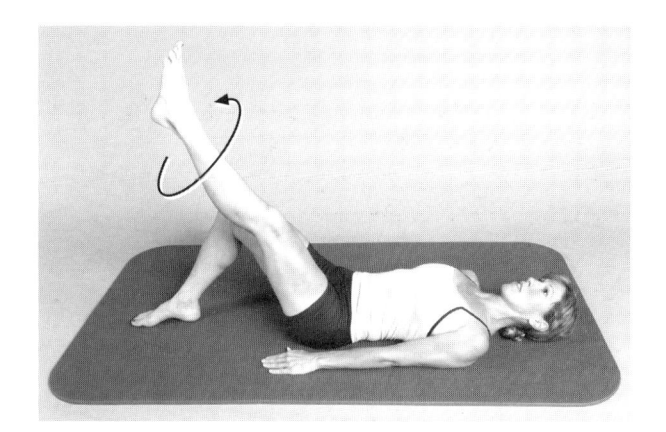

Inhale, maintain neutral pelvis, and make a half circle toward the midline by adducting the hip across the midline and then extending. Exhale to complete the circle, abducting the hip away from the midline and flexing it to the starting position. Pause slightly at the top of the circle. Reverse directions.

Purpose:

- To isolate hip movement independent of the pelvis and spine in the sagittal and frontal planes

Clinical Application:

- Use this movement pattern when dissociation of the hip from the pelvis and spine is not occurring
- Suggested patient pulations: Patients with hip osteoarthritis, hip adductor strain, hip flexor tendonitis, patellofemoral syndrome, and to enhance approximation for an unstable hip via approximation with specific cueing (see Single-Leg Knee Stirs in Chapter 6); sport-specific training for soccer players, dancers, and skiers

Teaching tips:

1. Ask your patient to initially draw a large circle to feel the available range of hip motion and how the pelvis and lumbar spine follow the movement. To progress, ask your patient to palpate the ASIS bilaterally while performing the exercise. Next, introduce the concept of core stabilization and ask the patient to draw the circle while maintaining pelvic stabilization. If the patient is stabilizing the core adequately, the ASIS will not move.

2. Cue your patient to move through the hip versus the foot to assist with feeling the hip muscles and to keep the knee from hyperextending.

Repetitions: 5 times in each direction

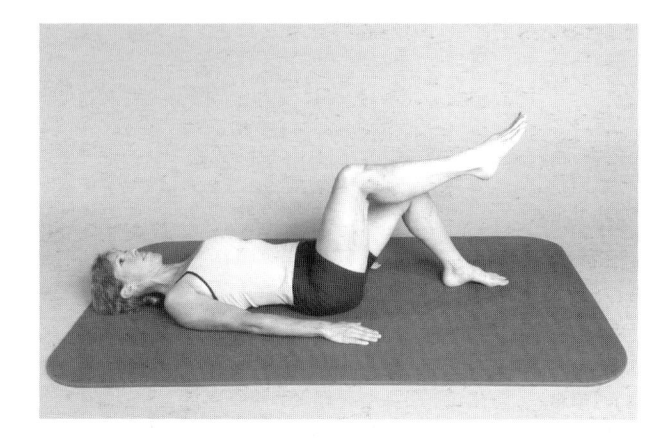

Variations: Leg in the air, knee bent (shown); leg on the floor long, leg in the air long.

Faulty Movement Patterns: Not maintaining neutral pelvis secondary to tight hip flexors or weak abdominals; inability to stabilize the pelvis, resulting in weight shifting from side to side or pelvic rotation; inability to isolate the hip from the pelvis; hyperextended knee(s); hip rotation of the leg on the mat; pressing the hands into the mat; upper body tension; Valsalva; inability to coordinate breath with movement

Shoulder Bridge Variations

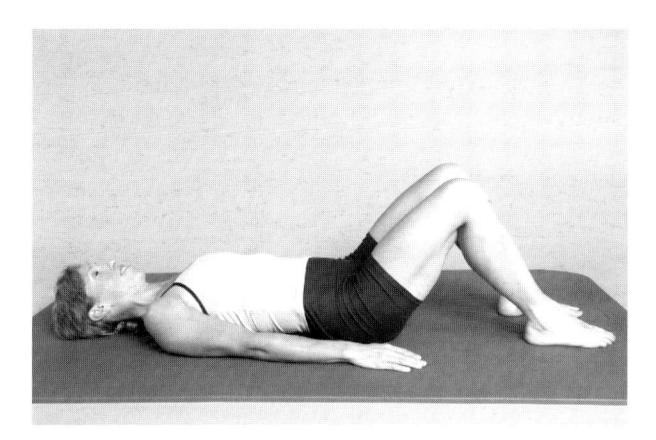

Start in hooklying with neutral pelvis, head, and neck alignment, the knees bent, hips distance apart, the arms alongside the body, elbows slightly bent, with the palms down.

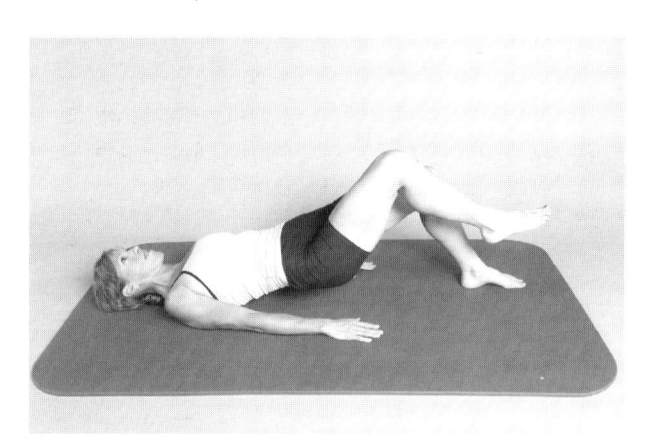

Inhale to stay; refocus breathing. Exhale and lift the torso off the floor while keeping the pelvis and spine in neutral, extending the hips to create a bridge position from the scapulae to the knees. Gently push the feet into the floor to increase hip extensor involvement. Inhale, keeping the hips square to the ceiling.

Flex the hip and knee to lift the leg off the floor. Exhale to return the leg to the floor. Repeat with the other leg.

Practitioner's tips:

1. To progress patients to the original Shoulder Bridge, perform the above exercise three times on each leg. For further challenge, extend the knee of the lifted leg and perform as above.

2. Avoid using a pillow beneath the head as it will increase pressure on the cervical spine.

Purpose:

- Maintain neutral spine and pelvis with rhythm of the leg
- Mobilize the hip joint through flexion and extension
- Coordination of the primary and secondary stabilizers (TrA, obliques, multifidus, hip adductors/abductors/hip extensors)

Clinical Application:

- Performed correctly, this exercise teaches individuals to stabilize the torso with asymmetrical lower extremity movement.
- Useful in teaching patients to isolate hip movement from the pelvis.
- Excellent advanced lumbar stabilization exercise to strengthen the hip extensors and hip abductors/adductors on the weight-bearing leg, the abdominals and lumbar stabilizers, and lengthen the one-joint hip flexors via concentric/eccentric contractions with open kinetic chain movement.
- Suggested patient populations: Advanced functional training for hamstring strain, patellofemoral syndrome, hip adductor strain, SI joint/anterior innominate dysfunction, and sport-specific training for runners, cross-country skiers, etc.

Repetitions: 5-10, depending on patient goals

Variation:

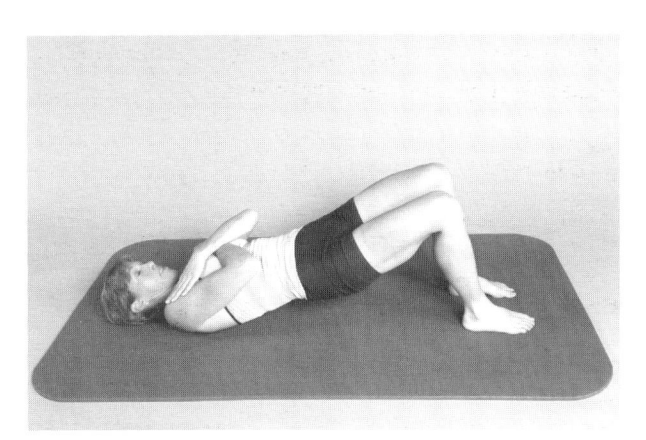

Hands crossed on the chest or placed at the ASIS and ribs for tactile feedback; opposite arm and leg lift.

Faulty Movement Patterns: Inability to stabilize the pelvis, resulting in anterior or posterior tilting; unilateral pelvic rotation; pelvis rising and lowering with the rhythm of the hip; femoral rotation; pressure on the cervical spine; abdominal popping; Valsalva; inability to coordinate breath with movement

Prone Hip Extension

Practitioner's tips:

1. Before concluding that this is an appropriate exercise for your patient, first assess the muscle recruitment pattern. Janda identified the normal firing pattern as follows: The gluteus maximus and hamstring muscles are recruited first, followed by the contralateral erector spinae and ipsilateral erector spinae muscles, followed by the contralateral and ipsilateral thoraco-lumbar erector spinae (1,2,3). If a faulty recruitment pattern is present, see Movement Patterns 1 and 2 in Chapter 6 to reeducate a normal firing sequence.

2. Use a pad beneath the ASIS to support neutral pelvis with patients who demonstrate excessive lumbar lordosis and cannot maintain neutral. Progress to no pad.

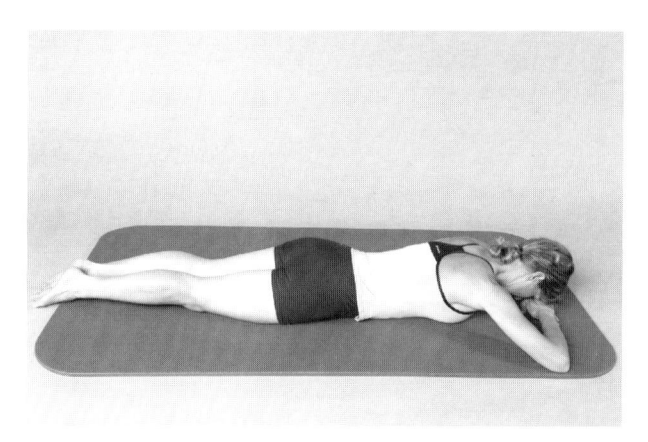

Start prone on the mat, hands beneath the forehead, the head, spine, and pelvis in neutral. The legs are extended long, hip-distance apart. The ankles are plantar flexeds.

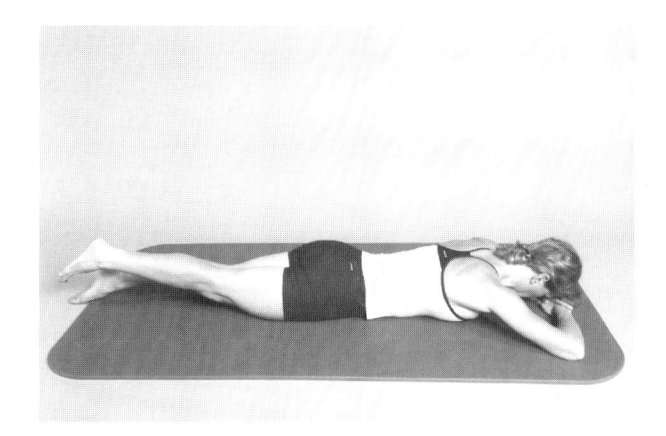

Inhale to stabilize the spine and pelvis. Exhale and extend the hip, lifting one leg off the floor. Inhale to flex the hip, returning to the floor. Exhale and repeat on the opposite side.

Variation: Hips exterally rotated; standing. Once mastered on the floor, challenge your patient by performing this exercise prone on a stability ball or in standing with the hips neutral.

Purpose:

- To challenge pelvic and spinal stability with unilateral movement
- Mobilizing the hip joint into extension
- Normalizing the hip extensor firing pattern
- Hip extensor strengthening

Clinical Application:

- Coordinates lumbo-pelvic stability with hip mobility
- Essential lumbar stabilization exercise
- Hip extensor strengthening
- Challenging unilateral movement
- Suggested patient populations: Use with rehabilitation of post-hamstring strains; hip osteoarthritis; SI joint/anterior innominate dysfunction; ACL reconstruction; gait training, retraining running mechanics, or as an adjunct to mobilization of the anterior hip capsule and/or manual techniques for tight hip flexors.

Repetitions: 5-10, depending on patient goals

Faulty Movement Patterns: Anterior tilting of the pelvis as a result of decreased hip extension secondary to one-joint hip flexor tightness/anterior hip capsule tightness, or not stabilizing the spine/pelvis with the abdominals; segmental hinging at the lumbar spine (thoraco-lumbar junction); pelvic rotation as a result of not stabilizing with the TrA and/or multifidus/obliques, resulting in body weight shifting unilaterally; faulty hip extensor muscle recruitment pattern; Valsalva; inability to coordinate breath with movement; upper body tension

"Frog"

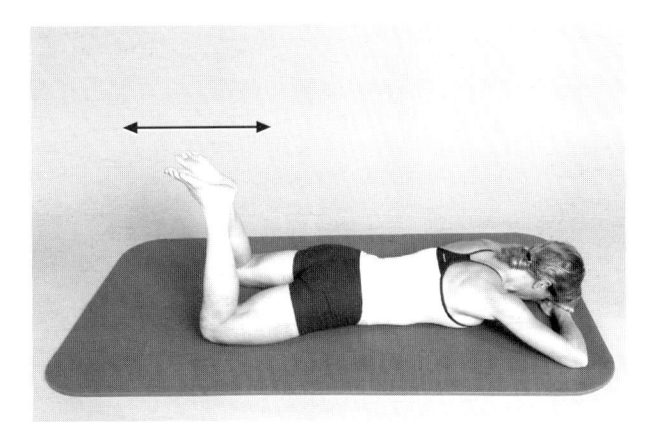

Start prone with the head lying on the hands, palms down. The pelvis and spine are in neutral. The hips are externally rotated to create a V-shape, the knees are flexed to 90 degrees, and the ankles are dorsiflexed, with heels together, toes apart.

Inhale and stabilize the pelvis, spine, and scapulae. Exhale, squeeze the heels together, and extend the knees bilaterally from 90 to about 40 degrees, keeping even pressure on the heels. Inhale to return to the starting position.

Practitioner's tip: Use a pad beneath the ASIS to support neutral pelvis with excessive lumbar lordosis when the patient is unable to maintain neutral with use of the abdominals. Progress to no pad.

Variation: Isometric contraction (4,5)

Purpose:

- Lumbo-pelvic stability with knee flexion and hip external rotation
- Concentric/eccentric strengthening of the hip external rotators and knee flexors and isometric strengthening of the abdominals

Clinical Application:

- Hamstring strengthening via concentric/eccentric contraction with emphasis on the biceps femoris
- Use as an adjunct to manual therapy for a tight anterior hip capsule
- Suggested patient populations include hamstring/adductor/quadriceps muscle strains

Repetitions: 5-10, depending on patient goals

Faulty Movement Patterns: Overflexing at the knee; anterior tilt or hips lifting; abdominal popping; weight shifting from side to side; Valsalva; inability to coordinate breath with movement; upper body tension

Hip Abduction/Adduction Progressions in Sidelying and Standing

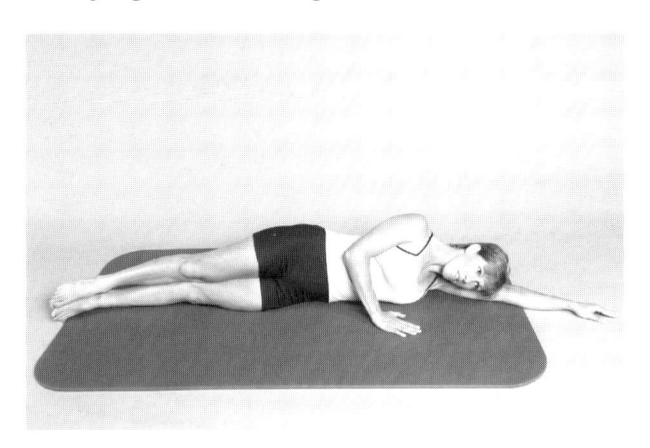

Starting Position for All Exercises: Sidelying with the pelvis and spine in neutral. The hips are adducted and in line with the ankles and shoulders, and the ASIS are aligned. The shoulder on the floor is flexed, providing support for the head; the arm on top is positioned in front of the sternum. The scapulae are stabilized.

Faulty Movement Patterns: Inability to maintain pelvic/spinal stability; hip flexion; inability to fire the hip abductors/adductors; weight shifting forward or back; femoral rotation; hip hiking; upper extremity tension; faulty muscle recruitment pattern

Repetitions for all exercises: 10 on each side, depending on patient goals. Layer exercises of choice one after another. Repeat on the other side.

Practitioner's tips:

1. To enhance stability in Movement Patterns 1 to 3, flex the bottom knee and hip. Progress to hip neutral and extended knee.

2. Cue the patient to lift from the hip versus the foot to enhance muscle activation at the hip and decrease compensatory strategies through the foot.

Movement Pattern 1: Hip Abduction

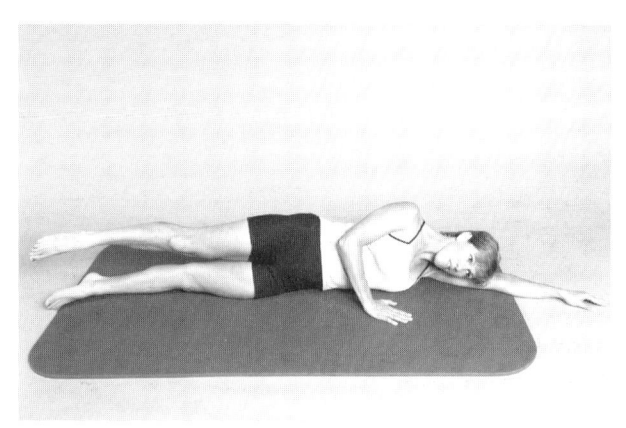

Inhale, maintain neutral pelvis, and abduct the hip on top to hip height. The ankle simultaneously plantar flexes. Exhale and adduct the hip on top to meet the leg on the bottom, dorsiflexing the ankle.

Variation: Extend and externally rotate the hip slightly. Research suggests that runners with IT bend syndrome had a significant decrease in symptoms with use of this exercise to strengthen weak hip abductors (6).

Hip Abduction in Standing

Follow the pattern above in standing position with emphasis on pelvic and hip stability. Be sure to cue your patient to keep the knee on the weight-bearing leg "soft." To enhance stability through the foot, press evenly onto the weight-bearing foot without flexing the toes. Avoid a lateral sway.

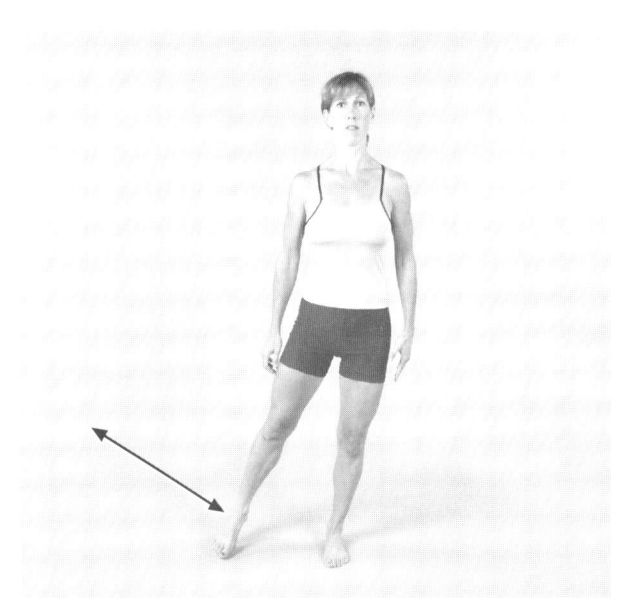

125

Purpose:

- Concentric/eccentric contraction of the hip abductors
- Hip mobility in the frontal plane
- Lumbo-pelvic stabilization
- Coordination

Clinical Application:

- Hip strengthening
- Neuromuscular reeducation of a normal firing pattern of the hip abductors. Janda identified the normal firing patterns as follows: gluteus medius/minimus and tensor fascia latae followed by the ipsilateral quadratus lumborum (2,3).
- Abdominal and multifidus strengthening through stabilization
- Mobility of the hip and ankle joints
- Suggested patient populations: ACL reconstruction; patellofemoral syndrome; total hip replacement; gluteus medius tendonitis; IT band syndrome; hip adductor strains; symphysis pubis dysfunction. This is an excellent exercise to enhance pelvic stabilization with gait, running, and athletic activities such as kickboxing, gymnastics, dance, cross-country skiing, etc.

Movement Pattern 2: Hot Potato

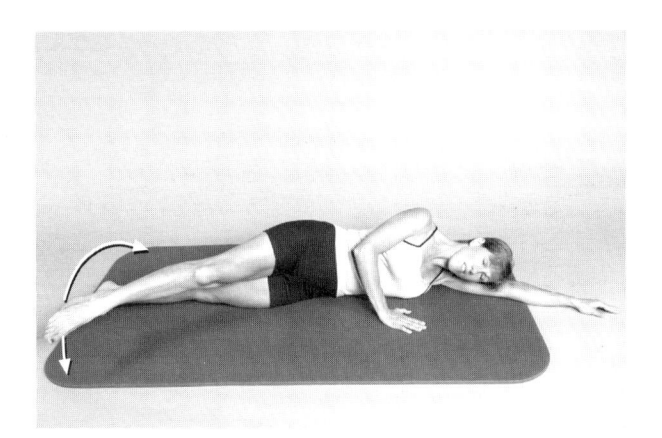

Inhale, maintain neutral pelvis, and abduct the hip on top to hip height. The ankle simultaneously plantar flexes. Exhale to flex the hip 30 to 45 degrees and "tap" the foot in front of the torso three times (may or may not touch floor/mat, depending on tightness). Inhale and extend the hip 20 degrees. Exhale and tap the foot behind the torso three times.

Purpose:

- Concentric/eccentric contraction of the hip abductors/adductors
- Hip mobility in the frontal plane
- Lumbo-pelvic stabilization
- Coordination

Clinical Application:

- Hip strengthening
- Abdominal and multifidus strengthening through stabilization
- Mobility of the hip and ankle joints
- Suggested patient populations: Hip adductor strains; symphysis pubis dysfunction; gluteus medius tendonitis. This is an excellent exercise to enhance pelvic stabilization in sport-specific training for soccer and dance.

Once your patient has mastered Hot Potato in sidelying, consider challenging him/her in standing. All principles and faulty movement patterns remain the same.

Teaching tip: When a patient lies on his/her side, the waist naturally relaxes to the mat, putting the trunk into a side bend position. To support the pelvis in neutral in the frontal plane, cue the patient to reach the top leg about one-quarter inch longer and then the bottom leg the same amount. Ask the patient to feel a small space under the waist and provide a visual cue, such as to think of the waist as a stone arch or cave, to maintain pelvic alignment in neutral.

Movement Pattern 3: Small and Giant Leg Circles

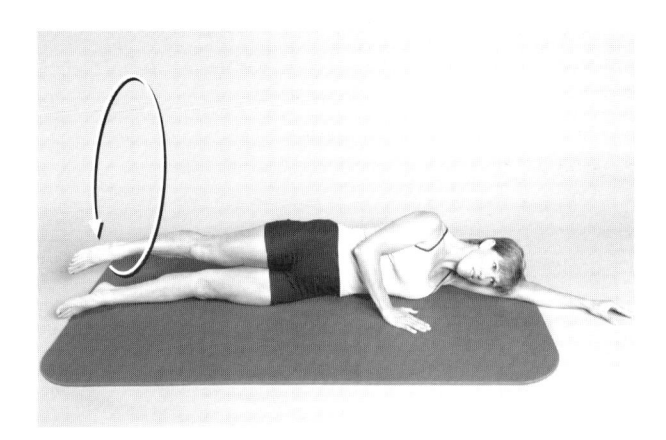

Inhale, maintain neutral pelvis, and abduct the hip on top to hip height. The ankle simultaneously plantar flexes. Exhale to begin a pattern of circling the top leg forward to create a half circle. Inhale halfway through the circle pattern, with the hip extending back to complete the circle. Reverse direction and dorsiflex the ankle.

Purpose:

- Concentric/eccentric contraction of the hip abductors/adductors and hip flexors/extensors with circumduction
- Use this exercise as a progression of the One-Leg Circle
- Hip mobility
- Pelvic/spinal stabilization
- Coordination

Clinical Application:

- See the One-Leg Circle
- Hip abductor/flexor/extensor strengthening
- Hip mobility
- Abdominal and multifidus strengthening through stabilization
- Pelvic and spinal stability

Practitioner's tip: If your patient can demonstrate control with a small circle, gradually increase the size of the circle until the patient no longer demonstrates control.

Movement Pattern 4: Split Leg Lifts

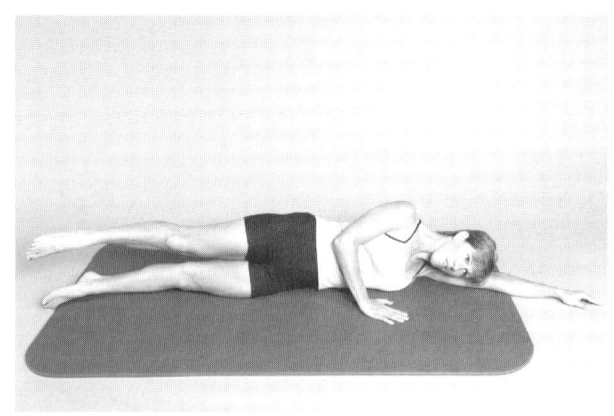

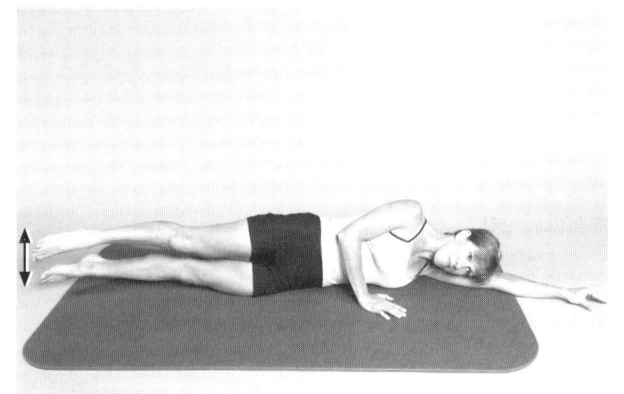

Inhale and abduct the leg on top to hip height, keeping the legs parallel. Exhale and adduct the bottom hip to meet the leg on top. Inhale, lowering the bottom leg to the floor.

Purpose:

- Isometric hip abduction and concentric/eccentric contraction of the adductors
- Hip mobility
- Lumbo-pelvic stabilization

Clinical Application:

- Suggested patient populations: Hip adductor strain; ACL rehabilitation; symphysis pubis dysfunction; hip flexor tendonitis; sport-specific training for dancing, soccer

Movement Pattern 5: Split Leg Lift and Lower

Inhale and abduct the hip on top to hip height, keeping the legs parallel. Exhale and adduct the bottom hip to meet the leg on top, lowering the legs together to the mat.

Purpose:

- Isometric hip abduction and concentric/eccentric contraction of the adductors
- Hip mobility
- Lumbo-pelvic stabilization

Clinical Application:

- Suggested patient populations: Use this exercise with patients who have a hip adductor strain, gluteus medius tendonitis, hip bursitis, symphysis pubis dysfunction, hip flexor tendonitis, and for sport-specific training for dancing, soccer, and basketball.

Movement Pattern 6: Double Leg Lift

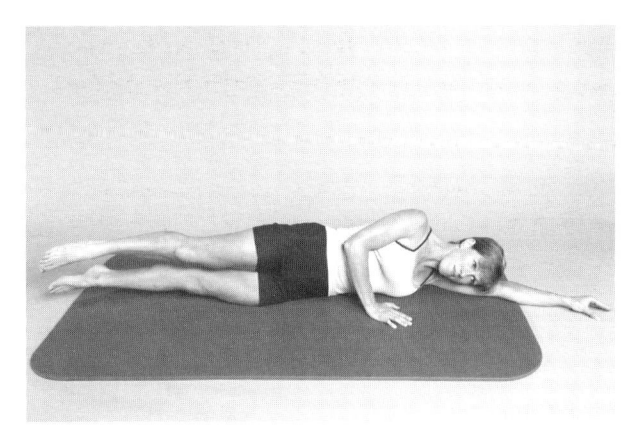

Inhale to lift both legs off the mat while maintaining neutral pelvis. Lift only as high as neutral pelvis can be maintained. Exhale to return the legs to the mat.

Purpose:

- Concentric/eccentric contraction of the hip adductors/abductors
- Hip mobility
- Lumbo-pelvic stabilization

Clinical Application:

- Advanced strengthening of the hip abductors/adductors
- Coordination
- Abdominal/multifidus strengthening through stabilization
- Hip mobility
- Suggested patient populations: hip adductor strain; symphysis pubis dysfunction; hip flexor tendonitis; gluteus medius tendonitis; hip bursitis; IT band syndrome; sport-specific training for dancing, soccer, and basketball.

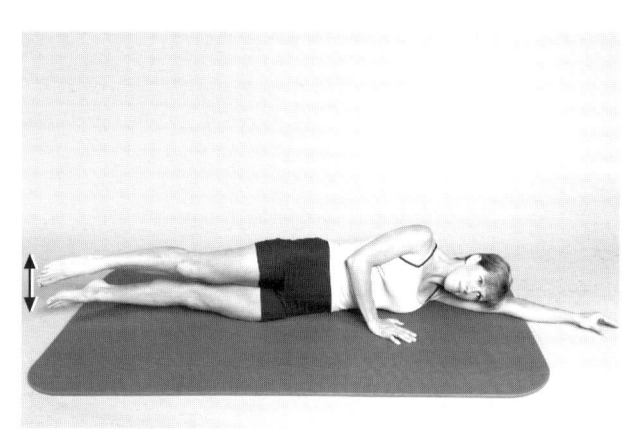

Variation: For further challenge, lift the legs together and follow with three quick "beats" in rapid succession, with emphasis on control.

Movement Pattern 7: Trunk Side Bend (also see Section 6)

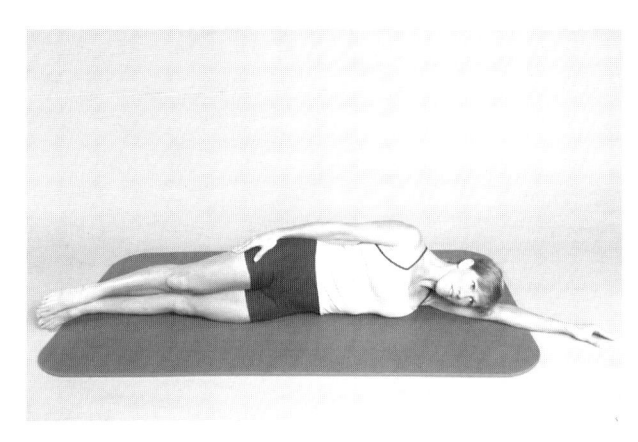

The starting position is the same as for the other movement patterns, but the hand in front is placed on top of the thigh. Inhale to connect with the abdominals.

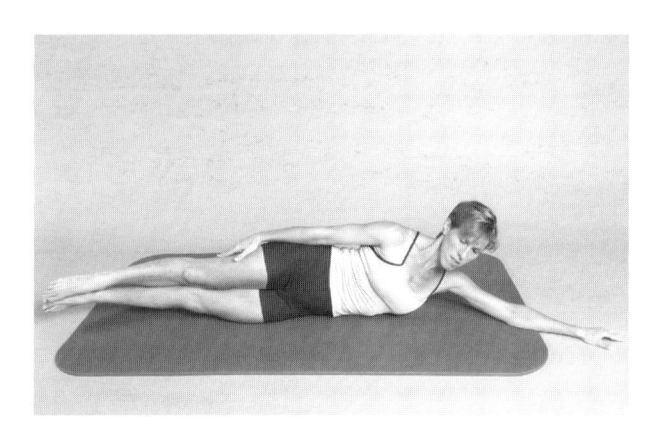

Exhale to lift the upper and lower extremities off the mat at the same time, moving sequentially from the top of the head to the toes. The arm reaches long down the thigh. The waistline will gently press into the mat. The head follows the line of the spine. Inhale to return to the starting position.

Purpose:

- Concentric/eccentric contraction of the hip adductors/abductors/lateral spine flexors
- Trunk side bend via ipsilateral contraction of the internal/external obliques, multifidus, paraspinals
- Challenge pelvic/spinal stability in the sagittal and transverse planes
- Hip mobility

Clinical Application:

- Lengthening and strengthening of the lateral spine flexors
- Strengthening of the hip abductors/adductors, lateral spinal flexors
- Scapular stabilization
- Balance and coordination
- Hip mobility
- A nice adjunct to conventional exercises for patients with scoliosis, sport-specific training for dancers and other sports that require lateral flexion, such as volleyball

Variation: Follow the exercise as above, holding the trunk in side flexion and adding two breaths. Inhale as the arm is raised overhead; exhale to return to the hip.

Helpful hint: As with the other exercises in this section, the starting position for the Trunk Side Bend is the same but the trunk will go into lateral flexion and the natural waistline will lower to the floor in the movement pattern.

Clam in Sidelying (4,7)

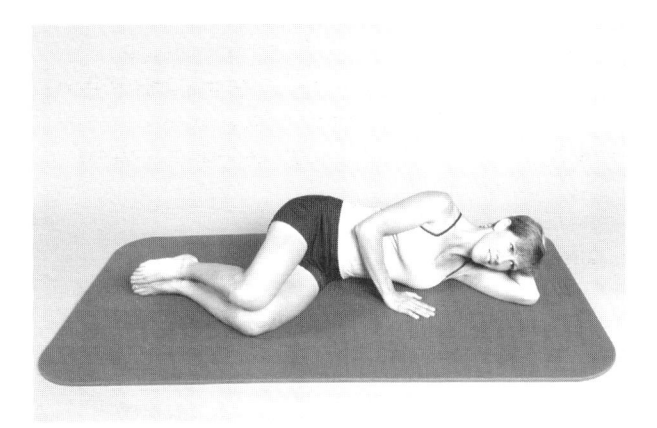

Start in sidelying with the pelvis and spine in neutral. The hips are adducted, and the hips and knees are flexed to 45-60 degrees. The shoulder on the mat is flexed, providing support for the head. The arm on top is positioned in front of the sternum. The scapulae are stabilized.

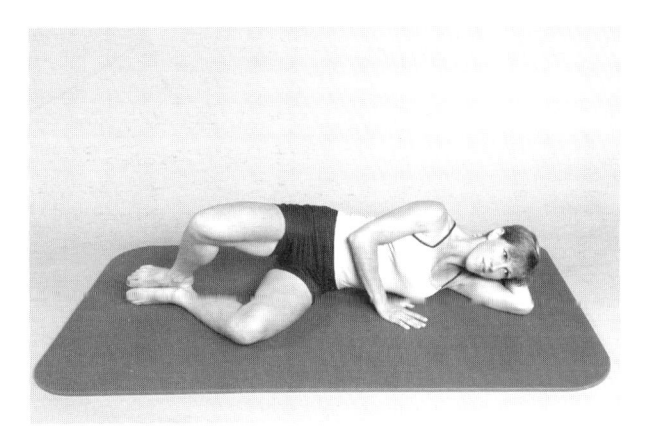

Inhale to maintain neutral and refocus breathing. Exhale and externally rotate at the hip just to the point where neutral pelvis/spine and weight distribution cannot be maintained. The opposite leg supports movement through stabilization. Inhale to return to the initial position.

Practitioner's tip: When patients lie on their side, their waist naturally relaxes to the mat, putting the trunk into a side bend position. To achieve a neutral position, cue your patients using visual imagery to stack the ASIS like a bookcase or manually assist neutral through movement of the pelvis.

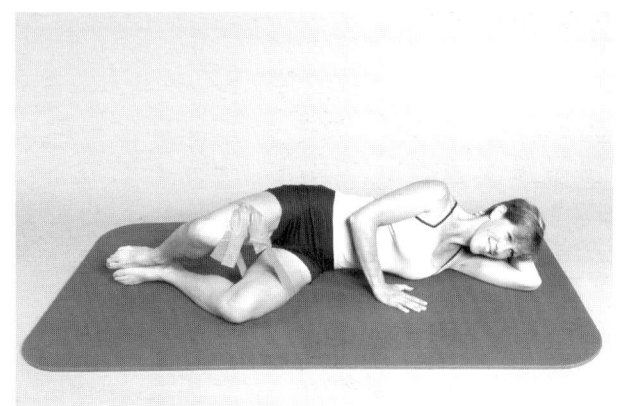

Variation: Tie an exercise band around the distal femurs to add resistance and challenge to this exercise.

Purpose:

- Challenging dissociation of the femur from the pelvis in the transverse plane
- Hip strengthening
- Hip mobility

Clinical Application:

- Challenges movement of the femur from the pelvis
- Lumbo-pelvic stabilization via IM contraction of the TrA, obliques, and multifidus
- Concentric/eccentric strengthening of the gluteus medius
- Suggested patient populations: Use this exercise for patients who have a total hip replacement, when appropriate, a tight anterior hip capsule, or tight adductor muscles; patellofemoral syndrome; IT band syndrome; gluteus medius tendonitis

Repetitions: 5-10 each side, depending on patient goals

Faulty Movement Patterns: Inability to maintain pelvic/spinal stability; increased lumbar lordosis when externally rotating at the hip; weight shifting back with external rotation, leading to a posterior pelvic tilt; not maintaining the natural curve of the waist (trunk side bend); hip hiking or flexing; upper extremity tension; abdominal popping; Valsalva; inability to coordinate breath with movement

Clam in Standing (7)

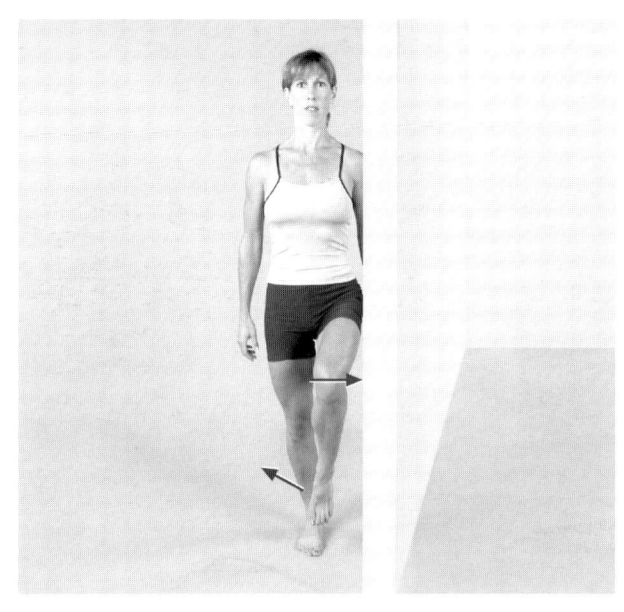

Stand next to a wall with neutral pelvis, the left hip and knee flexed to 90 degrees and the right knee slightly flexed. Inhale, maintaining lumbo-pelvic stabilization. Exhale to abduct and externally rotate the left hip into the wall. Inhale, maintaining lumbo-pelvic stabilization, and perform 5 to10 repetitions. Repeat on the other side.

Teaching tip: To enhance hip external rotator contraction, cue the patient to push the outside of the foot into the outer border of the shoe without flexing the toes.

Purpose:

- Lumbo-pelvic stabilization in standing in multiple planes
- Isometric gluteal medius strengthening in weight bearing

Clinical Application:

- Use this exercise to challenge lumbo-pelvic stabilization via IM contraction of the TrA, obliques, and multifidus while strengthening the gluteus medius in standing
- Suggested patient populations: Use for patients who experience IT band syndrome, patellofemoral syndrome, or a tight anterior hip capsule. Use as advanced neuromuscular training for pelvic instability noted with Trendelenburg gait/running mechanics.

Repetitions: 5-10, depending on patient goals

Faulty Movement Patterns: Inability to maintain pelvic/spinal stability; femoral rotation; hip flexion or lateral pelvic tilt; upper extremity tension; Valsalva; abdominal popping; hyperextend knee on weight-bearing leg

Section References

1. Janda, V. Rational Therapeutic Approach of Chronic Back Pain Syndromes. *Janda Compendium*, Volume I. Minneapolis, MN: OPTP. 1998.

2. Janda, V. *Janda Compendium*, Volume II. Minneapolis, MN: OPTP. 1998.

3. Page, P. 2003. In: Lardner, R., *The Janda Approach to Musculoskeletal Pain Syndromes*. Thera-Band Academy.com. Course Manual, Bloomington, MN, June 14-15.

4. Sahrmann, S.A. 1992. In: McDonnell, K., *Diagnosis and Treatment of Muscle Imbalances and Associated Regional Pain Syndromes*. Course Manual, Minneapolis, MN, February 28, 29, and March 1.

5. *STOTT Pilates Comprehensive Matwork Manual.* 2001. Toronto, Canada: Merrithew Corporation.

6. Fredericson, F., Cookingham, C.L., Chaudhari, A.M., Dowdell, B.C., Oestreicher, N., Sahrmann, S.A. 2000. Hip abductor weakness in distance runners with iliotibial band syndrome. *Clinical Journal of Sports Medicine* 10(3): 169-175.

7. Bookhout, M.R. 2002. *Exercise as an Adjunct to Manual Medicine*. Course notes, Minnesota APTA Spring Conference, Brooklyn Park, MN, April.

Upper Body Strengthening and Stabilization

The entire body must work together for quality movement: the upper and lower body—torso and extremities—support each other's work in both an integrated and isolative manner. Case in point: Perform a standing biceps curl with no attempt to stabilize the shoulder girdle, torso, or legs. Repeat the effort applying the Pilates principles. Can you tell the difference?

Unfortunately, unless your patient is in a weight training program or in a physically active occupation, the upper body is often neglected. This neglect can lead to a weak shoulder girdle, or secondary stabilization system, affecting the rest of the kinetic chain.

This section describes introductory to advanced closed kinetic chain exercises for the shoulder girdle and coordinates the Pilates principles and fundamentals in many ways. No longer are the exercises simply upper body strengthening, but exercises that work the entire body, tip to tail. Consider the role of the abdominals, lower back, and gluteals while performing these exercises yourself and as you observe your patients' movements.

Use your creativity and skill to add equipment or modify these exercises as appropriate for your patient.

Leg Pull Front Warm-up

Practitioner's Tip: Use this exercise as preparation for teaching the Pushup.

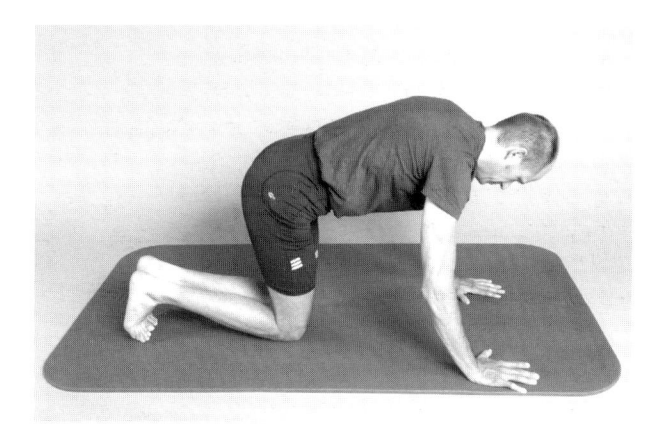

Start in quadruped, with the hands aligned just outside the shoulders, the knees beneath adducted hips, the pelvis and spine in neutral. The toes are extended, and the hands are opened like a starfish, with equal weight distribution front to back.

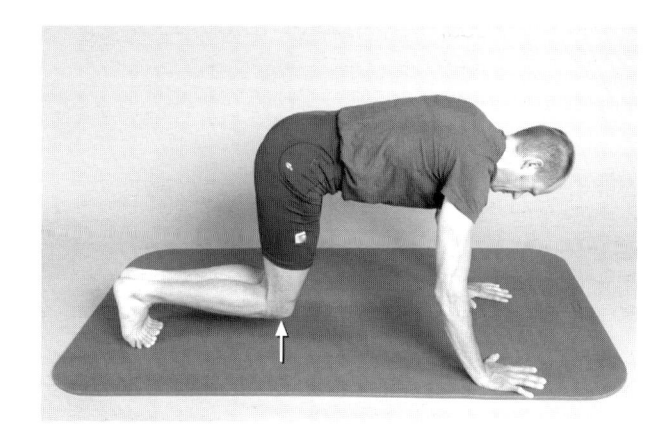

Inhale to connect with the abdominals. Exhale, keeping the spine and pelvis neutral and the scapulae stabilized, and lift the knees about 2 inches off the mat. Inhale to stay. Exhale to return the knees to the mat.

Purpose:

- First exercise to introduce closed kinetic chain training of the upper extremity
- Torso, scapular, and shoulder stabilization

Clinical Application:

- Preparatory exercise to teaching the Pushup
- Upper extremity strengthening
- Glenohumeral joint approximation
- Stimulation of joint proprioceptors
- Decreasing glenohumeral joint translation
- Enhancing muscle co-activation patterns of the glenohumeral joint and scapulae
- Strengthening of the external obliques, upper fibers
- Torso stabilization through the abdominals (TrA, obliques), multifidus, preventing pelvic/spinal rotation, flexion/extension; isometric quadriceps strengthening; toe mobilization

Repetitions: 6-10, depending on patient goals

Variations: Lifting one foot off the mat or lifting the knees and extending to the plank position

Faulty Movement Patterns: Not maintaining neutral pelvis/spine; scapular winging, elevation, and/or adduction; elbow hyperextension; Valsalva; abdominal popping; inability to coordinate breath with movement

Teaching tips:

1. *Hand variation can make a difference in the stability base as well as in recruitment of the serratus anterior. Positioning the hands outside the shoulder joint is a nice starting point for enhancing scapular stability. Change the hand placement to increase challenge once your patient is ready.*

2. *Have your patient wear shoes when there is a lack of mobility in the great toe or it isn't comfortable for the patient.*

3. *If wrist tension presents, there are a number of strategies you can use:*

   a. *Ensure sufficient stabilization at the shoulder girdle by encouraging the patient to stabilize the scapulae in slight protraction and depression.*

   b. *Cue the patient to increase pressure through the fingers or the hypothenar eminence.*

   c. *Check the elbows for hyperextension, as that will effect scapular stabilization.*

Pushups: Knees Down or Plank

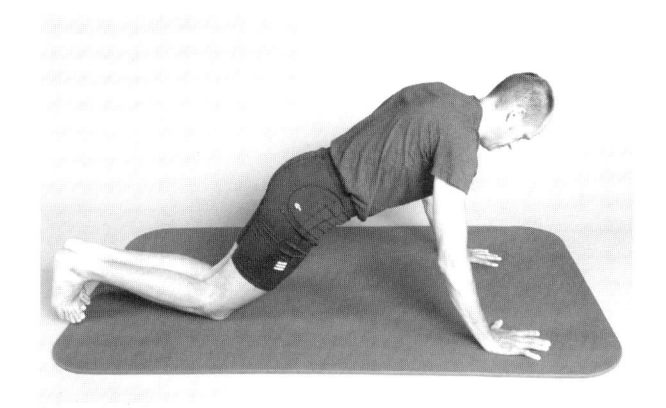

Start in plank position with the spine and pelvis in neutral, the legs parallel, and the hips adducted. The hands are positioned just outside the shoulders. The knees can be on or off the mat. The toes are extended.

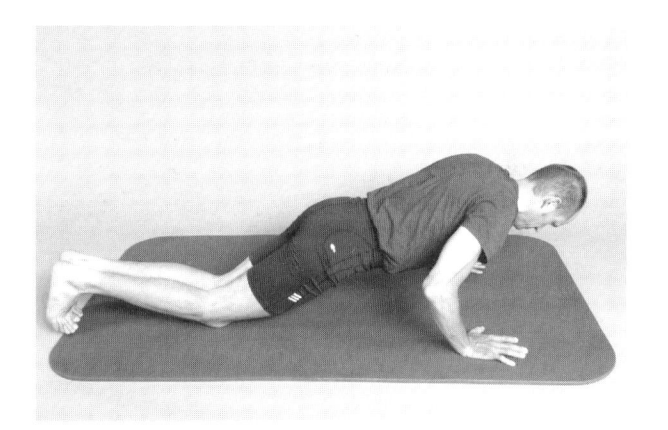

Bend at the elbows/shoulders, and while stabilizing the torso, lower the body toward the mat for a count of three inhales. Exhale once to push away from the mat by extending at the elbows.

Teaching tips:

1. *If wrist tension presents, there are a number of strategies you can use:*

   a. *Cue your patient to increase pressure through the fingers or through the hypothenar eminence.*

   b. *Ensure sufficient stabilization at the shoulder girdle by encouraging the patient to stabilize the scapulae in slight protraction and depression.*

   c. *Check the elbows for hyperextension, as that will effect scapular stabilization.*

   If wrist pain continues, an option is to use a stability ball if appropriate stabilization skills have been demonstrated. See the Teaching tips under Leg Pull Front Warm-up. A second option is to hold onto dumbbells greater than 5 pounds to encourage neutral wrist and prevent slipping.

2. *Remember that the hips are in neutral when in a semi-plank position. Use a mirror to enhance your patient's kinesthetic awareness of hip positioning. Once awareness is demonstrated, remove the mirror.*

Although the Pushup isn't a new exercise, applying the Pilates principles to this exercise can increase its efficacy. Progress patients from the wall to the floor with the knees down, then to the plank with the knees off the mat. More challenging positions include varying the hand position or taking a foot away.

Variations: Stability ball; small ball

Purpose:

- To strengthen the secondary stabilizers of the upper extremities
- Shoulder and abdominal strengthening
- Mobilization of the shoulders and elbows
- To increase the ability to maintain neutral spine and pelvis

Clinical Application:

- Advanced closed kinetic chain training
- Strengthening of the shoulder, scapular, and torso stabilizers, including the serratus anterior and upper fibers of the external obliques
- Upper extremity mobilization
- Hip and cervical spine stabilization
- Balance
- See Leg Pull Front Warm-up for additional benefits

Repetitions: Dependent on patient goals

Faulty Movement Patterns: Not maintaining neutral pelvis/spine; leading with the head, resulting in cervical protraction; neck hyperextension; scapular winging, elevation, and/or adduction; elbow hyperextension; Valsalva; abdominal popping; inability to coordinate breath with movement

chapter 8

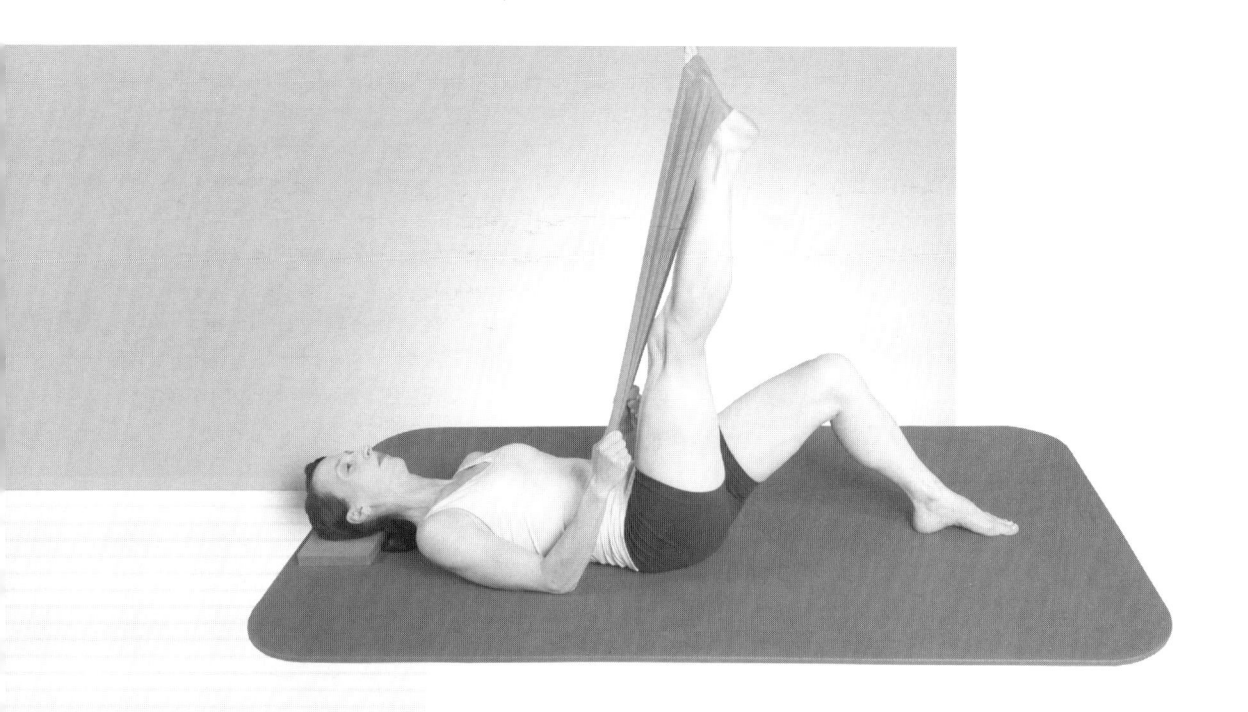

Using Equipment to Teach and Challenge

The focus of Pilates training is first stability, then mobility. The challenge of functional training of the body starts with mastering stabilization via isometric, concentric, eccentric, and co-contraction of muscles while moving the upper and lower extremities in all planes of movement. This generally occurs in supine and prone positions where the body has the most contact with the floor.

Ideally, as your patients' strength and kinesthetic awareness increase, you will move them into less stable positions: sitting, standing, etc. Increased core stabilization leads to improved use of the upper and lower extremities in uniplanar and multiplanar movement patterns that are essential to activities of daily living, sport, and quality of movement.

Adding Equipment

Once a patient masters the principles of core stabilization in fundamental Pilates mat exercises, add equipment to increase challenge, variety, or focus on target muscles. Depending on your patient's musculoskeletal dysfunction and rehabilitation goals, add equipment first with basic or fundamental exercises and progress to those that are more difficult.

Equipment can also help rehabilitation providers to enhance or modify exercises based on the patient's capabilities or identified faulty movement patterns and to make the most of a patient's alignment.

Benefits of Using Equipment

Using equipment can transfer to functional movement in these ways:

- Enhanced kinesthetic or proprioceptive awareness—provides focus or neuromuscular feedback, allowing patients to recruit intended muscles, recruit new muscles, or correct faulty movement patterns.
- Reinforcement of core stabilization principles—equipment can reinforce scapular, elbow, and wrist placement and neutral pelvis/spine through proprioceptive awareness. Often patients perceive correct motion when, in fact, it is less than ideal.
- Isolation of deep core muscles—enhances muscle fiber recruitment of deep muscles. Often core muscles are forced to stabilize the torso against the resistance of equipment or an unstable surface that challenges body position and lever length.
- Neuromuscular reeducation—equipment can help to "reteach" muscles via sensory feedback or proper alignment
- Improved strength—choose equipment that first offers light resistance and focus on maintaining pelvic and torso stabilization. Use it as a static (nonmoving) piece of equipment or as a tool to facilitate movement. Once the patient has mastered light resistance, it is appropriate to increase the resistance or lever length.
- Increased flexibility—can help restore proper alignment and increase joint range of motion.
- Increased balance—contraction of the core is necessary to progress from non-weight-bearing to weight-bearing patterns to unstable surfaces that include stability balls and balance boards. Patients should master less stable positions on stable surfaces before moving to unstable surfaces.
- Restored postural alignment—towels, pillows, and pads help patients to perform exercises in neutral alignment, the body's strongest position, leading to improved muscle balance and ultimately enhanced function.
- New exercises that resemble Reformer-based Pilates exercises—as patients demonstrate mastery of stabilization with static or facilitated movement, gradually increase challenge by adding exercises that draw on the Pilates Reformer regimen. Balls and exercise bands are most suited to the Pilates Reformer regimen.
- Simulated functional movement required for ADLs and athletic activities—many ADLs are performed against the resistance of the body (rising from a chair, getting out of bed) or against the resistance of a physical object (i.e., lifting a bag of groceries or child, hitting a baseball).

What Types of Equipment Should You Use?

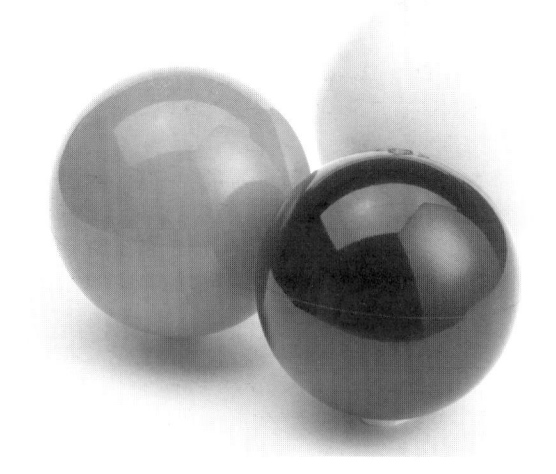

There are many types of equipment to choose from. Here's a brief list to get your creative juices flowing.

Small and large balls: Balls of any size or weight can help improve alignment or add challenge by having patients sit, hold, balance, or lay on top of them in supine, prone, or sidelying positions. Be sure to size the stability ball to your patient.

Exercise bands and tubing: Exercise bands or tubing give you the flexibility to customize the resistance to your patient's capabilities and movement awareness and can be used as a stabilization teaching tool. Moreover, these products are inexpensive and portable; most patients can take them home to complete their home exercise program.

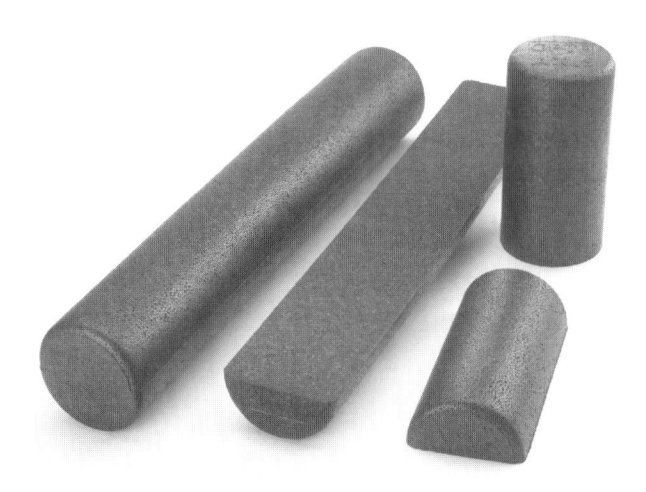

Foam rollers: Today's foam rollers come in a variety of sizes, lengths, textures, and material. We prefer rollers that are 6 inches in diameter and about 4 feet in length. Start patients with a more stable "half" roll and progress to the less stable full roll. Newer products include those that are textured, which can enhance sensory feedback, and those that look like an elongated stability ball. The latter is relatively new to the market and offers patients a "kinder, softer" surface on which to work and clinicians the ability to customize the firmness/stability of the roller to the patient.

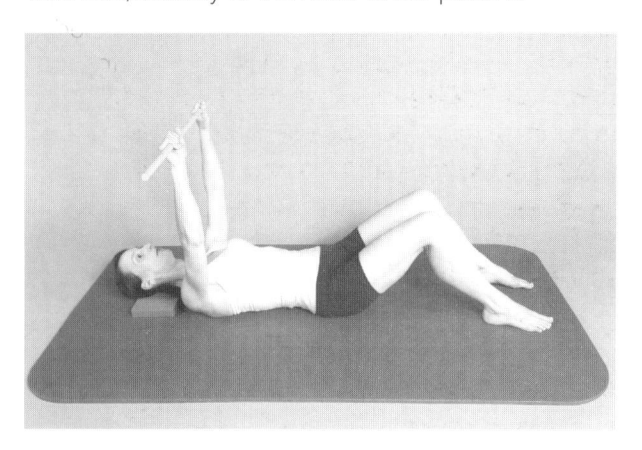

Wooden dowel: We particularly like wooden doweling to enhance cervical, scapular, and rib cage alignment. This small, lightweight tool can prove invaluable as a teaching aid and can be purchased inexpensively at craft stores.

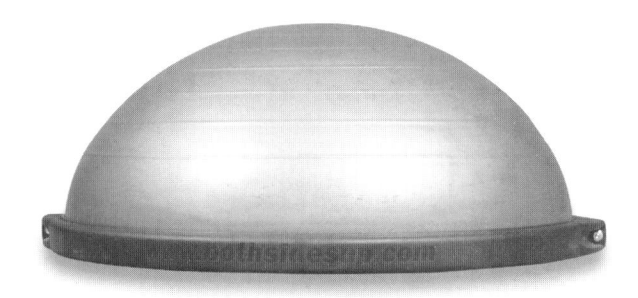

Balance boards, BOSU®, Reebok Core Board®: Balance boards are nothing new to rehabilitation providers; the BOSU® and the Reebok Core Board® are. BOSU® stands for Both Sides Up and is the brainchild of a physical therapist. When using this half stability ball on a flat surface, patients are challenged to lie, sit, kneel, or stand on it. Many Pilates exercises can be modified to accommodate this unique piece of equipment or made more challenging. The Reebok Core Board®

is essentially a balance board that moves in all planes of movement—sagittal, frontal, and transverse—by pivoting on an axis. As with the BOSU®, a number of Pilates exercises can be customized to this equipment. It is particularly helpful as your patient moves from prone, supine, and sitting positions to standing.

Towels of any thickness can help improve alignment in many ways. Place beneath your patient's head to support cervical alignment. Place beneath the ASIS to support neutral pelvis. Place between the knees to support the femurs in parallel and/or facilitate a hip adductor contraction.

Yoga blocks: Although you might think it strange to mix mind-body practices, yoga blocks are an effective tool for creating interest and challenge in your patient's exercise prescription. We've used it to help support upper extremity exercises, as a tool to sit on, or as a way to support hip alignment during particular exercises.

Chairs or benches: Chairs or benches can be easily accessed anywhere: at home, the office, or a nearby park. Use this equipment for patients who can't sit on the floor or who have a disabling condition. You can increase patient compliance by providing a framework for exercises that can be done anywhere, at your patient's convenience.

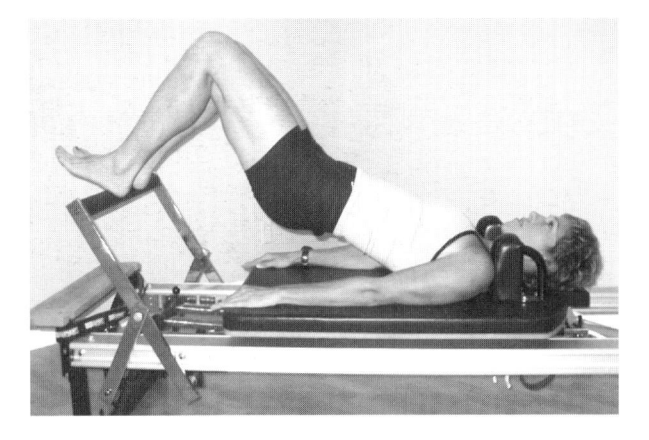

Specialized Pilates equipment: Reformers fitness/magic circles, stability chairs, arc barrels, and long/short boxes are among the many types of specialized equipment you can add to your practices toolbox. Myriad Pilates vendors and training centers can provide helpful suggestions and training in how to use these products with your specialized patient base.

Not all patients respond to the same types of cues, exercises, or tactile feedback. That's why we included the following sample exercises using equipment. In this chapter, we provide you with variations or modifications of exercises previously highlighted. Sample from these exercises to further challenge your patients or find an alternative method of education and movement repatterning.

Tips to working on a Stability Ball, Foam Roller, or BOSU®

- *Use a textured surface to provide more sensory feedback and reduce the patient's risk of slipping off the rounded surface.*
- *Perform exercises with bare feet to enhance sensory feedback and stability.*
- *Use a yoga mat under the ball/roller or BOSU® and the feet to increase surface stability, if needed.*
- *Choose clothing that is not tight, restrictive, or slippery that may affect joint range of motion or decrease an individual's ability to stabilize on the equipment. Patients should always wear a shirt when working on equipment.*
- *Demonstrate mounting positions and exercises first to increase your patients' safety and understanding of them*
- *The firmer the stability ball/roller/BOSU®, the greater the challenge. A slightly underinflated surface can also be used for the novice, deconditioned people, and older adults. A less-inflated surface increases the surface size of the ball, thereby enhancing stability.*

A Word about Stability Balls

Once a patient can demonstrate correct ball mounting procedures, introduce Pilates-based core stabilization principles. The focus of the principles is the same as on the mat. An advantage to using a ball is that it can further enhance a patient's movement awareness and postural alignment through feedback and stimulate key torso stabilization muscles with its unstable surface.

Mounting Balls

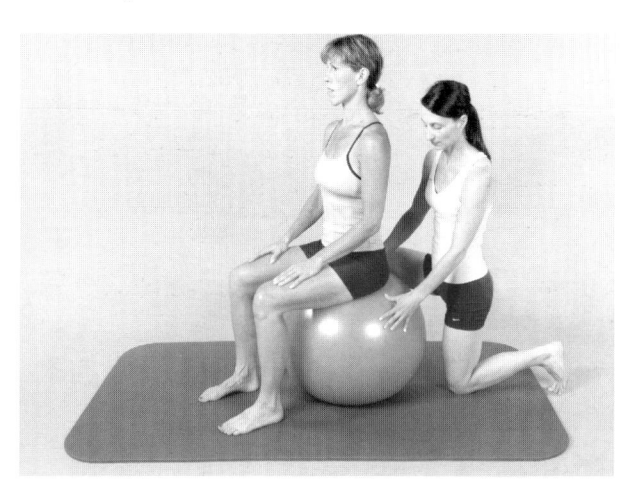

Initially, the clinician should stabilize the ball on either side while the patient gets on it. The patient should stand as close to the ball (behind the body) as possible with feet hip-width apart and transition to sitting while reaching the hands simultaneously to the sides of the ball and tightening the abdominals to support the lumbo-pelvic region. Progress the patient to independent transitioning from standing to sitting following the procedure above without clinician assistance.

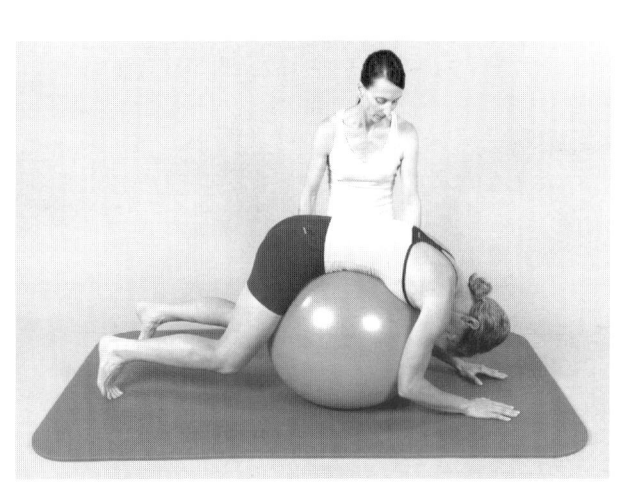

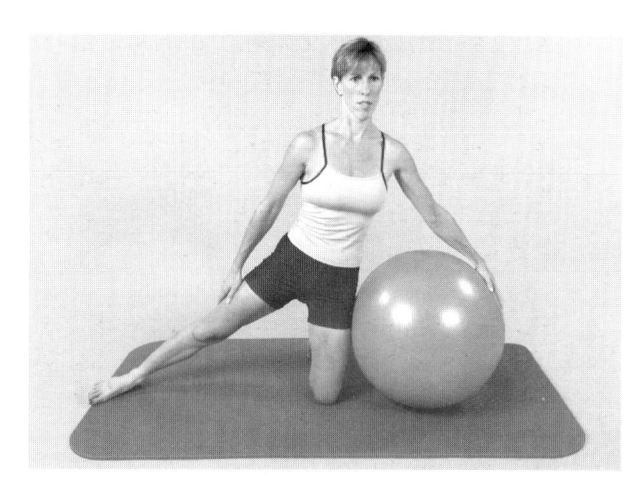

Initially, the clinician should stabilize the ball on either side as the patient kneels next to one side of the ball (i.e., left side) with the pelvis facing straight ahead. The patient's left hand is placed on the outside of the ball and pulled toward the left hip. Instruct the patient to drive the left hip into the ball as he/she lowers the torso and left elbow to the ball and simultaneously extends the right knee, positioning the right foot on the floor. Progress to place the right hand on top of the ball in front of the sternum with the hip and pelvis in neutral. Progress the patient to independent transition on the ball.

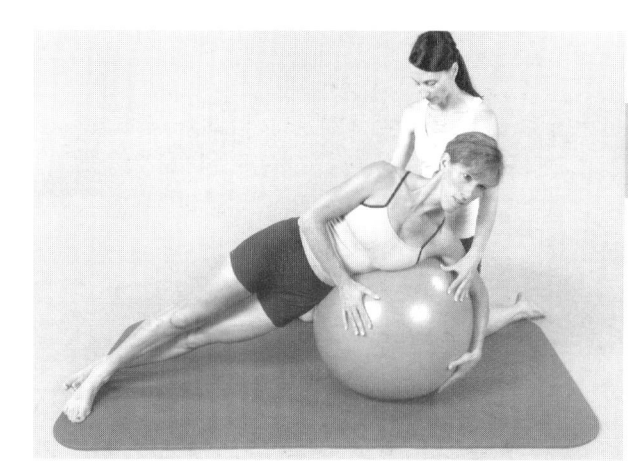

Prone positions vary from having the pelvis centered on the ball to having the thighs, toes, or sternum on the ball. To begin, the clinician should stabilize the ball on either side while the patient assumes a kneeling position as close as possible behind ball with the knees hip-width apart, the toes extended, and the hands supporting along the sides of ball (wider than shoulder width). The clinician removes his/her hands from the ball and instructs the patient to apply firm downward pressure on the ball with the hands to stabilize the ball as the body is lowered on top of it.

Sidelying positions are similar to the side-kneeling position with one exception: the hips and knees are extended, effectively taking away a stability point for your patient and challenging dynamic equilibrium. Follow the mounting procedures as described. The legs may be scissored or progressed to legs stacked one on top of the other or one in front of the other to assist with bracing. Patients who are capable of sidelying positions often appreciate the assistance of a wall to brace the feet initially. To advance, move the feet away from the wall.

The Pilates Principles Using Equipment

Breathing

Use breathing as an adjunct to manual therapy of the ribs, thoracic spine, and/or diaphragm, to restore normal breathing mechanics, and to enhance flexibility and strengthening exercises, and transitional movements, ADLs, and sport-specific drills. See Chapters 4 and 5 to reference breathing assessment, breathing as a Pilates principle, and strategies to correct or enhance faulty breathing.

Supine Breathing on the Foam Roller

Helpful tip: Use the foam roller when you want to facilitate spinal extension.

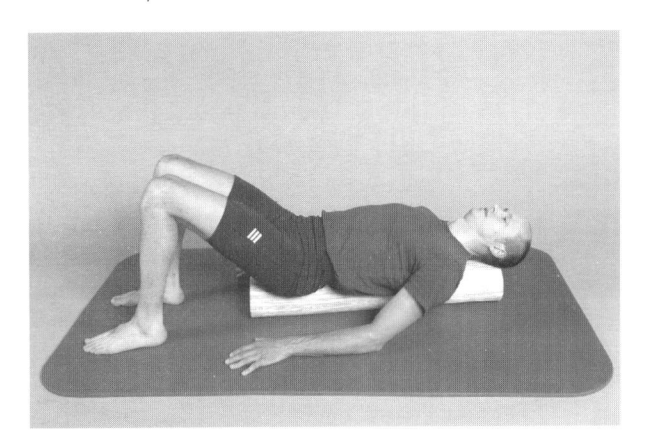

Start in supine with neutral pelvis/spine centered on the roller, neutral head and neck alignment, the legs in hooklying, and heels hip-width apart. Place the hands bilaterally along the anterior and lateral portions of the rib cage.

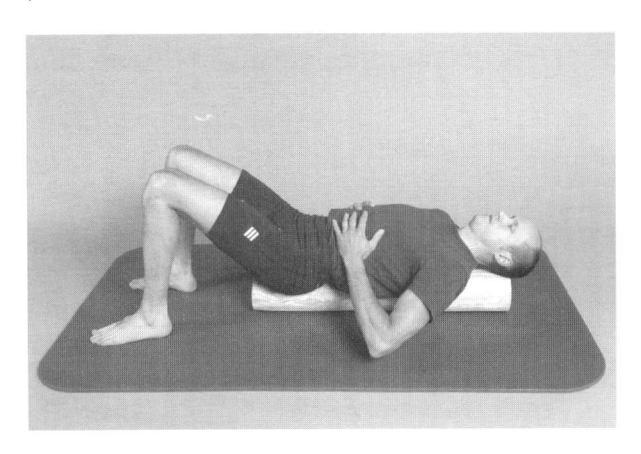

Inhale into the posterolateral ribs bilaterally to enhance mobilization of the thoracic spine into extension. With exhalation, feel the ribs move medially and inferior while maintaining lumbo-pelvic stability on this unstable surface. *Option:* Use a small ball to support neutral cervical alignment.

Prone Breathing on the Stability Ball

Teaching tips:

1. Use sensory feedback from the ball's surface to help reeducate your patient's breathing pattern.

2. To maximize the length of the torso on the ball and increase chest comfort with breathing, have the patient practice getting on the ball sequentially, moving from the lumbar to the thoracic spine.

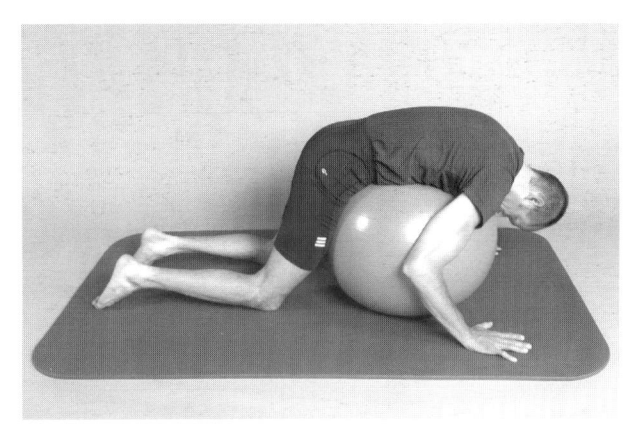

Start by kneeling behind the ball with the hands alongside of it. Lower the torso over the ball while holding it still. Rest the head on the ball with the arms relaxed along the sides of the ball.

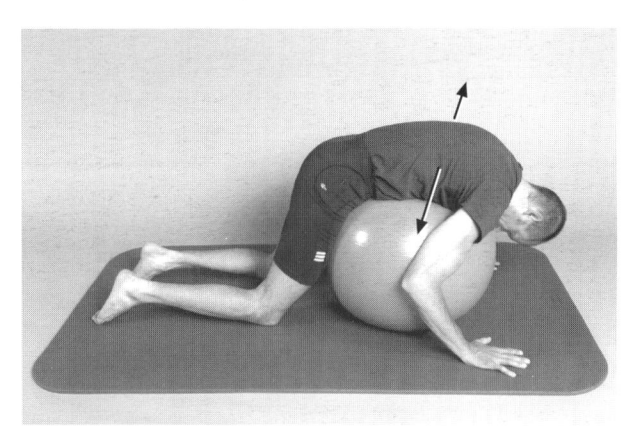

Inhale into the posterolateral ribs, feeling them move laterally and superior with the breath. With exhalation, feel the ribs move medially and inferior while maintaining lumbo-pelvic stability on the unstable surface. Prone positioning on the ball can help enhance the inspiration phase of breathing, increase rib mobility, and reeducate rib cage breathing via sensory feedback on the anterior portion of the torso. *Variation: Use the BOSU®.*

Breathing Using an Exercise Band

An exercise band helps enhance the inspiration phase of breathing, increases rib mobility, reeducates rib cage breathing, and strengthens/stretches the obliques and intercostals via sensory feedback and resistance.

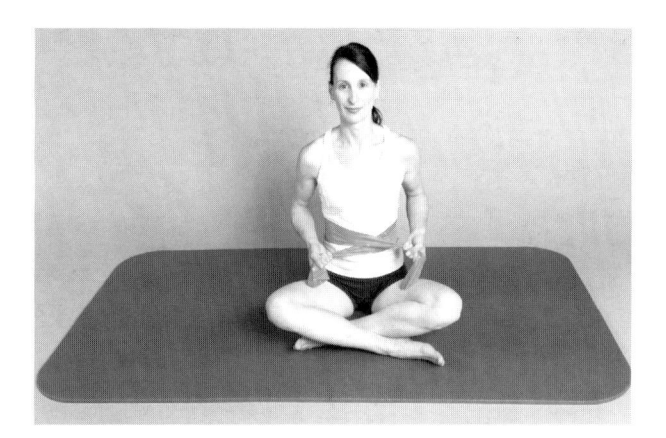

Start by sitting in a chair or on a mat with neutral pelvis and spine and the ribs aligned over the pelvis. Position the exercise band across the back, just beneath the scapulae. Cross the band in front of the body with the hands applying slight tension on the band until it is taut against the ribs.

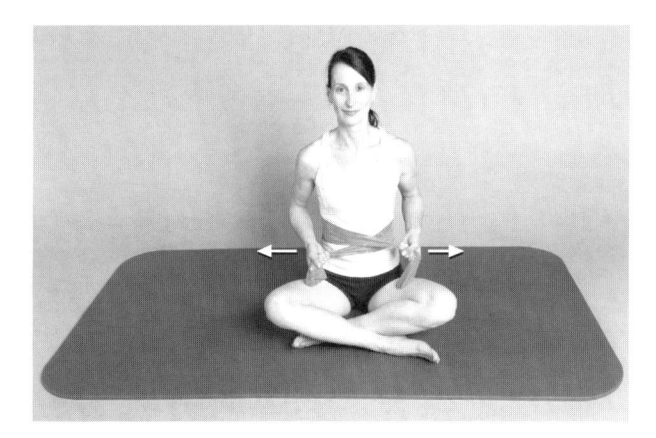

Inhale and breathe into the lateral and posterior ribs bilaterally. Cue the patient to feel the ribs expand into the band. Then cue the patient to exhale and feel the ribs naturally move away from the band as the oblique abdominals contract.

Helpful tip: The focus of mastering Pilates is first stability, then mobility. Less is more. Once a patient has mastered the principles of core stabilization in isolation and in combination with the Pilates mat rehabilitation exercises, add intensity and challenge by using the stability ball and a little creativity. Have the patient put the ball between the knees to enhance pelvic floor firing, hold the ball overhead to create resistance with supine or sitting positions, sit, kneel, or sidelie on the ball to simulate unstable surfaces, and so on.

Pelvic Position

The pelvis moves in all planes and ranges of movement. Many people are unaware of these ranges. If there is some awareness, it usually occurs with a posterior tilt during the traditional abdominal crunch exercise. Having knowledge of how the pelvis moves anteriorly or laterally and tilts or rotates is important to maintaining stability of the pelvis with movement of the upper and lower extremities when on an unstable surface such as the ball or a roller. This series of movement patterns develops kinesthetic awareness of pelvic mechanics and its relationship to the lumbar spine and hips.

Neutral Pelvis: Supine on Foam Roller

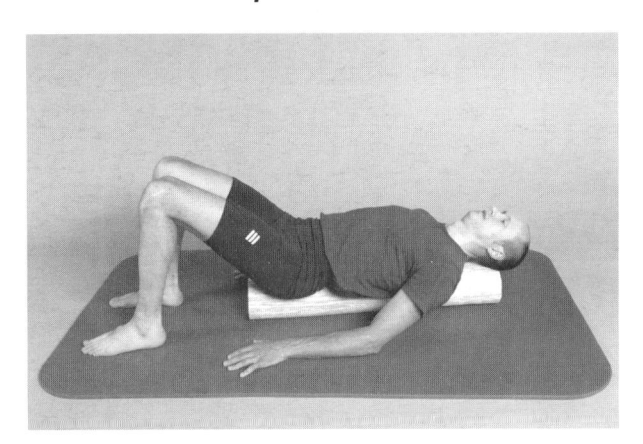

Start supine on the roller with neutral pelvis, the heels hip-width apart. Tilt the pelvis anteriorly and posteriorly and feel the degree of movement between the two ranges while maintaining balance on the unstable surface. Find neutral pelvis by locating the midpoint between the anterior and posterior pelvic tilt. Be sure to apply even pressure with the feet. *Option:* Use a small ball to support neutral cervical alignment.

Pelvic Position: Direct Method Sitting on a Stability Ball

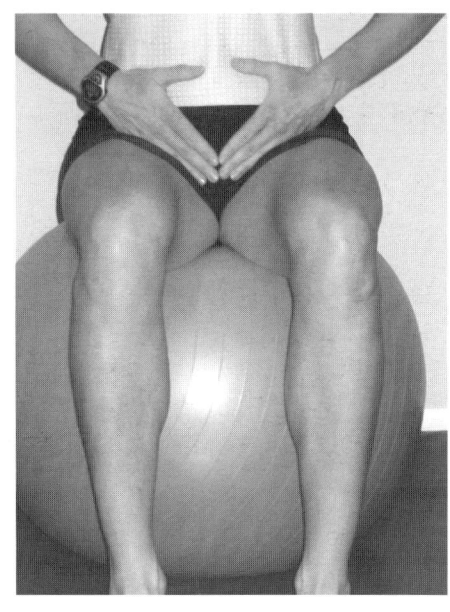

Sit on the ball with the pelvis directed straight ahead, in neutral head and neck alignment, with the feet hip-width apart and the arms alongside the body with the option of gently holding onto the sides of the ball.

Find the neutral pelvis position using anatomical landmarks. Place the hypothenar eminence on the ASIS bilaterally and angle the second fingers toward the midline to form a triangle. Keeping the second fingers perpendicular to the floor, slide them toward the symphysis pubis. Once the pubis is located, determine the position of the pelvis.

If the pelvis is in an anterior or imprinted position, move the pelvis to neutral. If low back pain or strain is felt in neutral, back off slightly.

Purpose:

- To teach kinesthetic awareness of neutral pelvis and its relationship to the lumbar spine
- To create safe and efficient movement through neutral spine and pelvis

Clinical Application:

- Apply to all types of exercise to reduce faulty movement patterns that may result in acute or overuse injuries and in degenerative changes over time. Neutral pelvis encourages the core muscles to work optimally and prepares the lower and upper extremities for more efficient movement.

Equipment Variations: Practice pelvic positioning on a BOSU® or foam roller. The BOSU® offers patients a more stable surface than the stability ball and is an excellent starting point for working on a ball.

Faulty Movement Patterns: Overactive gluteals in beginners; inability to maintain pelvic position; inability to stabilize the pelvis independent of hip movement; rib cage popping; upper body tension; weight shifting; the ball not rolling in a straight line

Initially, when sitting on a ball and performing exercises, the feet should be hip-width apart to achieve optimal stability. Once your patient demonstrates the ability to maintain good alignment and apply core stabilization principles with exercises, challenge balance by having the patient adduct the hips to decrease the base of support. This may result in a smaller range of motion within each exercise as the patient tries to maintain alignment and stabilization.

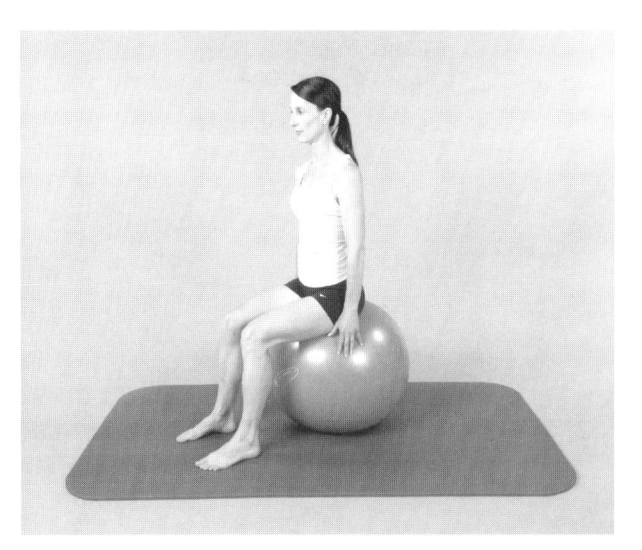

Pelvic Position: Indirect Method

Anterior and Posterior (Imprinted) Tilts. While sitting on the ball, tilt the symphysis pubis moving up and away from the ball, allowing the ball to roll/pull forward for posterior tilt, and then reverse to the starting position. Anteriorly tilt the pelvis by moving the symphysis pubis down toward the ball, allowing the ball to move backward, and then reverse to the starting position. Feel the degree of movement that occurs between the two ranges and how the low back follows the movement of the pelvis.

Posterior

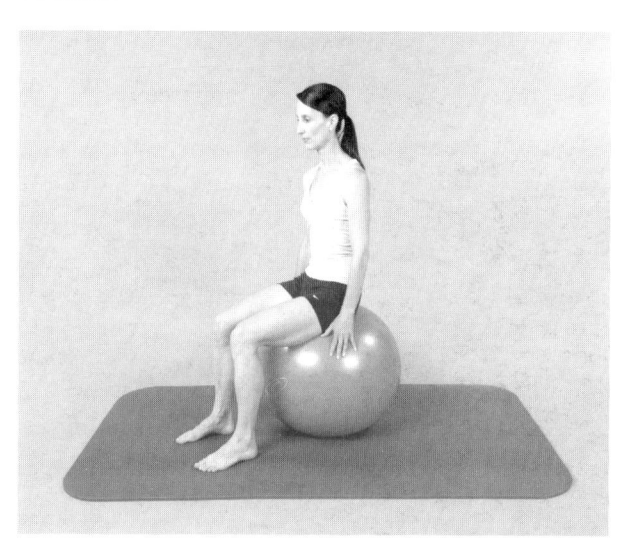

Anterior

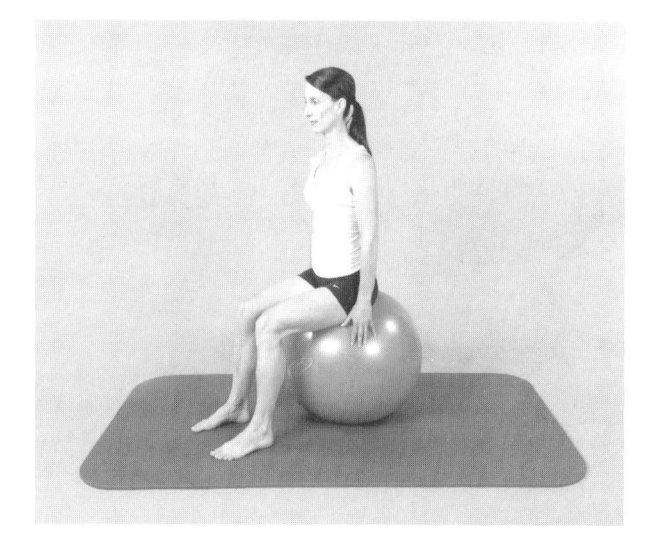

Practitioner's tips:

1. *This is an excellent exercise to use when a patient has difficulty articulating the spine in supine. The ball helps facilitate spinal articulation.*

2. *Practice pelvic positioning in supine on a BOSU® or foam roller. The BOSU® and roller offer patients a more stable surface than the stability ball and are excellent starting points for working on a ball.*

Lateral Pelvic Tilt

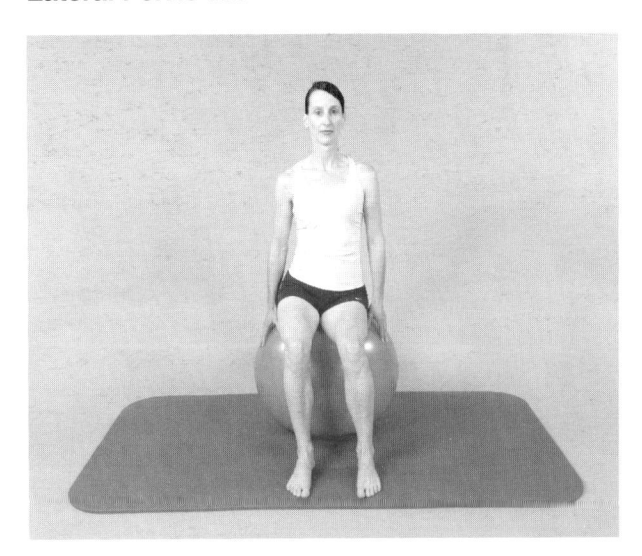

While sitting on the ball, shift weight to the left ischial tuberosity (IT), allowing the ball to roll right for a right lateral pelvic tilt. Keep the upper extremities still. Change directions to find a left lateral pelvic tilt. Feel the degree of movement that occurs between the two ranges and how the lower back follows the movement of the pelvis to create a right side bend.

Pelvic Circles

Helpful tip: This movement combines anterior, posterior, and lateral pelvic tilts and is a natural progression to teaching patients all movements of the pelvis in a dynamic fashion. This is an excellent exercise for teaching patients the relationship between the pelvis, the lower back, and the hip.

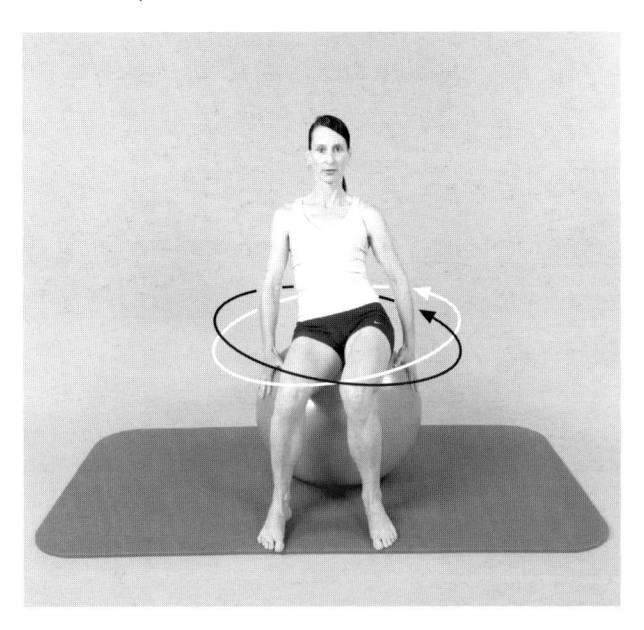

While sitting on a ball, tilt the pelvis posteriorly by moving the pubis symphysis up and away the ball, allowing the ball to roll forward, then shift weight to the right IT, allowing the ball to roll left. Next, tilt the pelvis anteriorly by moving the symphysis pubis down from ball, allowing the ball to move backward, and then shift weight to the left IT, allowing the ball to move right.

Focus on creating a smooth circle without stopping. Allow the legs to move. Reverse the direction of the circle and observe movement awareness. Repeat the counterclockwise and clockwise patterns, keeping the upper extremities still. Notice how the pelvic range of motion decreases to maintain stabilization through the hip: too large of a circle causes compensatory hip movement.

Ball Bouncing

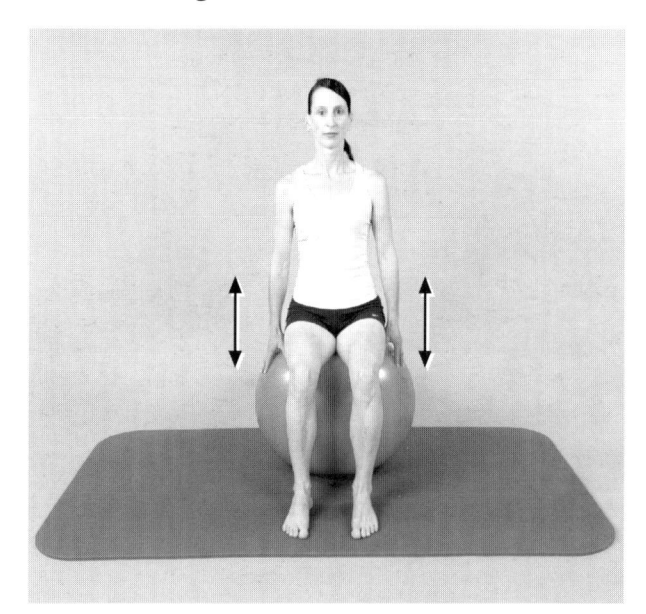

Sit on a ball with the feet hip-width apart, the arms held along the sides, with the palms facing toward the midline. Gently press the feet into the floor and bounce up and down on the ball using the muscles of the lower extremities for motion. The abdominals/lower back muscles contract to stabilize the torso on the ball. Keep the pelvis neutral.

Helpful tip: While the patient is bouncing, instruct him/her to relax the abdominals. The patient will be surprised that they will be unable to relax the abdominals secondary to the bouncing, helping to facilitate abdominal muscle contraction or bracing.

This is a great way to introduce an indirect method of finding neutral pelvis on an unstable base of support. Patients activate the core stabilizers and muscles of the lower extremities via movement of the ball to keep the body stable over the center of the ball. It also introduces an element of play. Be on the lookout for curling toes, an inability to fire the quadriceps and hamstring muscles, and femoral rotation.

Neutral Pelvis with Leg Patterns on a Foam Roller

Practitioner tips: Refer to Chapter 4 for extended movement descriptions and breath pattern.
Option: Use a small ball to support neutral cervical alignment.

Supine Heel Slide

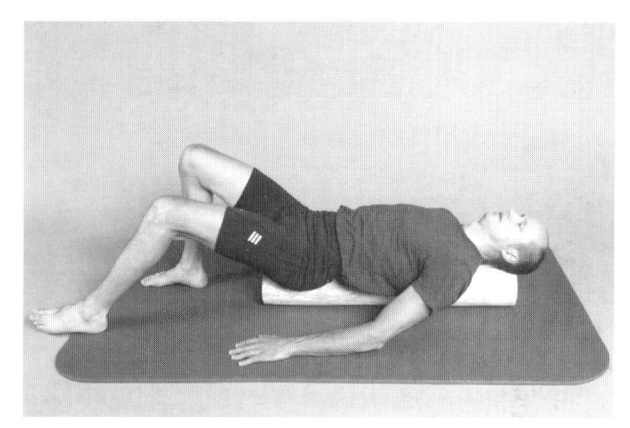

Start supine on the roller with neutral pelvis, the heels hip-width apart. Maintain stabilization on the unstable surface via the primary and secondary core stabilizers while extending the hip and knee. Flex the hip and knee to the starting position. Follow the breath pattern in Chapter 4.

Single Tabletop (knee and hip flexed to 90 degrees)

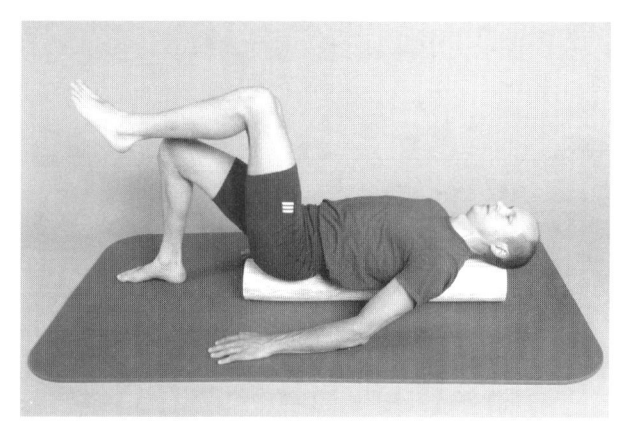

Start supine with neutral pelvis and neutral head and neck alignment. Exhale, maintain neutral, and lift one leg up into tabletop position. Inhale and lower the foot back to the mat. Repeat on the other side. To increase challenge, add Single Leg in Tabletop with arm patterns of your choosing.

Single Tabletop with Knee Extension Supine

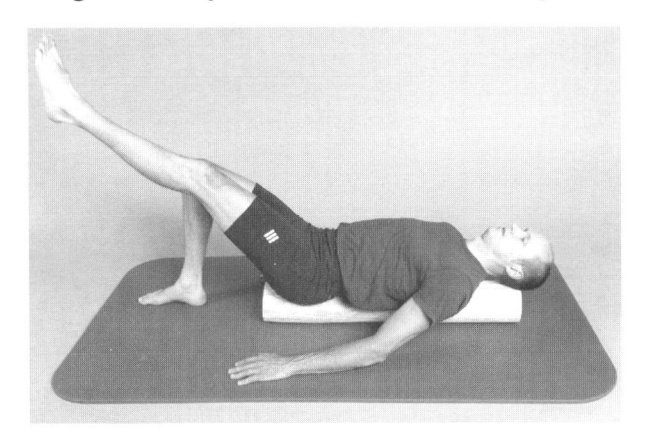

Start supine with neutral pelvis, the heels hip-width apart. Maintain stabilization on the unstable surface via the primary and secondary core stabilizers while flexing one hip to 90 degrees and by keeping the other foot on the floor. Extend the knee in the air while holding the hip still. Flex the knee to 90 degrees. Return to the starting position. Follow the breath pattern in Chapter 4. Option: Use a small ball to support neutral cervical alignment.

Variations: Lower/lift with the hip/knee extended.

Single-Leg Knee Stirs

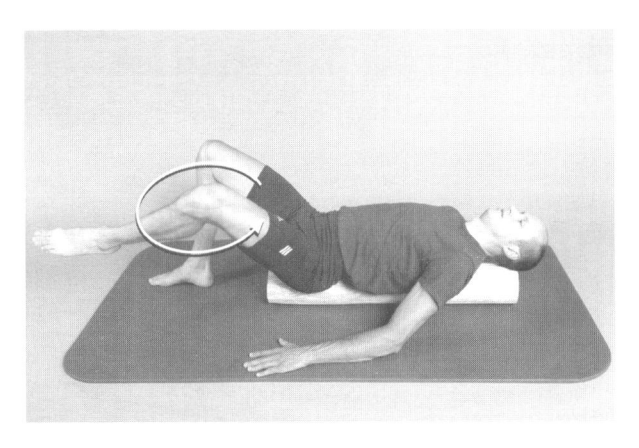

Start in hooklying with neutral pelvis, neutral head and neck alignment, one leg in tabletop and the other aligned with the ASIS, the arms alongside the body, and the elbows slightly bent, with the palms facing down on the floor. Inhale and start to "draw" a half circle (hip circumduction) with the patella, adducting the hip across the midline and then extending it. Exhale to complete the circle, abducting the hip away from the midline and flexing it to the starting position. Maintain neutral with the movement. Repeat with the other leg.

Bent-Knee Fallout

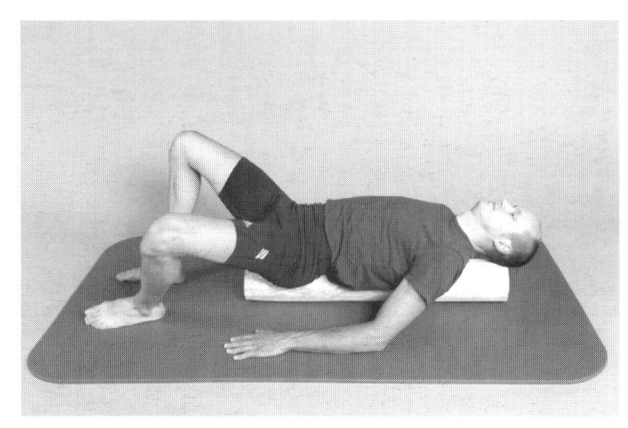

Start in hooklying with neutral pelvis/spine, head, and neck alignment, the heels hip-width apart, the arms alongside the body, and the elbows slightly bent, with the palms facing down on the floor. Inhale, maintain neutral, and externally rotate the hip, letting the knee fall to the side with control. The opposite leg on the floor supports the movement through stabilization. Exhale and internally rotate the hip to the initial position.

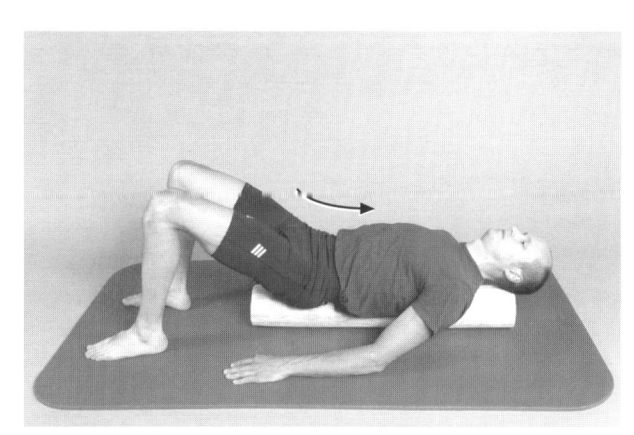

Imprinted Pelvis on a Foam Roller

Start supine on the roller with neutral pelvis, the heels hip-width apart. Tip the ASIS bilaterally toward the ribs while maintaining balance on the unstable surface. Follow the breath pattern in Chapter 4.

Scapular Retraction and Protraction on a Foam Roller

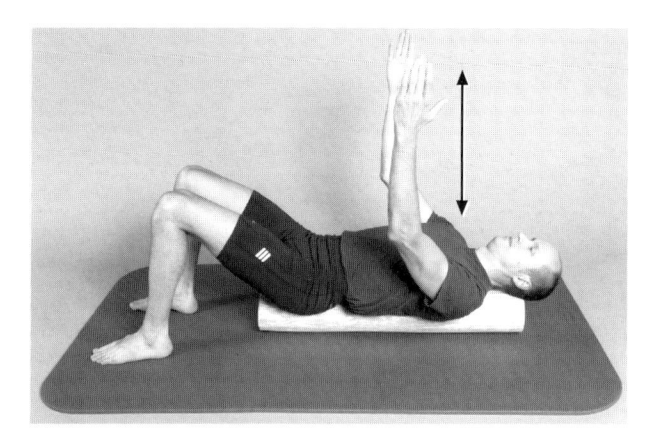

Start supine on the roller with neutral pelvis, the legs hip-width apart. Flex the shoulders to 90 degrees. Protract the scapulae and retract them, maintaining torso stabilization on the unstable surface. Follow the breath pattern in Chapter 4.

Variation: Place resistance tubing under the roller and hold it with the hands.

Spinal/Thoracic Flexion

Quarter Rollup in Neutral with Stability Ball
Start supine with neutral pelvis, neutral head and cervical alignment, the calves on the ball.

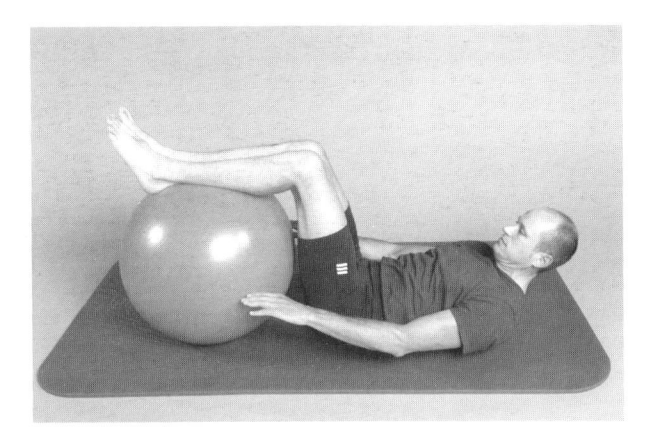

Maintaining neutral, flex the craniovertebral/thoracic spine and reach to the kneecaps. Sequentially roll the thoracic to cervical spine back to the mat and return the shoulders to the initial position. Follow the breath pattern in Chapter 6.

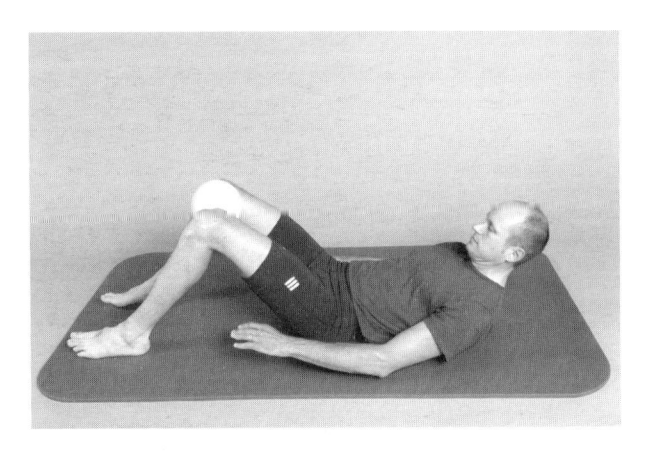

Equipment Variations: Small ball between the knees; isometric holds with varied ball patterns; semi-sitting on the ball with the ball positioned beneath the lumbar spine.

Rollup with Wooden Dowel
Start supine with neutral pelvis, the legs extended and the hips adducted, the ankles dorsiflexed, and the shoulders flexed to 180 degrees with the dowel in the hands.

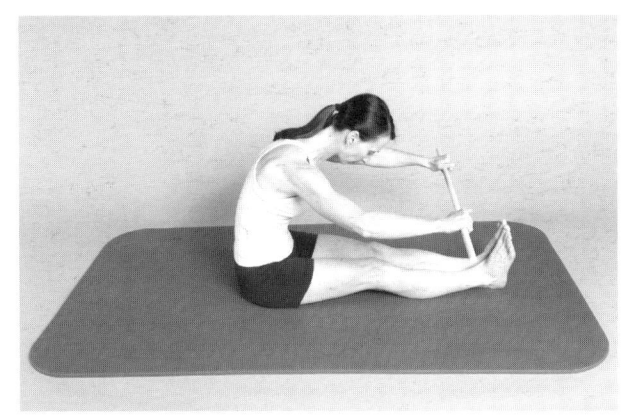

Maintaining neutral, flex the craniovertebral/thoracic spine and reach the dowel to the kneecaps. Sequentially unroll the thoracic to cervical spine back to the mat and return the shoulders/dowel to the initial position. Follow the breath pattern in Chapter 6.

Equipment Variations: Small ball between the knees; stability ball in the hands; Quarter/Half Rollup with the knees flexed; Half Rollup with the legs extended; Full Rollup with the legs flexed; arms held next to the ears; two breaths

Helpful tips:

1. Patients who require transversus abdominis training benefit from using a small ball between the knees to recruit the TrA via hip adductor contraction.

2. A wooden dowel helps reinforce alignment principles.

The Hundred with Stability Ball
Start supine with imprinted pelvis, the hips and knees flexed to 90 degrees, and a stability ball placed beneath the lower legs.

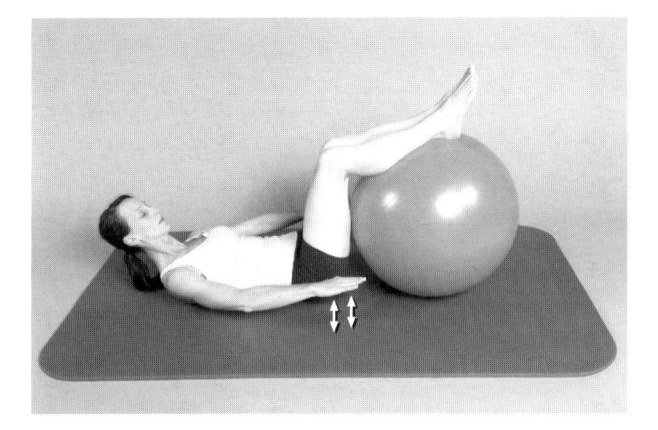

Maintaining imprint, sequentially flex the craniovertebral/thoracic spine. Hold the flexed position while pulsing the arms and maintaining torso stabilization against the weight of the ball. Follow the breath pattern in Chapter 6. *Variations:* Isometric holds in varied positions; lower/lift legs, ball between ankles.

Single-Leg Stretch with Stability Ball

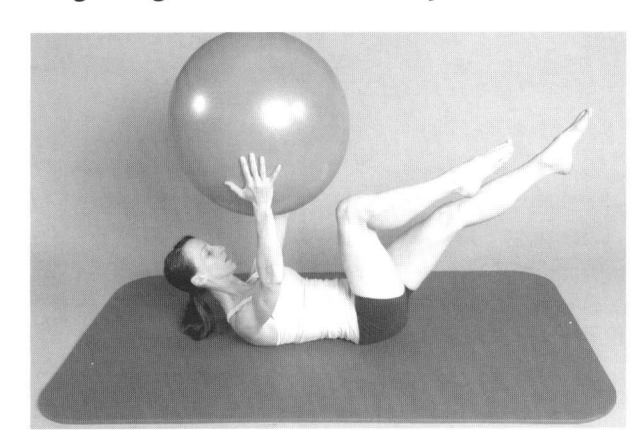

Start supine in craniovertebral/thoracic flexion with a posterior pelvic tilt, the hips adducted in tabletop with the hips and knees flexed and the ankles plantar flexed. Hold onto the ball with the hands, the shoulders flexed to 90 degrees. Maintaining neutral, extend one leg on the diagonal, maintaining imprint while touching the ball to the opposite knee.

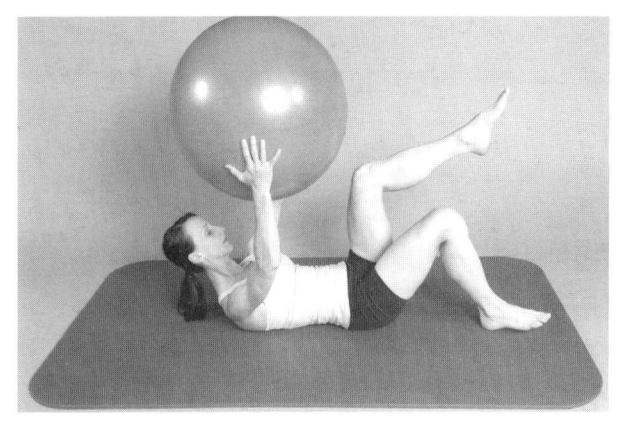

Variations: Alternating touching one heel to the floor (or as low as possible while maintaining a posterior tilt); raising the head off the mat in spinal/thoracic flexion, with the knees remaining flexed. *Option:* Keep the head on the mat.

Spine Stretch Forward on BOSU® or Chair
Start by sitting with neutral pelvis on a chair. Extend the legs and abduct the hips to shoulder-width apart. The ankles are neutral, and the hands are placed along the lateral hips bilaterally.

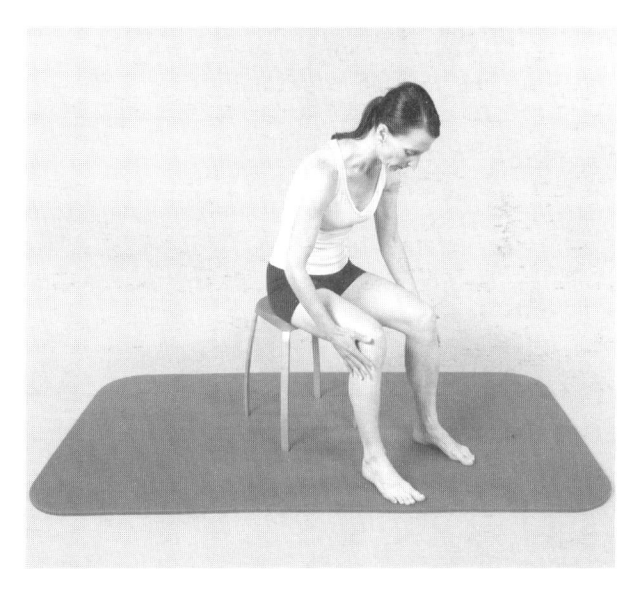

Sequentially flex the cervical to lumbar spine with transition from neutral pelvis to a posterior pelvic tilt when moving into the lumbar spine, maintaining balance on the unstable surface. Reverse the articulation from the lumbar to the cervical spine with transition to neutral pelvis when moving into the thoracic spine. Follow the breath pattern in Chapter 6.

Variations: Sit on a BOSU® with the flat side up. Place a stability or small ball between the legs and roll the ball forward/backward with the movement pattern.

Helpful hint: This is a nice exercise to use when a patient has difficulty finding neutral pelvis secondary to tight hamstring muscles. Remember that balance is challenged unless sitting on a firm surface.

Criss Cross with Stability Ball

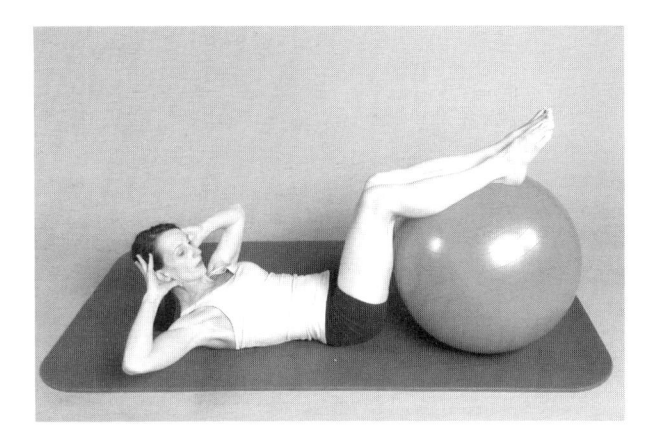

Start supine with a posterior pelvic tilt, the hips adducted in tabletop, the ankles plantar flexed, and the calves/ankles resting on the ball. Both hands behind the head. Exhale and flex the cervical/thoracic spine. Rotate the thoracic spine, left shoulder to right hip, keeping the shoulders open and stabilized. Repeat on the opposite side.

Equipment Variations: Ball between ankles/calves; standing with ball

Standing Criss Cross with Small Ball

Stand with the ball elevated to the right diagonal, the legs in "athletic-ready, supportive position," and the pelvis neutral.

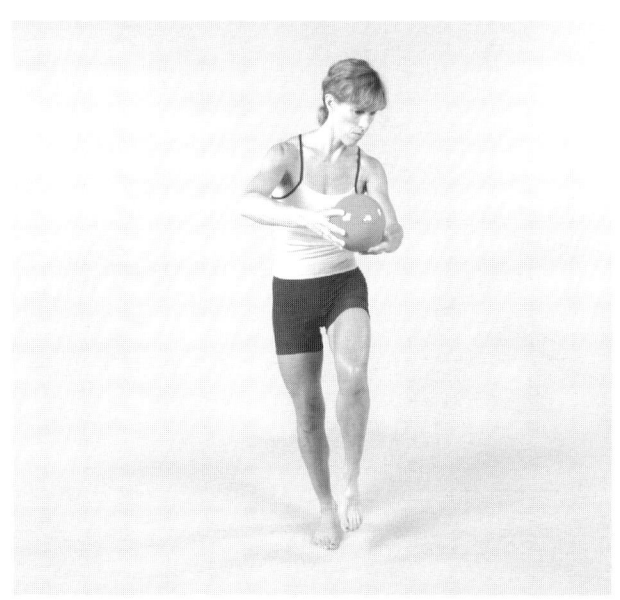

Inhale to prepare; exhale, draw the ball down to the left hip while flexing and rotating the thoracic spine, maintaining neutral pelvis. To further challenge, draw the left leg into tabletop while simultaneously flexing and rotating. Repeat other side.

Equipment Variation: Stability or medicine ball

Teaching tip: First teach your patient rotation in standing without equipment. Add a lightweight ball and perform upper extremity motion only. Once mastered, add spine rotation/flexion and hip flexion, progressing one to the other as appropriate.

Double-Leg Stretch with Ball

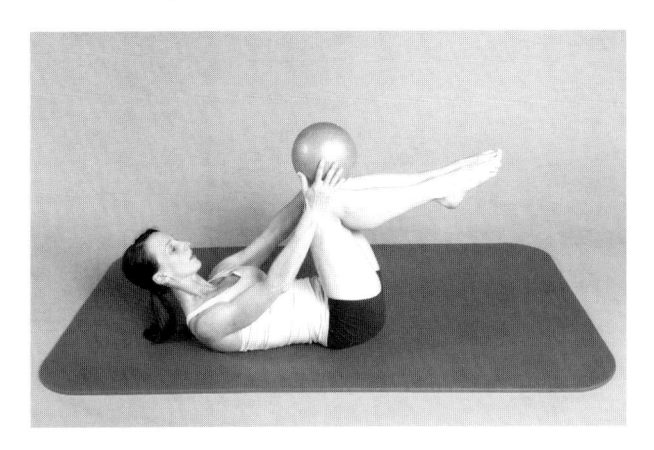

Start supine in craniovertebral/thoracic flexion with a posterior pelvic tilt, the hips adducted in tabletop with the hips and knees flexed and the ankles plantar flexed. The ball is resting on top of the kneecaps, firmly held in the hands, with the elbows bent. Inhale to prepare and deepen the connection to the abdominals.

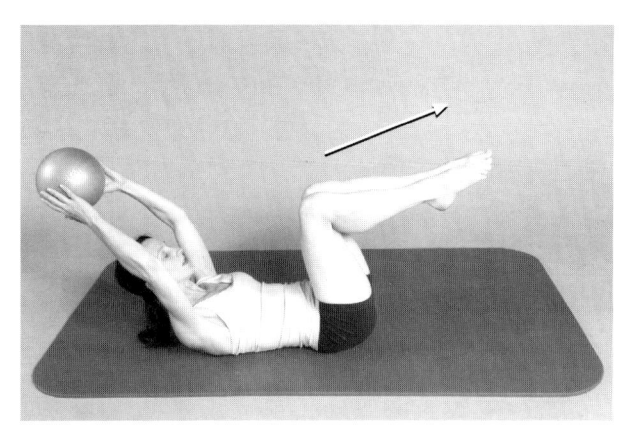

Exhale, maintain spinal flexion, and stretch the legs on the diagonal as low as the posterior tilt can be maintained. The arms and ball simultaneously arc 180 degrees overhead.

Variation on BOSU®, Arms Only: Semi-recline on the dome, the lower back supported by the BOSU® with neutral pelvis and spine. Inhale to prepare. Exhale and extend the arms overhead and circle around.

Spinal/Thoracic Extension

Trunk Extension on a BOSU® or Stability Ball

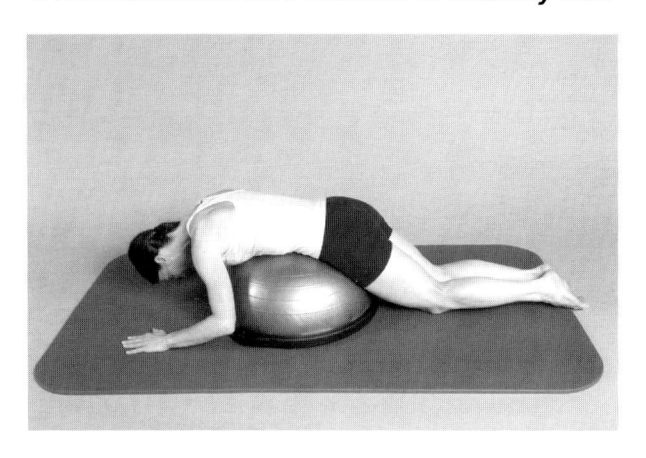

Start kneeling behind the BOSU®. Flex the torso over the BOSU®, maintaining neutral pelvis and keeping the knees near or on the floor. The hands and elbows are positioned on the ball just outside the shoulders with the hips abducted to hip-width apart.

Helpful tips:

1. To find neutral pelvis, position the knees a few inches away from the BOSU®.

2. For more challenge, choose the plank option, knees off the floor.

Prepatory Exercise 1

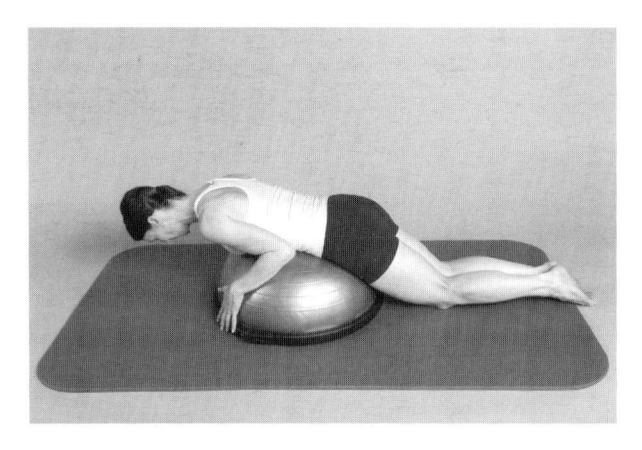

Sequentially extend the cervical to thoracic spine, maintaining neutral pelvis. The hands/forearms remain on the floor or BOSU® with minimal pressure.

Prepatory Exercise 2

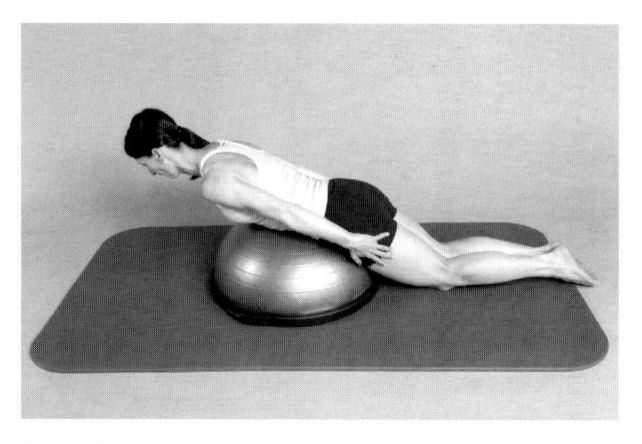

Extended shoulders with hands (palms) against the thigh or the back of the BOSU® or ball.

Prepatory Exercise 3

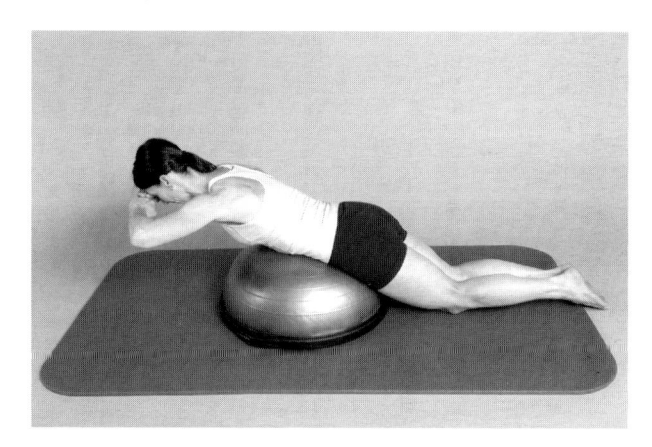

Shoulders abducted with the elbows bent, the hands beneath the forehead, and the thoracic spine extended.

Prepatory Exercise 4

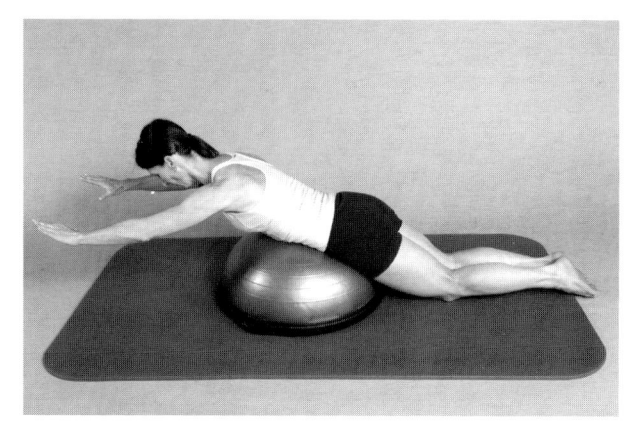

Shoulders flexed to 180 degrees and the arms/hands on the floor. The arms and head will lift as the spine is extended.

Trunk Extension with Wooden Dowel

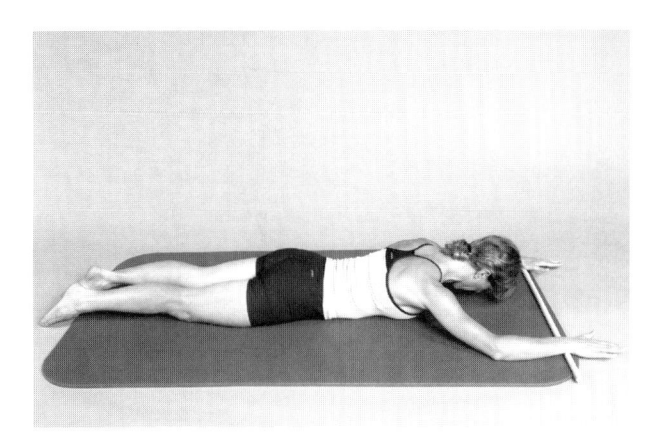

Start prone with neutral pelvis, hips adducted, and shoulders flexed to 180 degrees. Place the hypothenar and thenar eminences on top of the wooden dowel with the hands aligned outside the shoulders and the elbows slightly flexed.

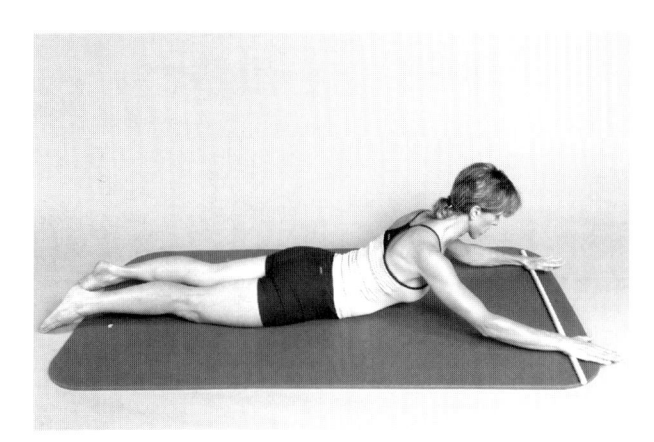

Retract and depress the scapula. Inhale to prepare; exhale and extend the cervical and thoracic spine, then simultaneously roll the dowel toward the body to assist with thoracic extension while maintaining neutral pelvic alignment. Return to the starting position, maintaining torso stabilization and rolling the dowel away from the body with inhalation. Follow the breath pattern in Chapter 6.

Variation: Add resistance with a Body Bar®, thumbs positioned up to emphasize the lower trapezius muscles.

Helpful tip: This is an excellent exercise to use when there is loss of scapular stabilization and/or anterior rib popping secondary to weak external oblique muscles with Prepatory Exercise 4.

Swimming Progressions on BOSU® or Ball
Progression 1

Start prone on the BOSU® with the arms overhead, the spine and pelvis neutral, the legs extended hip-width apart, the hips neutral, and the ankles plantar flexed.

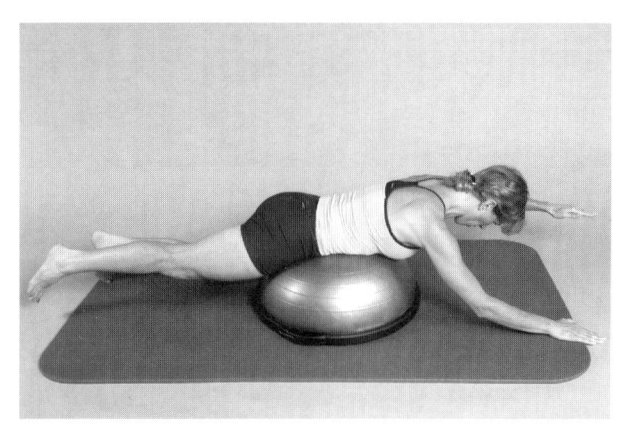

Inhale to prepare; exhale and extend the right hip/left arm off the floor (lift the opposite arm/leg), maintaining neutral spine and pelvis and scapular stabilization. *Option:* The knees may remain on the floor or in a plank position with the unilateral arm lift.

Progression 2

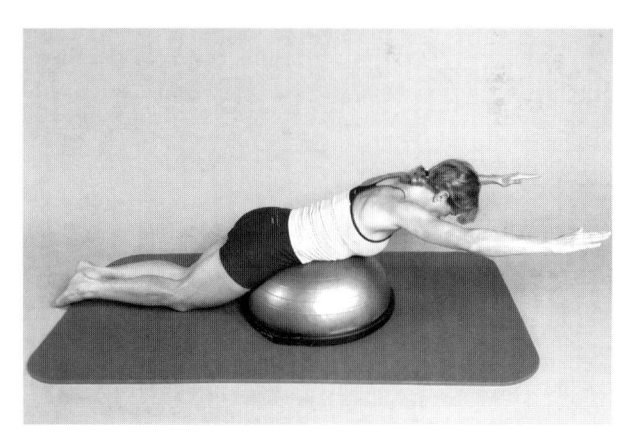

Start prone on the BOSU® with the arms overhead, the spine and pelvis neutral, the legs extended hip-width apart, hips neutral (knee on or off), and the ankles plantar flexed. Inhale to prepare; exhale, extend the cervical and thoracic spine sequentially, and lift the upper extremities off the floor, maintaining neutral spine and pelvis, legs on the floor.

Progression 3

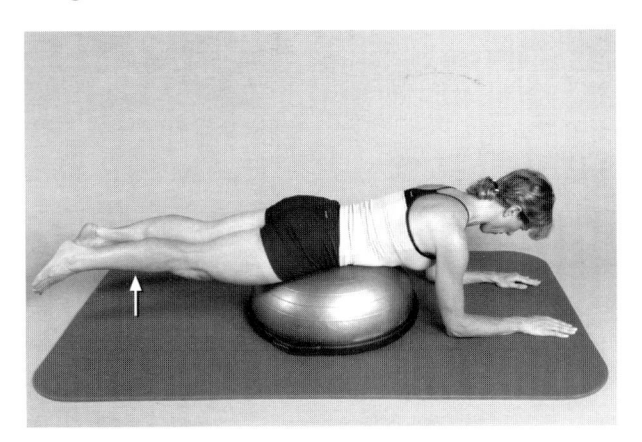

Start prone on the BOSU® with the arms positioned on the floor and the elbows beneath the shoulders, the spine and pelvis neutral, the legs extended hip-width apart, hips neutral, and the ankles plantar flexed. Inhale to prepare; exhale and extend the hips to lift the lower extremities off the floor, maintaining neutral spine and pelvis, hands on the floor.

Progression 4

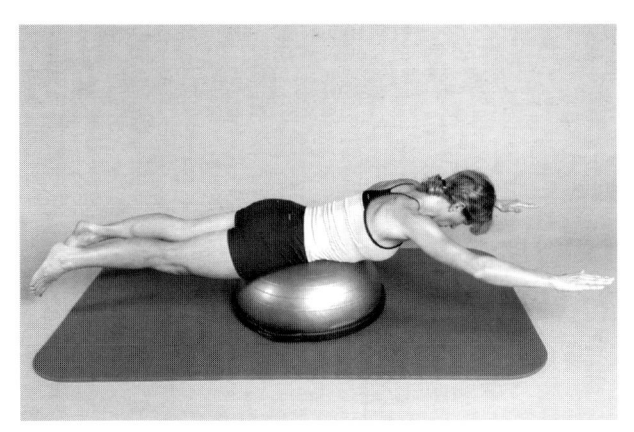

Start prone on the BOSU® with arms overhead, the spine and pelvis neutral, the legs extended hip-width apart, and the ankles plantar flexed. Inhale to prepare; exhale and extend the cervical/thoracic spine and hips, lifting the upper and lower extremities off the floor, maintaining neutral spine and pelvis.

Editor's note: Avoid performing Progression 4 on a stability ball. Progressions 1-3 modified on ball.

Torso: Stabilization, Rotation, and Lateral Flexion

Knee Sways, Heels on Ball

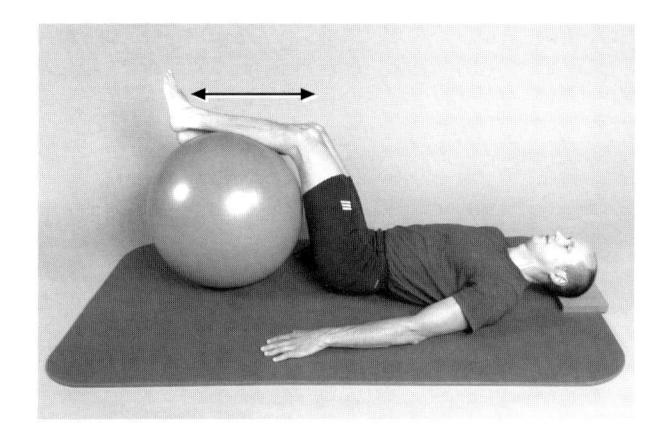

This is a great exercise for initially teaching your patient what rotation feels like. Start supine with neutral pelvis, the ankles plantar flexed with the feet resting on the ball, the hips adducted and the hips/knees flexed to 90 degrees, the arms alongside the body, the scapulae stabilized, and the elbows slightly bent, palms down on the mat.

Inhale to prepare. Exhale and sway the hips/legs to the right, maintaining neutral and keeping the upper extremities still, with emphasis on sequential rotation at the thoracic spine. Inhale to return the knees to the center.

Helpful tip: This exercise provides an opportunity to observe/challenge/teach spinal rotation and pelvic stabilization capabilities. It is a good exercise to introduce prior to oblique strengthening and the Spine Twist in sitting.

Spine Twist with Exercise Band

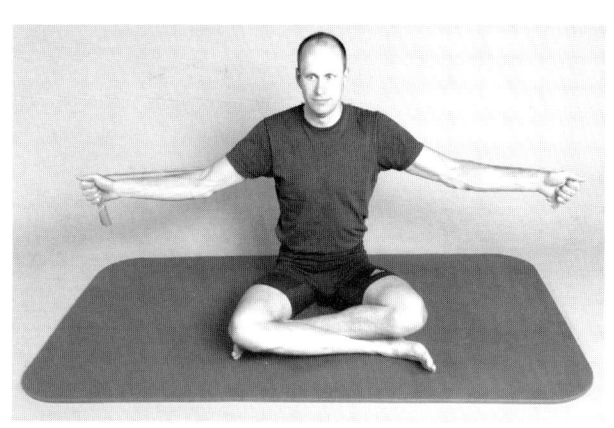

Progress from Knee Sways to the Spine Twist once your patient "feels" rotation in a supine position. Sit in a chair or on a mat with neutral pelvis, spine, and neck and the shoulders aligned over the pelvis. Position the exercise band across the back, just beneath the scapulae, hands on the ends of the band. Abduct the shoulders to 90 degrees with the palms forward. Inhale to prepare.

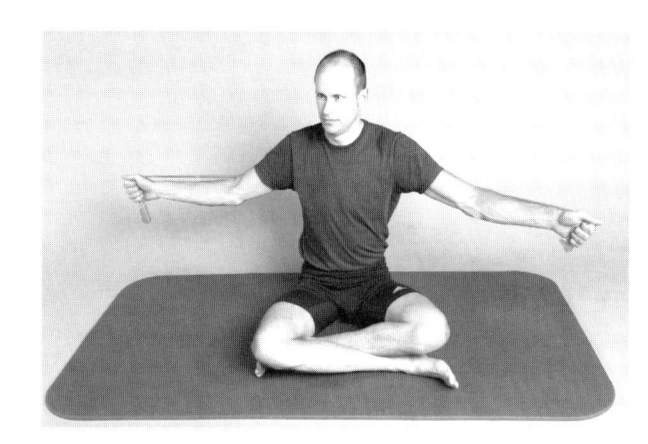

Exhale; rotate to the right one to three times, increasing rotational range with each exhale. Inhale and return to the center.

This exercise challenges scapular and lumbo-pelvic stabilization with spinal rotation; the band enhances kinesthetic awareness and strengthens the middle deltoid muscles.

Equipment Variations:

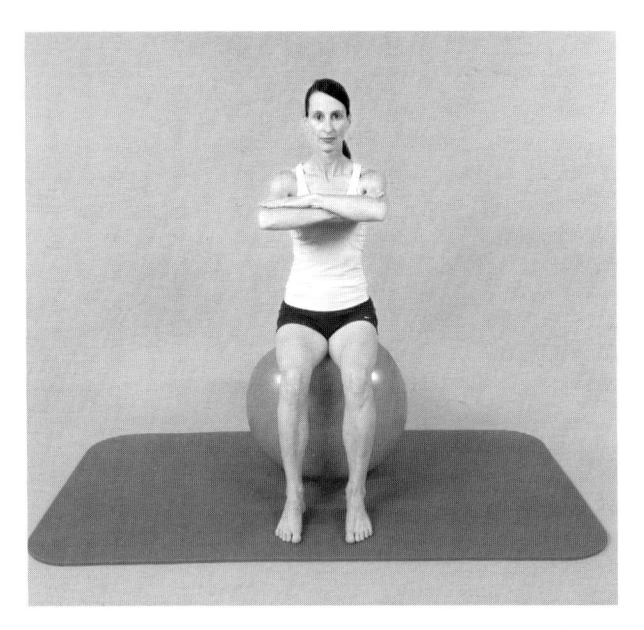

Sit on a stability ball with the arms crossed in front of the body; kneel on a BOSU®; stand holding tubing or a stability ball in the hands

Spine Twist: Standing Lunge on BOSU®

Start in lunge position with neutral spine and pelvis, with the right foot on the BOSU® and the shoulders aligned over the pelvis. The shoulders are abducted to 90 degrees with the palms down. The left foot is aligned with the left ASIS behind the body, with the weight centered over the metatarsals. Slowly lower into the lunge (left knee dropping toward the floor and right knee moving forward), maintaining balance via the primary and secondary core stabilizers.

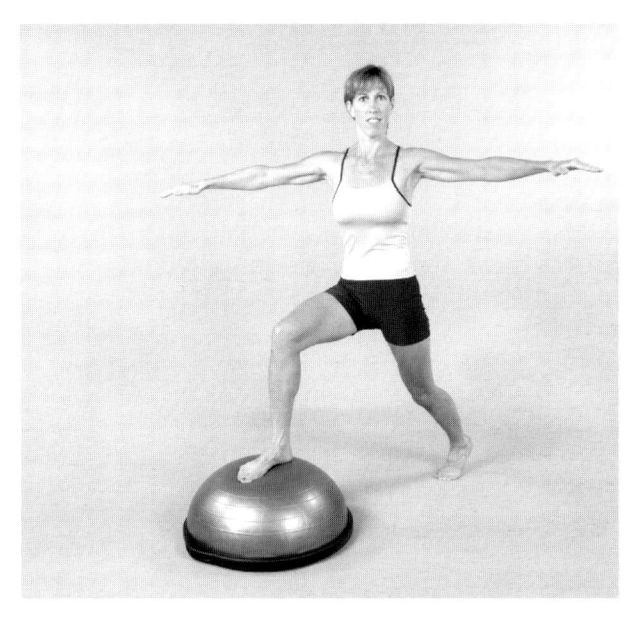

Hold the lunge position. Inhale to prepare. Exhale; rotate to the left one to three times, increasing rotational range with each exhale. Inhale and return to the center. Repeat on the opposite side. *Variations:* Simultaneous lunge with spinal rotation; hold a lightweight Body Bar or medicine ball.

Helpful tips: Use this exercise to simulate sport-specific movement patterns such as running, ice skating, basketball, and cross-country or telemark skiing. This advanced movement pattern challenges dynamic stabilization on unstable surfaces while simultaneously mobilizing the thoracic spine in the transverse plane and the lower extremities in the sagittal plane.

Mermaid: Lateral Flexion in Sitting

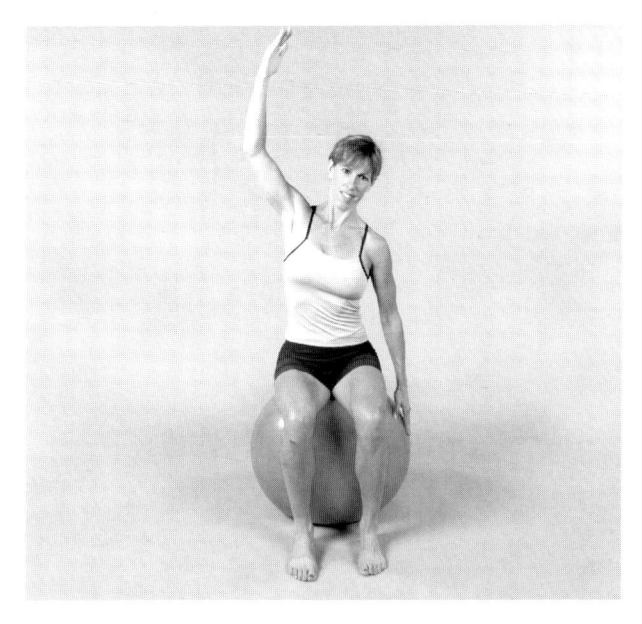

Sit on a chair or ball in neutral spine and pelvis, the ribs aligned over the pelvis, with the knees flexed 90 degrees and the hips abducted to shoulder-width apart. The hands are on the outside of the ball with the right palm facing up. Inhale to prepare, then abduct the right shoulder to 180 degrees. Exhale and left trunk side bend while maintaining neutral pelvis.

Helpful tip: Use this and other exercises that emphasize lateral flexion with patients who require lengthening and strengthening of the lateral torso flexors and for sport-specific training for dancers and others whose sports require lateral flexion, such as volleyball players or figure skaters.

Trunk Side Bend on a Ball or BOSU®

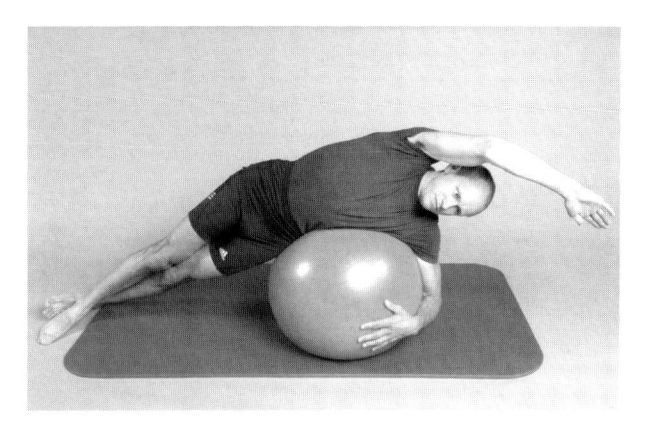

Lie sideways on a ball or BOSU® with the pelvis/lumbar spine centered on it, the left hip resting on the decline of the surface. The hips/knees are extended and may be stacked on each other or scissored one in front of the other for bracing. The left hand is placed on the floor or ball. The right shoulder is abducted to 180 degrees, and the scapulae are stabilized.

Inhale and abduct the right shoulder to 90 degrees. Exhale, adduct the shoulder another 90 degrees, and laterally flex the spine right while lifting the torso off the ball at the same time, moving sequentially from the top of the head to the lumbar spine. The arm reaches long down the thigh; the head follows the line of the spine. Inhale and abduct the shoulder to 90 degrees, exhale, and sequentially articulate the spine onto the ball and abduct the shoulder to the starting position.

Hips: Joint Mobilization and Strengthening

Leg Press with Ball or Foam Roller

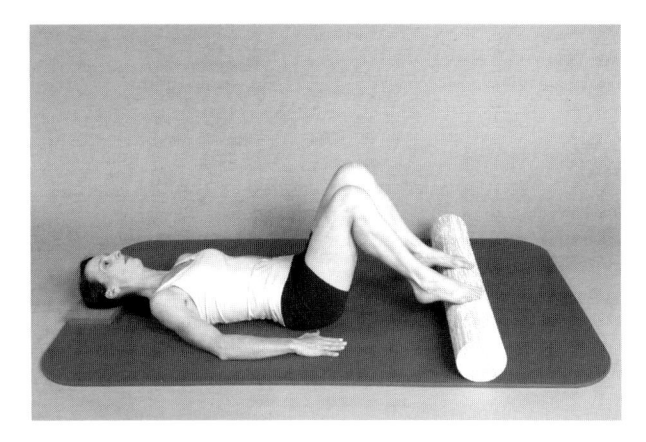

Start supine with neutral pelvis, neutral head and cervical alignment, the hips and knees flexed to 90 degrees, the feet hip-width apart on the ball or roller, the ankles plantar flexed with the feet flat on the surface. The arms are alongside the body, and the elbows are slightly bent, with the palms facing down on the floor.

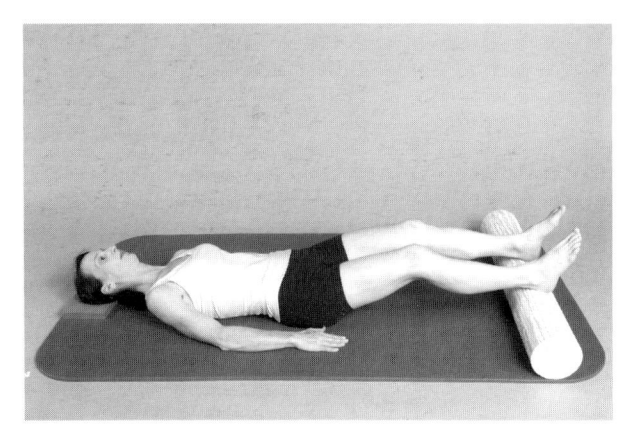

Inhale to prepare. Exhale and extend the hips and knees to roll the ball or roller away from the torso while maintaining neutral pelvis. Inhale and flex the hips and knees, drawing the ball or roller toward the torso.

Helpful tips:

1. When using a foam roller, start with the toes on the edge of the roller and evenly press through the feet as the roller moves forward, and then reverse heel to toe.

2. When using the stability ball, as the hips and knees extend, press the heels as the ankles move to neutral onto the surface. Maintain heel pressure on ball throughout the exercise.

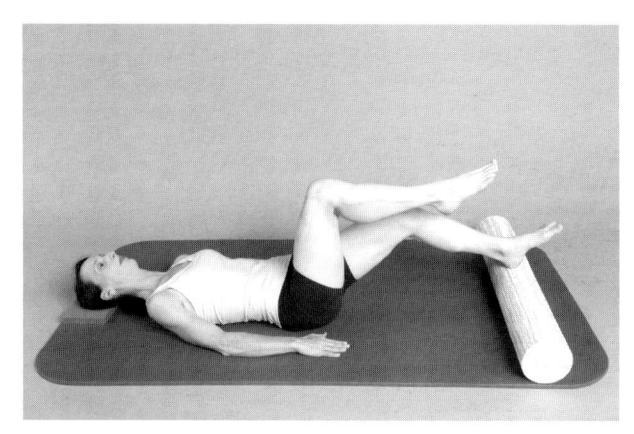

Variations: Single-Leg Press (as shown) with the contralateral foot on the floor, in tabletop, or in diagonal position in the air; combine with simultaneous Shoulder Bridge

One-Leg Circle with Exercise Band

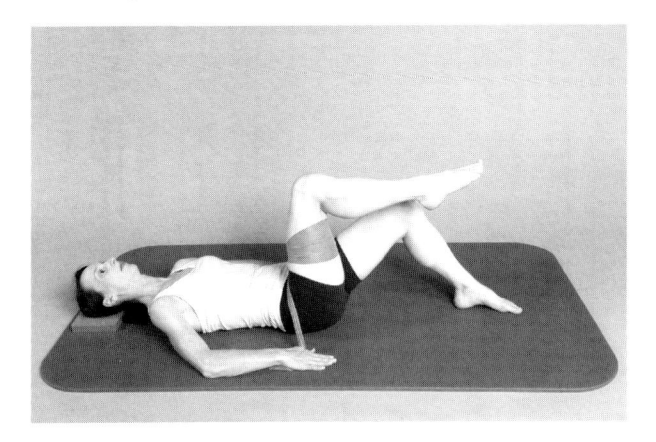

Start supine with neutral pelvis, one leg in the air with the hip flexed to 90 degrees. Place the band behind the thigh in the air, then wrap it around the sides of the thigh and cross it in front of the thigh. The shoulders are abducted to 45 degrees and the wrists are neutral, with the hands stabilizing the tubing with slight tension on the mat. The other leg is flexed at the knee and hip, the arms alongside the body, the scapulae stabilized. The ankles are plantar flexed.

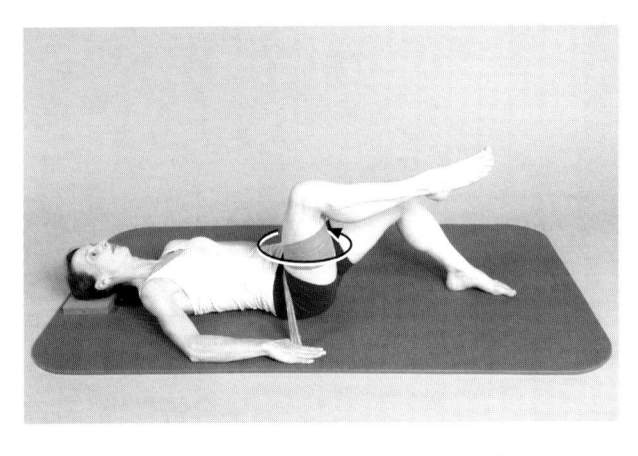

Inhale, maintain neutral, and make a half circle into the band with the leg in the air moving toward the midline. Exhale and complete the circle, moving the leg away from the midline into the band; pause at the top of the circle. Repeat five times in each direction.

Teaching tip: To facilitate neuromuscular reeducation of the hip muscles with the exercise band. Break down the exercise into the following movement patterns and feel the muscles: abduction, extension, adduction, and flexion. Now have the patient try the full exercise with the band, feeling the muscles within each movement.

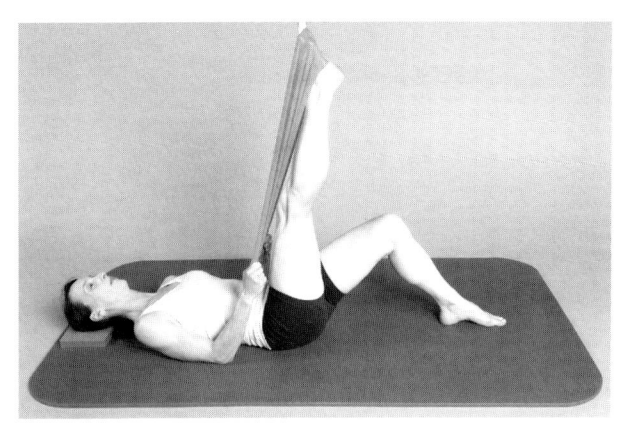

Variation: Band or tube placed across the plantar surface at the base of the metatarsals, the leg long.

One-Leg Circle on Foam Roller

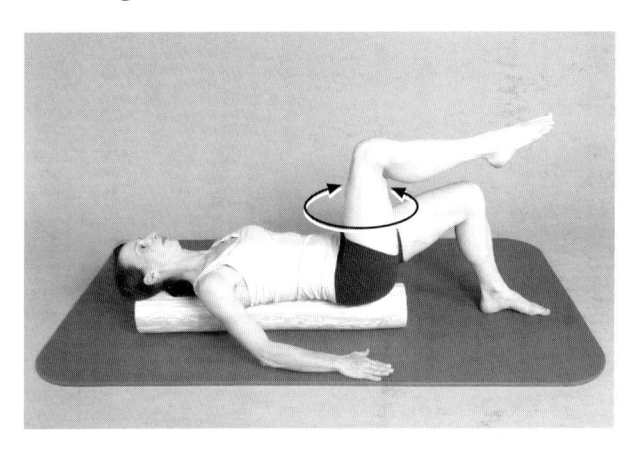

Start supine on a roller with neutral pelvis, one leg extended in the air with the hip flexed to 90 degrees. Align the other leg with the ASIS and flex the knee to 90 degrees. Maintain spinal stabilization on the roller while simultaneously making a half circle toward the midline with the inhale and a half circle away from the midline with the exhale. Repeat five times and reverse direction.

Variation: Flex shoulders to 90 degrees.

Helpful hints: Stabilize through the foot on the floor and begin with a small circle. Remember, the focus is stability before mobility.

Bend and Stretch with Ball

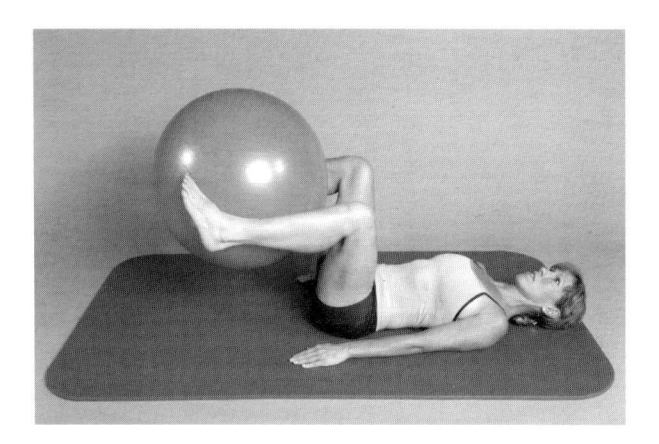

Start supine with neutral pelvis/spine, head, and cervical alignment, the knees and hips flexed, the hips externally rotated outside the shoulders, the ankles dorsiflexed, and a small or large ball held gently between the ankles or calves. The arms are alongside the body, the elbows slightly bent, with the palms facing down. Inhale and breathe into the back and sides of the ribs, maintaining neutral pelvis.

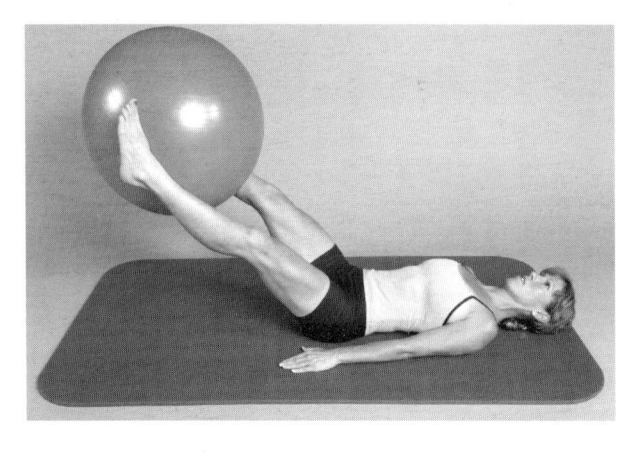

Exhale and imprint the pelvis/spine, then extend the hips/knees to move the ball toward the ceiling. Maintain the hips in external rotation. Inhale and return to the initial position and neutral pelvis. For more challenge, extend the hips and knees with the ball on the diagonal. Repeat 5 to 10 times.

Variations: Limited range of motion (knees/hips in external rotation).

Spine Rolls, Feet on Ball or Foam Roller

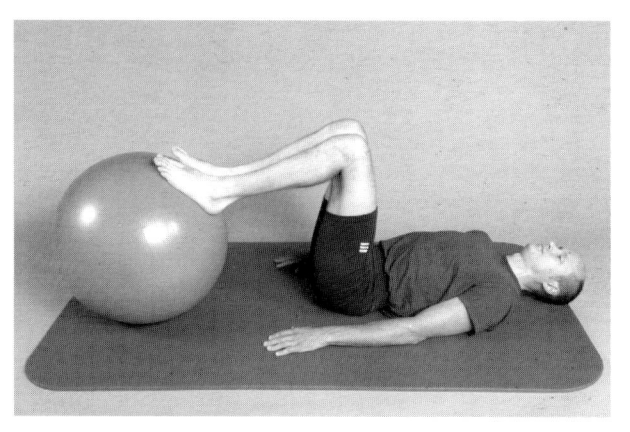

Start supine with neutral spine, head, and cervical alignment, the hips/knees bent to 90 degrees, the ankles plantar flexed, the feet flat on the ball or roller, and the hips adducted. The arms are alongside the body, the elbows slightly bent, with the palms facing down on the floor. Inhale to prepare.

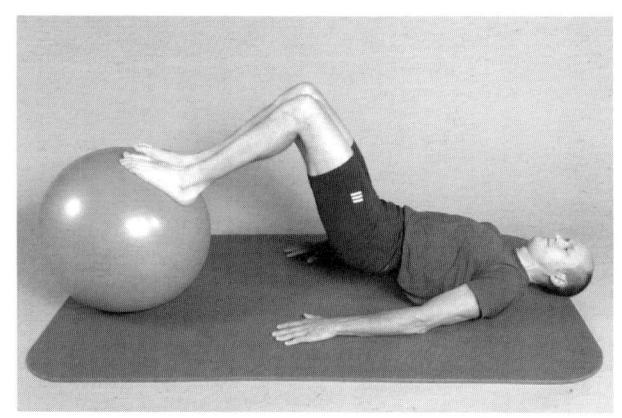

Exhale, imprint the pelvis, press the feet into the ball or roller, and sequentially lift the spine off the mat, leading with the tailbone and progressing to the upper thoracic region. Avoid putting pressure on the cervical spine.

Variation: Hips abducted.

Shoulder Bridge Modification, Feet on Ball or Roller

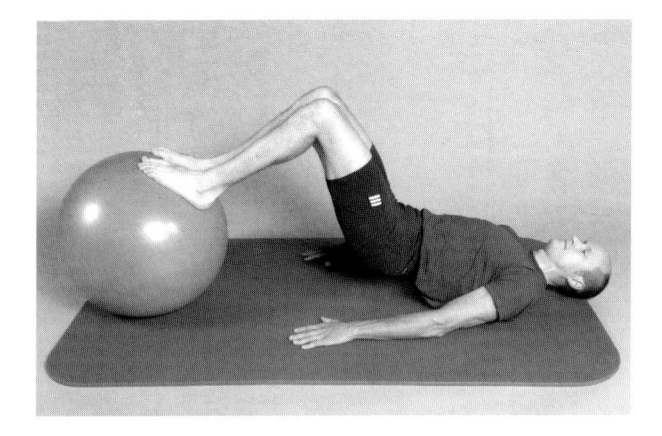

Start supine with neutral spine, head, and cervical alignment, the hips/knees bent to 90 degrees, the ankles plantar flexed, the feet flat on the ball, and the hips adducted. The arms are alongside the body, the elbows slightly bent, with the palms facing down on the floor.

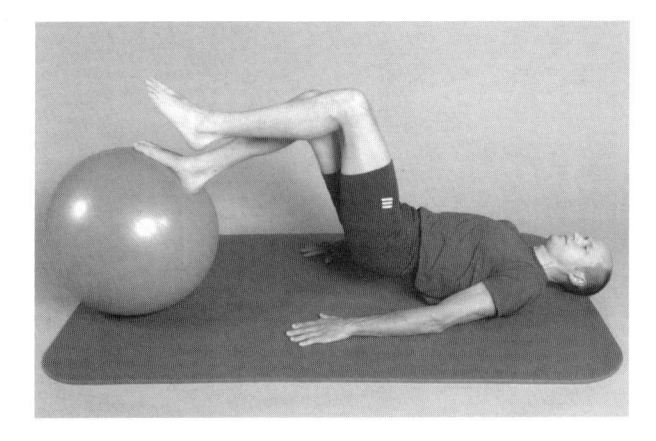

Exhale, lift the torso off the floor, keeping the pelvis and spine in neutral and extending the hips to create a Bridge position from the scapulae to the knees (pressure on the upper thoracic spine); push the feet into the ball or roller to increase hip extensor involvement. Inhale, keep the pelvis level, flex at the knee and hip, and lift one foot off the ball or roller. Exhale and put the foot back on the ball or roller, and switch legs.

Variations: Hips abducted; hip or knee extension.

Hip Abduction/Adduction Progressions

Practitioner's tip: Layer exercises of choice one after another; repeat on the other side.

Side kneel on the left side of the ball with the pelvis, spine, and hips in neutral. Place the left hand on the side of the ball. The scapulae are stabilized.

Hip Abduction

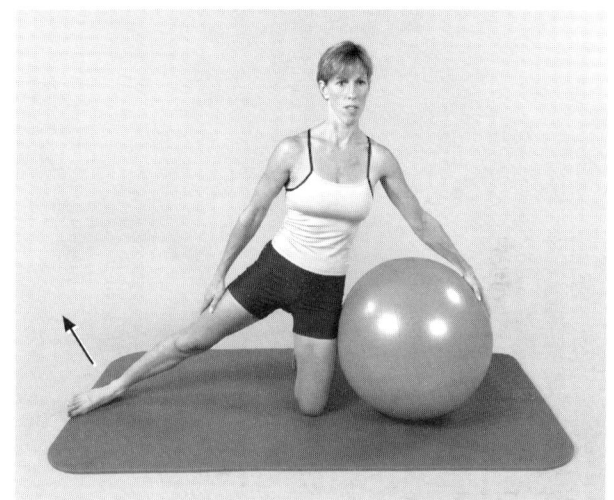

Inhale and plantar flex the right ankle and abduct the right hip, maintaining neutral pelvis, and spine. Exhale, adduct hip to the initial position.

Equipment Variations:

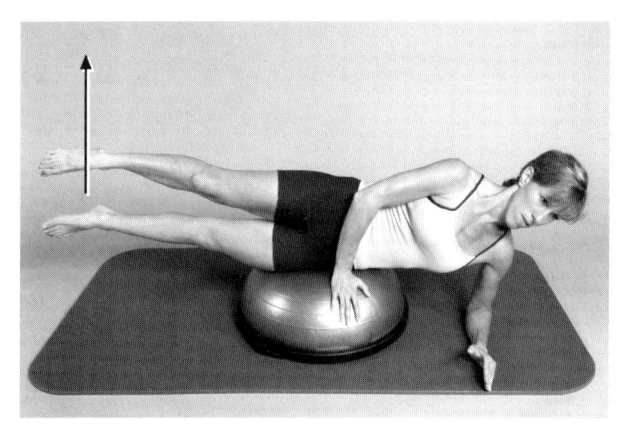

Lie on one side with the hip placed on the middle of the BOSU®, the torso supported by placing the arm/elbow beneath the shoulder.

161

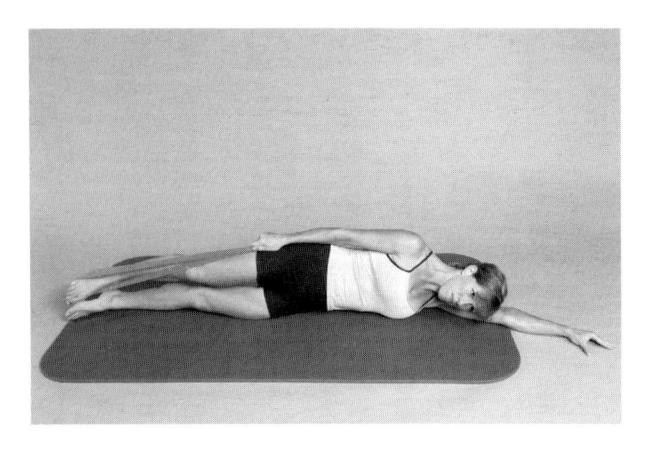

Exercise band or resistance tubing (advanced).

Leg Circles

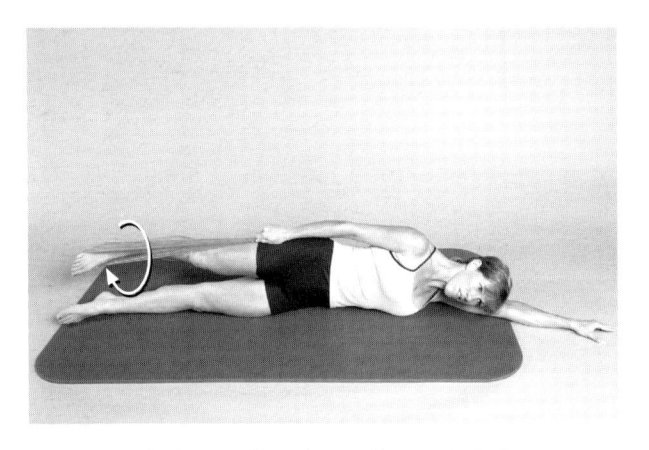

Inhale and plantar flex the ankle and abduct the hip on top to hip height with neutral pelvis. Exhale and begin a pattern of circling the top leg forward. Inhale halfway through the pattern, with the leg moving back to complete the circle.

Clam with Exercise Band

Start lying on one side with the pelvis and spine in neutral. The hips are adducted and the hips and knees are flexed to 45 to 60 degrees with the band wrapped taut around the distal thighs. The shoulder on the mat is flexed, providing support for the head. The arm on top is positioned in front of the sternum. The scapulae are stabilized.

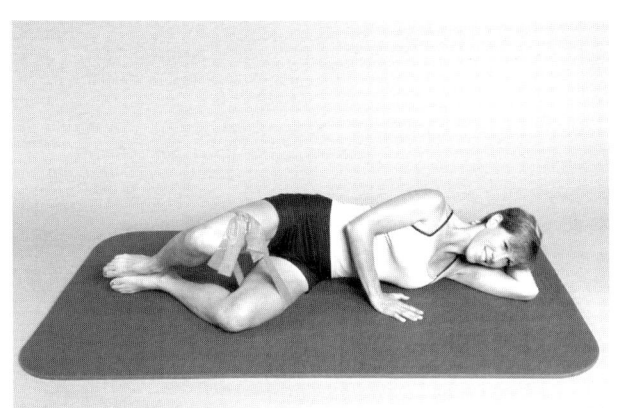

Inhale to prepare. Exhale and externally rotate the top hip, and stop just before the point where the patient cannot maintain neutral pelvis/spine. The opposite leg supports the movement through stabilization. Layer the exercise with the addition of Hip Abduction.

Variations: Bent-Knee Fallout in supine.

Purpose:

- Challenging dissociation of the femur from the pelvis in the transverse plane against the resistance of tubing
- Hip strengthening
- Hip mobility

Clinical Application:

- Use this advanced movement pattern to challenge movement of the femur from the pelvis against resistance
- Lumbo-pelvic stabilization via IM contraction of the TrA, obliques, and multifidus
- Concentric/eccentric strengthening of the gluteus medius
- Suggested patient populations: Total hip replacement per guidelines; tight anterior hip capsule; tight hip adductor muscles; advanced neuromuscular training for pelvic instability noted with gait/running mechanics

Faulty Movement Patterns: Inability to maintain pelvic/spinal stability; increased posterior tilt when externally rotating at the hip; inability to fire the hip abductors; weight shifting back; not maintaining the natural curve of the waist (trunk side bend); hip hiking or flexing; upper body tension

Hip Extension on Ball or BOSU®

Start prone on a BOSU® with the pelvis centered and neutral, the elbows positioned below the shoulder joints, and the legs extended long, hip-distance apart. The ankles are slightly plantar flexed. Stabilize the scapulae and position the cervical spine in neutral.

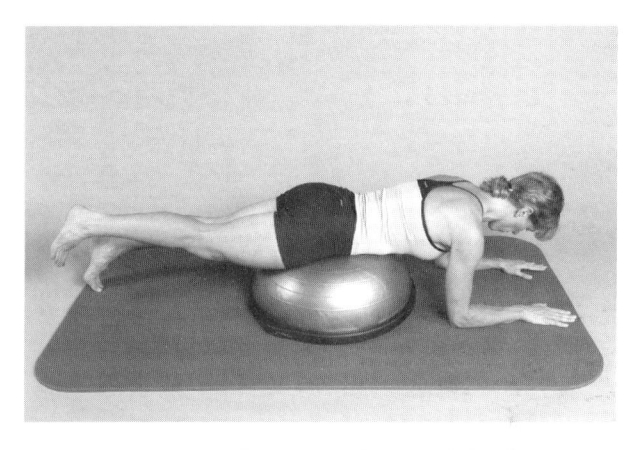

Inhale to prepare. Exhale and extend the hip, lifting one leg off the BOSU® while keeping the pelvis neutral and still. Inhale and flex the hip, returning the leg to the BOSU®.

Helpful tip: Advance this exercise to the Opposite Arm/Leg Lift with the feet/hands on the floor, with a focus on lumbo-pelvic and shoulder stabilization.

Upper Extremity Strengthening and Mobilization

Rolling Plank on Stability Ball

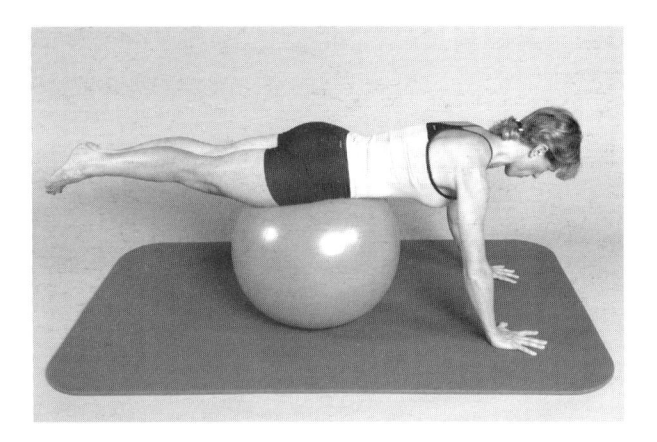

Start prone on the ball with the pelvis centered and neutral, the hands positioned just outside the shoulders, the legs extended long, the hips adducted, and the ankles slightly plantar flexed. Stabilize the scapulae and cervical spine in neutral.

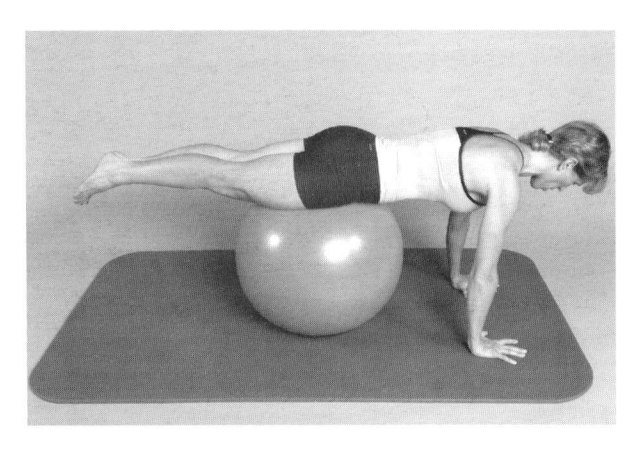

Inhale to stabilize the spine, pelvis, and shoulders. Exhale and extend the shoulders to pull the torso forward over the ball, maintaining neutral pelvis. Inhale and flex the shoulders, pulling the torso backward over the ball, maintaining neutral pelvis.

Leg Pull Front Warm-up with Exercise Band

Start in quadruped position with an exercise band placed at the base of the scapulae, the hands aligned just outside the shoulders and holding onto the ends of the band. The hips are adducted with the knees beneath the hips, the pelvis and spine in neutral, and the scapulae slightly protracted and depressed. The toes are extended, the hands opened like a starfish, with equal weight distribution front to back.

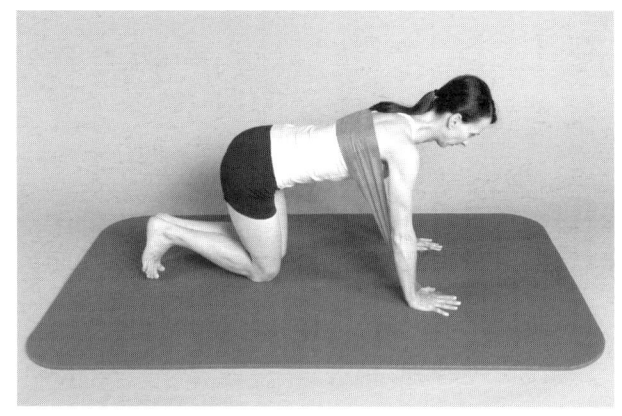

Inhale to further connect with the deep lumbo-pelvic stabilizers. Exhale, keeping the spine and pelvis neutral, and lift the knees off the mat about 2 inches. This is a good exercise to teach prior to Pushups to enhance scapular awareness and muscle endurance.

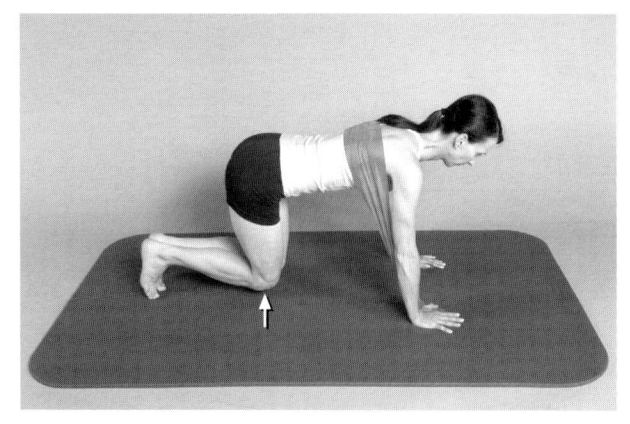

Helpful hint: The exercise band can be used in two ways: first, to help maintain scapular stabilization via sensory feedback; second, to enhance co-activation of the shoulder and scapulae muscles and increase their strength via the band's resistance.

Leg Pull Front Warm-up on BOSU®

Start in quadruped position with neutral pelvis/cervical alignment and place the hands along the sides of the BOSU® with the dome side down. The scapulae are slightly protracted/depressed, the hips adducted, and the toes extended.

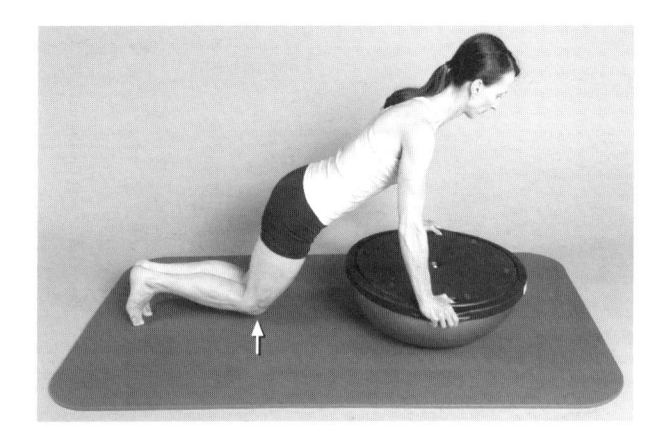

While maintaining stability with the primary and secondary stabilizers, lift the knees off the mat about 2 inches. Return the knees to the mat. Follow the breath pattern in Chapter 6. *Variations:* Lift to plank position; foam roller under hands; hips abducted.

Helpful hints: To start with optimal neutral alignment of the spine, begin by aligning the spine and torso sequentially from the cervical to the lumbar spine. This advanced closed chain exercise challenges dynamic stabilization on an unstable surface and offers sport-specific training for activities such as gymnastics, wrestling, and football.

Pushups in Plank on the Ball or BOSU®

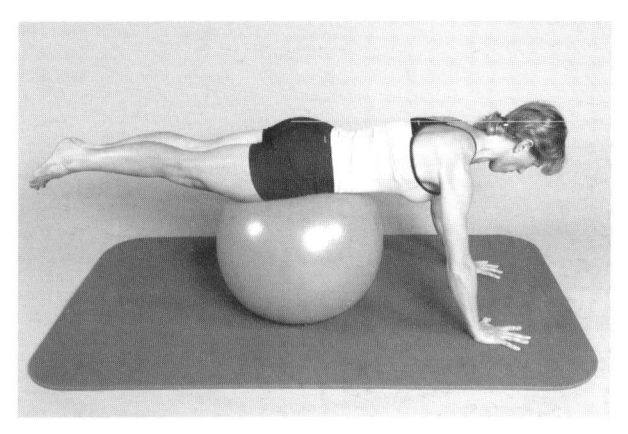

Start prone on the ball with the pelvis centered and neutral, the hands positioned just outside the shoulder joints, the legs extended long, the hips adducted, and the ankles slightly plantar flexed. Stabilize the scapulae and cervical spine in neutral.

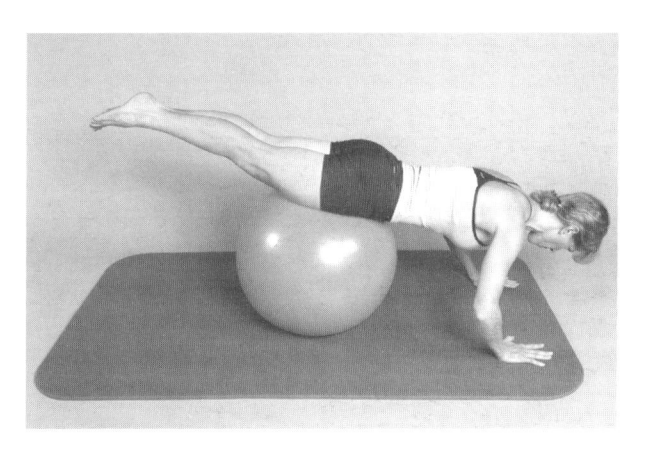

Inhale, stabilize the torso, and bend at the elbows/shoulders to lower the body toward the floor for a count of three inhales. Exhale once and push up from the floor by extending the elbows.

Variations: Change the lever length of the lower extremities (move the pelvis off the ball to more challenging positions; for example, hip to ankle); change hand positions (together, beneath the shoulder joint, elbows at sides, staggered)

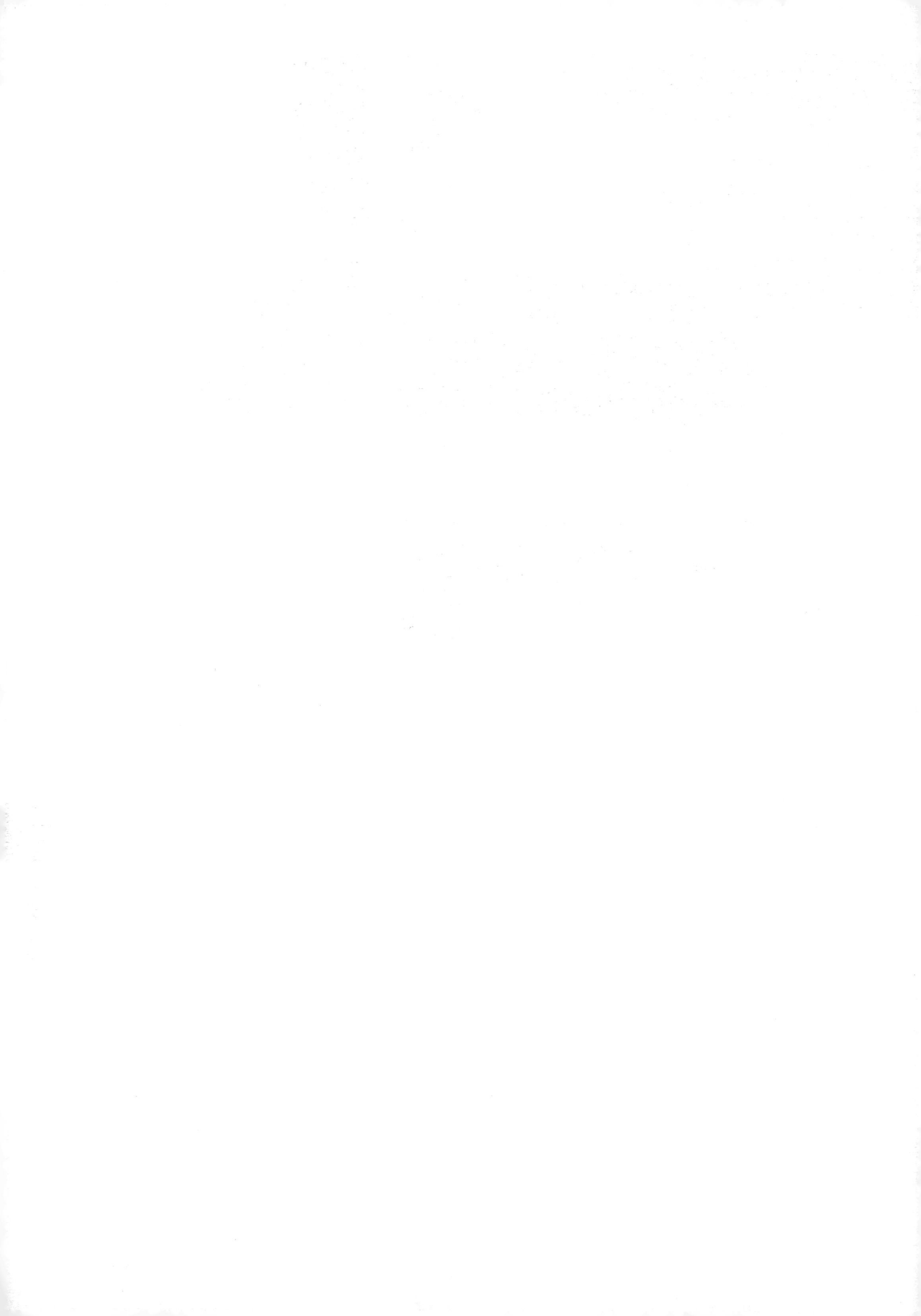

chapter 9

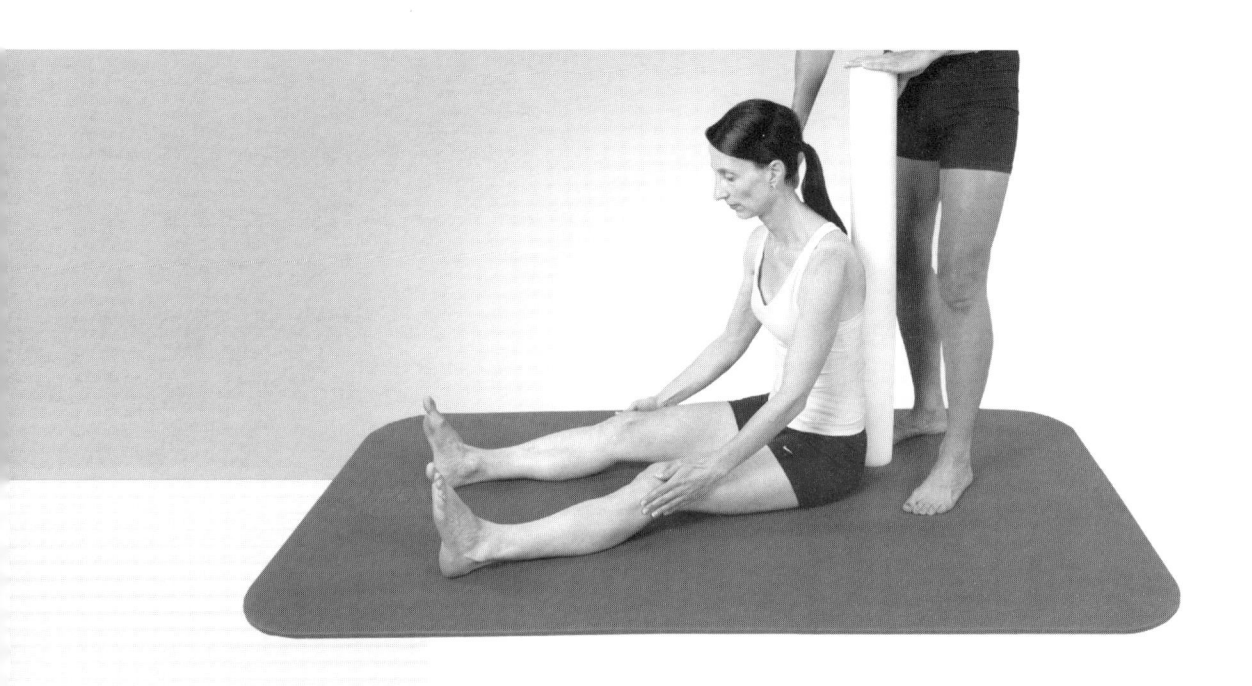

THE ART OF
TEACHING

Rehabilitation and fitness professionals are movement educators. We observe our patients' movement patterns, teach them about how their bodies move, and train them to improve their proprioceptive skills so that they can improve their function. *We help them to help themselves heal.* Key to our teaching is our communication: how we talk—verbally and nonverbally—to our patients to put them on the road to health and wellness.

Unfortunately, most clinicians don't learn patient communication strategies in the classroom. Once in practice, some clinicians will successfully learn how to best inspire patients to heal through well-honed communication skills, while others will continue to experience less than satisfactory patient outcomes and wonder why.

Teaching patients is an art form that is carefully cultivated over time with practice, additional training, and a desire to reach patients on a different level. Effective communication with your patient can reap these benefits:

- Create a mind-body connection to improve concentration, control, and quality movement
- Increase knowledge of the body and how it functions
- Engage key muscles
- Improve kinesthetic awareness
- Assist coordination
- Achieve the desired motor response while avoiding fatigue
- Improve exercise program adherence

"The Art of Teaching" introduces you to some ideas to help you better communicate with your patients and suggests some strategies for progressing patients through hands-on and verbal cueing.

Teaching Fundamental Movement Patterns

Retraining motor patterns starts with assessing your patient's ability to perform the exercise or movement pattern you've given him or her. From the start, be alert for compensatory strategies and determine how you can best achieve the desired movement outcome and your patient's satisfaction using the strategies below.

- Breathing
- Pelvic positioning
- Scapular control
- Rib cage postioning
- Head and neck positioning

1. **Start with the Pilates principles to create the foundation for successful, effective movement.** Successfully teaching functional movement patterns begins with teaching your patient the Pilates-based principles of core stabilization at the cervical spine, scapulae, ribs, and pelvis and how to coordinate breath with movement.

   It isn't enough to go through the movement patterns and ask patients to perform them. Discuss why stabilization is important to their movement quality and how it may help prevent injury recurrence or contribute to the healing process. Demonstrate and explain the purpose and essential components of the exercise, what the patient should be feeling with the movement, and how stabilization with exercise and movement can help improve his or her daily function with ADLs, work, or sport. Break down each principle and work toward mastery. It can help to begin with technical instruction of the movement pattern and observe the movement before applying cueing techniques.

   If your patient doesn't have good body awareness, alignment, or the ability to perform the principles in isolation or in combination with each other, don't progress to more difficult exercises until he or she is ready. Increase the patient's awareness about faulty movement patterns. Does it have to be perfect? No, but practice is needed to continue to refine quality of movement. In our experience, most people, whether patient or athlete, will not perform the principles perfectly. Rely on your observational skills and intuition to advance patients when appropriate.

2. **Know the goal of each exercise.** Each Pilates-based exercise has a goal. Some exercises focus on mobilization and stabilization, while others add focus on sequential mobilization, coordination, balance, or muscle stamina. Some exercises have multiple goals. As exercises progress from basic and intermediate to advanced, be aware that exercise goals

change or become more complex. Generally, fundamental exercises focus on stabilization, mobilization, and uniplanar and unijoint movement patterns of the upper and lower extremities to develop the foundation for advanced exercises. More advanced exercises challenge muscle stamina, balance, and coordination.

3. **Introduce bite-size movement patterns.** The nuances of Pilates can be overwhelming for patients (and clinicians) to learn at first. Breathing, pelvis and scapular positioning—patients may feel they need an engineering degree just to get through the principles.

   Rehabilitation professionals can help make the task less daunting by introducing movement in bite-size patterns. Choose one movement or task on which to focus, such as breathing or pelvic placement. Demonstrate the movement first without technical instruction and ask the patient to mirror you. Create movement awareness by having your patient first experience incorrect movement and then self-correct through use of the principles.

4. **Practice the movement or task until it has been mastered.** Help the patient to become excited about feeling the muscle(s) working correctly. Introduce the nuances of technical instruction next: identify target muscles and their attachments and actions, sequential movement of joints, and proper alignment.

5. **Sharpen your communication skills.** The language you use to talk with your patient can help or hinder your success. Words you use to address body alignment, muscle facilitation/inhibition, and exercise execution should be tailored to your audience.

   Who is your audience? Think about the patients with whom you work: young, old, male, female, executive, line worker. Each will respond positively to you once you've identified the communication style that works best for him or her.

   From technical instruction and visual imagery to the use of equipment or touch, the savvy practitioner has many tools from which to choose. Some tools are commonly used in the rehabilitation setting. Others are not. From our perspective, the more tools you use, the more options. Remember, everyone learns differently; some tools will work better than others.

   a. *Technical, action-oriented skills.* Technical instruction that encourages a desired action is a teaching fundamental and can be used to refine an exercise or movement pattern. Used wisely, technical instruction can help to modify an exercise or to correct faulty movement pattern(s).

   Example: "More than 58 percent of your abdominal muscles connect to the rib cage. Action: "As you are lifting your arms overhead, keep your ribs centered over your pelvis to keep the abdominals working at their best."

   b. *Sensory skills.* Sensory awareness is essential to functional movement. Day to day, all of us use our visual, auditory, and kinesthetic senses to automatically experience movement for work, activities of daily living, and athletics. While all senses are used to some degree, each of us uses a "primary" sense to process information (2). In a clinical setting, use of imagery, touch, and voice can be called upon to help improve your patient's outcomes.

   - Imagery. Imagery is a sensory awareness technique that has been used successfully in neuromuscular retraining dating as far back as the early 1900s. Choose images that your patients can relate to and that are age-appropriate. For further information, see Chapter 10, "Imagery: Creating a Mind-Body Connection."
   - Touch and kinesthetic. Tactile and/or kinesthetic cueing is a powerful tool for providing information to specific portions of the body that are being mobilized or stabilized. Tactile feedback can enhance kinesthetic cueing through stimulation of skin exteroceptors to facilitate desired motor response(s). Skin-to-skin contact that is firm and localized to the area where you want to elicit a response is best. Avoid general contact because it can lead to muscle inhibition and faulty movement.
   - Auditory. Your voice is a great a communication tool. Talk with a voice that is resonant and well-

modulated in tone, rhythm, pacing, inflection, and volume to influence execution of an exercise, your patient's motivation, or the stress level of a patient when they are performing a movement pattern.

c. *Cueing skills:* Learning to "cue" an exercise allows you to take advantage of your technical and sensory expertise and to fine-tune your use of imagery and touch. Use these tips to advance your practice.

- Introduce only one cue at a time, and customize your cues based on your patient's learning style and what you feel is appropriate. Cues can be modified to facilitate a desired motor response. Change a visual cue to a kinesthetic cue if you aren't eliciting the desired response.
- Develop a library of cues to avoid monotony and enhance the mind-body connection. Some cues will work; others will not.
- Use inclusive statements such as "Let's," "We," or "Our." Avoid using "I" statements when you are teaching your patient: "I want you to . . ." (3).
- Use action- and image-oriented words to describe the movement patterns you want your patient to perform. Examples: "Painting a line," "Drawing a circle," or "Hinging at the hips" (3).
- Talk to your patient in the present tense. Examples: "Stand in an athletic-ready position," "Notice what muscles are working hardest," or "Pay attention to the position of your wrists" (2)
- Use mirrors for visual feedback. Ask patients to watch themselves in the mirror to see and feel ideal form and alignment. Eventually, discontinue the use of the mirror so they can advance their kinesthetic awareness skills.

Try This Exercise

Identify the senses you rely on to "feel" the world. Review the Three Sensing Modalities chart and identify your primary sensory learning modality (2). Now use the chart to strengthen your communication skills in other sensing areas. Try to identify your patient's primary sense to better understand how he or she learns and to enhance your communication skills.

Three Sensing Modalities

Primary Learning Sense	How You Learn	Responds Best	Cueing Suggestions
Kinesthetic	Trusts intuition; "feels" things	When information is routed through the body	"Feel the weight evenly distributed on your entire foot."
Visual	Observes the exercise before trying; pictures an image	To pictures and exercises in writing and to demonstration of exercises	"Look at how I am standing," or "Imagine you are drawing a straight line with your toe."
Auditory	Learns about world, activity, or person through sound of voice	To the tone, volume, and rhythm of voice when learning something new	Concentrate on how you say things: "Listen to how your breath sounds when you exhale."

Adapted from Sachs, L.D. 2003. Strategic communication. Idea Health and Fitness Source, February. Used by author permission (2).

- Teach patients about their unique movement patterns first and observe their movement. Then ask them how it feels when movement is correct and incorrect. Patients should be familiar with common bony landmarks and major muscles and should understand their muscle imbalances and how those imbalances impact their movement or may contribute to injury.

- Communicate to the level of your patients and clients. Identify their primary sensory modality for motor learning. Remember that some may not respond well to imagery techniques. Others won't respond well to kinesthetic cueing.

- Cueing should be clear, age-appropriate, and specific for desired movements.

- Cue a foundational movement first and then add cues and movement patterns to challenge stability, coordination, balance, etc.

Chapter References

1. *STOTT Pilates*. 2001. Supplementary Notes, *STOTT Pilates Certification Course*, St. Paul, MN.

2. Sachs, L.D. 2003. Strategic communication. *Idea Health and Fitness Source*, February.

3. Shaw, B. 2001. *YogaFit Training Manual*, Level 1 Certification Program, Winona, MN, February 10-11, 2002.

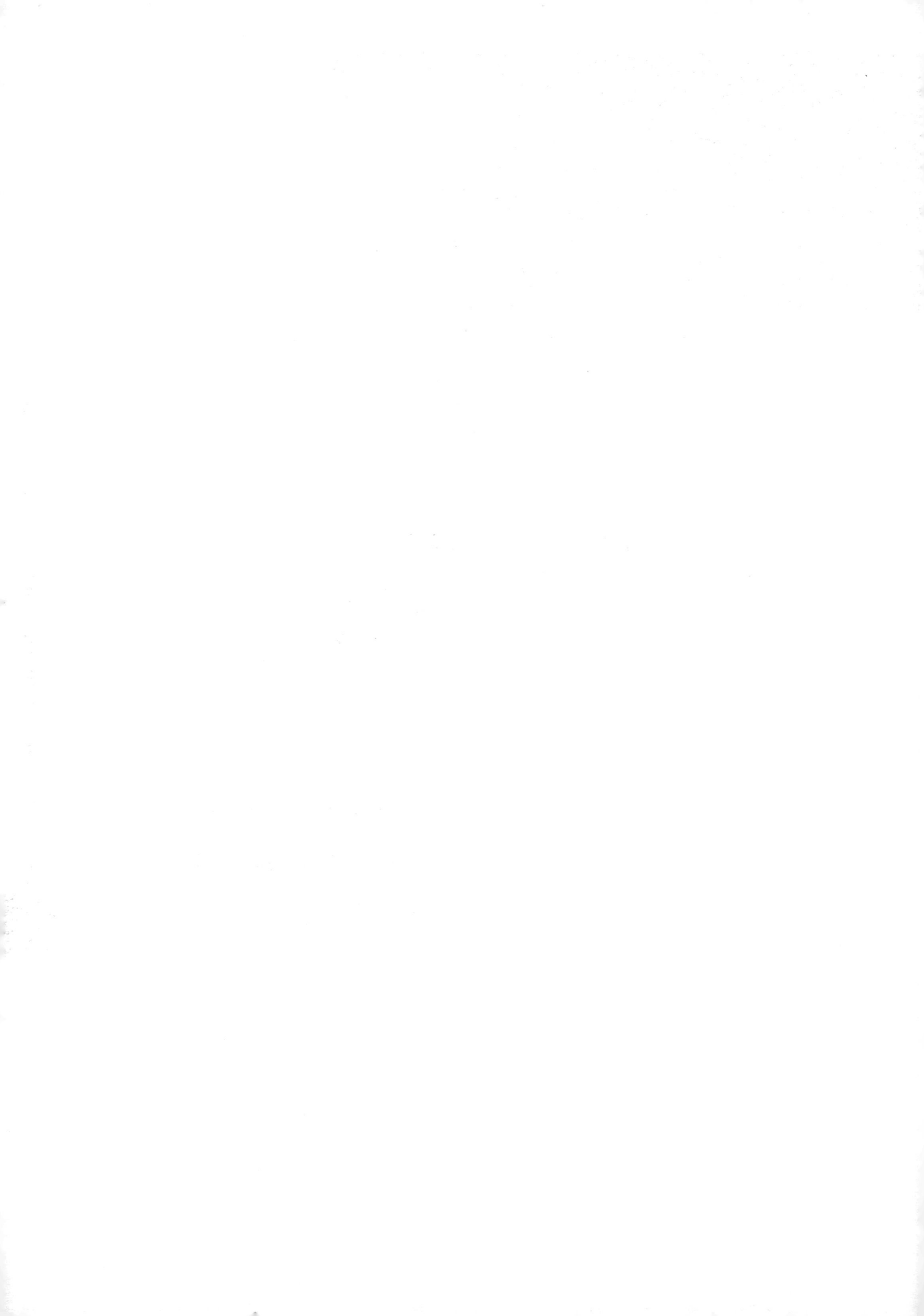

chapter 10

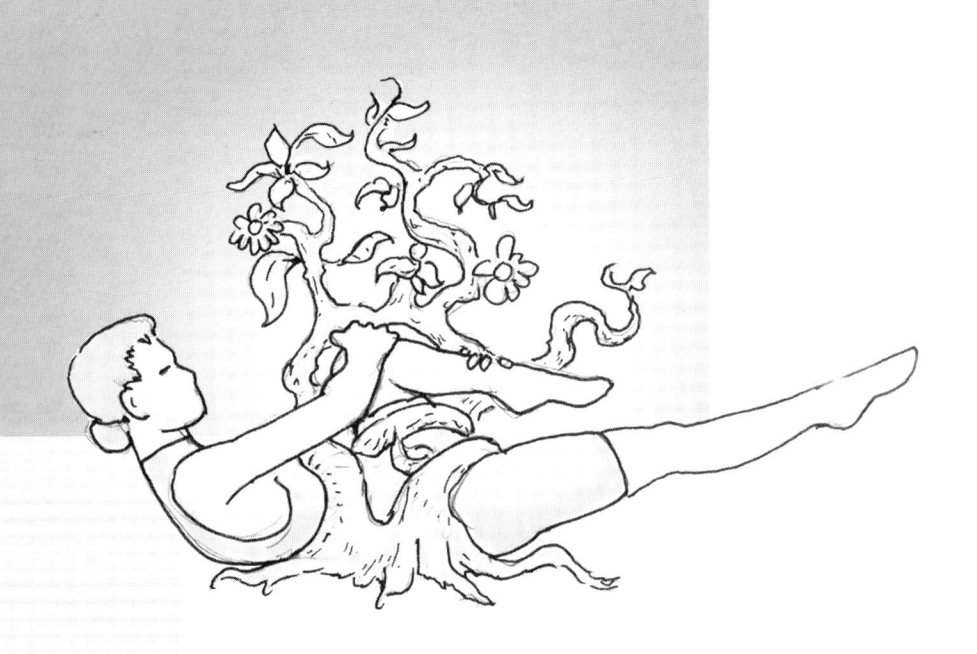

Using Imagery to
Improve Movement:
A Framework for
Physical Therapists

The use of imagery in functional and structural approaches to movement is long established. Movement artists, teachers, sports psychologists, and coaches have explored the use of imagery to enhance learning, skill, and performance since the turn of the century.

In her book *The Thinking Body*, teacher Mabel Todd detailed the link between mind and body through imagery to affect significant change in the body. Lulu Sweigard expanded Todd's theories in her work with dancers to improve their normal movements and performance and in the book *Human Movement Potential: Its Ideokinetic Facilitation*. Sweigard's imagery research, conducted as early as 1931 under the auspices of ideokinesis, supports "imagined movement" as an effective teaching method for reinforcing proper posture, alignment, and mechanical balance (1). Moshe Feldenkrais used imagery to develop quality movement in his Feldenkrais Method with emphasis on repetition and presenting "movement options" to encourage enhanced motion in activities of daily living.

Sports psychologists and coaches have used imagery, or visualization, to enhance sports performance since the '70s. Sports psychologist Jerry Lynch and author of *Running Within* discusses visual imagery as "an active, preplanned attempt to choose appropriate success images while in a deeply relaxed state of mind in order to influence how your body responds to a set of circumstances" (2). Studies of athletes have shown that visualizing a movement can lead to contractions in muscles needed for that movement and can impact body temperature, blood pressure, and heart rate.

From a neuromuscular perspective, Sweigard was one of the first to posit that imagery and imagined movement can be used to change nervous system patterning. Using this theory, she explored and demonstrated that postural alignment improved; research subjects reported ease of movement, reduced pain and fatigue, a taller carriage, and greater coordination (1).

Contemporary movement practitioners that include alternative medicine physicians, holistic nurses, movement therapists, Pilates and Feldenkrais instructors, and others have embraced the idea of neuromuscular repatterning using imagery in a way different from Sweigard's imagined movement, which deemphasizes volitional positioning and control of movement patterns. Rather, many alternative or nontraditional practitioners use imagery to encourage volitional control of movement. In practice, many attest to the power of this method in helping to change movement quality and reintroduce pain-free movement.

Using Imagery in a Rehabilitation Setting

Given the demonstrated success of imagery in influencing movement awareness, several logical questions arise. Can imagery be used by physical therapists and other musculoskeletal specialists to affect positive movement change? After all, physical therapists and other rehabilitation specialists are movement educators whose practices are devoted to increasing movement efficiencies and effectiveness in patients and clients. Physical therapists seek to restore normal function and improve quality of movement in activities of daily living and recreation. Neuromuscular reeducation, improved kinesthetic awareness, and proper alignment and mechanics are emphasized in a treatment setting. It seems natural that imagery may enhance patient outcomes.

Is imagery being used by physical therapists as a rehabilitation strategy, and what is the evidence base supporting its use clinically? Anecdotal evidence suggests imagery use by physical therapists is limited. A review of rehabilitation and motor learning literature reveals few studies suggesting the use of imagery as a rehabilitative care strategy. Those that have explored imagery or imagined movement are limited in scope and haven't demonstrated carryover into rehabilitation.

In one of the few studies done, Japanese researchers Oishi and Maeshima studied the autonomic nervous system in elite and non-elite speed skaters during performance and demonstrated that imagery improved performance and helped athletes to control autonomic responses that might inhibit performance. Based on their findings, they suggested that such training may be applied in a rehabilitation setting but provided no framework from which to work (3). Gandevia's research links mental imagery exercises to voluntary concentric contractions of muscles but doesn't suggest its use in a rehabilitation setting (4). Yue and Cole compared strength training with maximal voluntary and imagined muscle contractions in the fifth digit of the hand and showed strength increases in both training groups. On conclusion of their study, the authors suggest that the large strength increases observed in the imagined strength training group may indicate a therapeutic technique for treating loss of muscle strength after joint immobilization or peripheral nerve injuries but that more research is needed (5). Australian-based physical therapist Paul Hodges discusses use of imagery in his research with patients with chronic low back pain by using it to teach patients about back anatomy and to instruct patients in spinal stabilization (6). Like others, he does not offer a framework for its use outside of a vehicle for cueing and relaxation when appropriate.

Discussion Framework for Using Imagery in Rehabilitation

Physical therapists are not trained to incorporate imagery into their patient care paradigm, nor are they trained to use verbal cueing successfully to maximize patient outcomes. In school, physical therapists are trained to use technical instruction, and unless they are exposed to different methods of training postschooling, most will continue with this method of patient care despite the fact that it may be unsuccessful with many patients.

It is well demonstrated by movement- and body-oriented therapies and in athletics that imagery can promote a natural rhythm and energy to movement. It can help engage the mind, as opposed to letting it wander, and can help prevent boredom via focus and concentration. It can trigger such innate muscle reactions as concentric and eccentric muscle contractions, facilitate static and dynamic movement, and help individuals access specific muscles. The power of imagery makes a strong case for developing this skill clinically and integrating it into conventional physical therapy practice. As such, a framework for integrating imagery into physical therapy patient care is discussed here. For purposes of this guidebook, imagery and imagined movement are applied to volitional movement and muscle action, as opposed to Sweigard's proposed imagined movement where envisioning movement is purported to change neuromuscular coordination at a subcortical level.

Why use imagery clinically? Using imagery in a rehabilitation setting poses many benefits. First, it expands the physical therapy toolbox beyond one that focuses solely on the physical. Conventional physical therapy emphasizes healing the musculoskeletal dysfunction without consistently considering the necessary cognitive, emotional, or spiritual inputs that are also important to healing. This may be why some patients experience minimal improvement following physical therapy. While a discussion about mind-body pathways is beyond the scope of this guidebook, using imagery can help create a connection between mind and body in a nonthreatening manner for the physical therapist who explores supplementing conventional physical therapy models with imagery. Alternative and western medicine scientists alike have demonstrated that the mind and body respond as one unit, although the mechanisms remain unclear.

Second, imagery may help improve patient compliance. Traditional therapy calls for up to 30 repetitions of the same exercise, performed several times a day. Often patients don't understand the value of the exercise and its role in their recovery. Moreover, they can't feel their muscle(s) working, which leads them to believe the exercise isn't working. To improve compliance, imagery might be used in different ways. Patients might imagine unrestricted range of motion in the shoulder or the hip, or imagine the body healing a surgical incision in the knee, helping to facilitate the ability to walk without pain. One of the goals might be to change your patient's focus from pain or restriction to something more positive. Therapists might educate the patient in efficient movement using imagery based on language and images common to our culture, in addition to technical instruction, helping to enhance movement awareness and patient success, leading to improved compliance.

Last, imagery might help improve the quality of muscle contractions and contribute to neuromuscular reeducation. Therapists can choose language that either helps patients to feel muscles and joints working as they should or allows patients to self-visualize the desired action of the muscle or joint. Or, as Yue and Cole demonstrated, patients might imagine targeted muscle groups becoming stronger before resistance or greater challenge is added to the physical therapy regime.

This rehabilitation discussion includes critical success factors, some of which are detailed later. Among them are environment, body positioning, language choice, and self-teaching. To the latter, self-teaching is critical to using imagery clinically. Clinicians interested in using imagery to affect patient movement awareness, and ultimately favorable outcomes, should start by exposing themselves to basic imagery concepts and educating themselves about the types of imagery available to them.

Imagery literature in the dance or sports arenas can be confounding for the uninitiated but can provide some practical starting points for clinicians. Dancer, choreographer, and author Eric Franklin categorizes imagery through the senses: visual, kinesthetic, proprioceptive, olfactory, auditory, gustatory, and tactile (7). While he acknowledges that proprioception isn't technically considered a sense, he adds it to the sensory list because there is imagery that is proprioception-specific. According to Franklin, the most powerful images are those that combine as many senses as possible. Most of us are dominant in just a couple of these senses, and he suggests that we can learn to recognize our "preferred" sense(s) and to cultivate others through practice.

Sports psychologist and coach JoAnn Dahlkoetter presents another way of looking at imagery. "There's external imagery, which is like watching a movie of yourself, internal imagery, which can be thought of as having a camera mounted on your forehead and focused outward, and kinesthetic imagery, where you don't necessarily see anything, but very intensely feel the sensations. Different types of imagery works for different people and situations" (2).

Each patient will respond differently to imagery presented in a therapeutic setting. Because each of us learns about and experiences the world from diverse sensory perspectives, it is imperative that clinicians learn how to discern which patients will respond best to which type of imagery. One patient may prefer to visualize himself walking pain-free, an example of external imagery, while another might intensely feel the muscles around the joint becoming stronger and allowing her to walk pain-free, an example of kinesthetic imagery.

Exposure to imagery concepts and thinking should include observation of others using it in dance, movement, body, or fitness settings and practice in applying the observations to both self and patient. Changing one's own body alignment, balance, and individual movement patterns with visualization or kinesthetic imagery can be a powerful motivator in growing one's skills in this area. Seeing it used with success clinically is equally powerful.

Imagery use requires practice, often by trial and error. What constitutes practice? Practice on patients, coworkers, friends, and family. Practice helps the clinician learn to be concise, time-specific, fluid, and wide ranging in words or technique. It takes time and will be evolutionary. Knowing that patients will respond to different imagery techniques will come from experience and comfort in using imagery as a rehabilitation modality.

Success Factors to Using Imagery

There are general guidelines to successful use of imagery in a physical therapy setting, particularly when first introducing it as a method of eliciting certain movements, sensations, or outcomes. What does this mean? Practitioners who use imagery must consider myriad factors in facilitating concentration and relaxation that will promote successful use of imagery; body positioning, environment, audience age, language use, and learning styles are among them.

Body Positioning
While imagery can be performed in any position, activity, or environment, attention should be given initially to finding a comfortable, restful position that allows for concentration and practice. This can prove challenging in a clinical setting, where physical therapy is often conducted in large, gym-style spaces as opposed to private rooms. When privacy isn't an option, clinicians should choose a corner of a gym, away from others, and encourage patients to concentrate on the task at hand.

Sweigard suggested use of the constructive rest pose (CRP): subjects are positioned in a supine, or backlying position, with the knees flexed to 90 degrees and the arms crossed over the chest in a relaxed manner (1). In this position, the spine follows its natural curves and stress to the lumbar spine is reduced. Eric Franklin suggests the yoga-based "corpse pose" as an alternative. The legs are outstretched and the arms are at the sides (9). For many, this position is comfortable; for others, the weight of the legs can lead to increased lumbar lordosis or a sense of strain in the low back (3). Other positioning considerations include using towels, pillows, and other pieces of equipment to encourage comfort and proper alignment. For example, people who have a forward head, or cervical hyperextension, may require a small towel or pillow beneath the head to achieve cervical neutral. Others may have difficulty maintaining hip alignment in CRP. A small ball or towel between the knees may help enhance hip adductor involvement.

Environment, Language Use, Audience Age
Overhead and ambient lighting, background noise, air temperature, and therapeutic surface selection can all help or hinder concentration and relaxation. Most imagery practitioners discourage use of fluorescent overhead lighting and mute window shades during times of the day when the sun is at its strongest. Often, body positioning looking into harsh lighting can serve as a distraction.

Minimized background noise and a space warmed to the movers' comfort are ideal. Music and other soothing sounds, such as a water fountain, may help facilitate successful imagery use. Surface selection is important and should support the mover's spine in supine, prone, and sidelying positions. Some mats or plinths can absorb energy, inhibiting stabilization, proper alignment, and/or movement.

Common language and images that are part of our culture are effective imagery tools that can enhance movement awareness and help the clinician work more effectively with patients. Franklin writes: "Images based on childhood experiences are particularly powerful because everything is so new and fresh. The same image will evoke a different response from each person because each sensory cupboard is filled with a personal mix of experiences" (7).

Just as common language and images are important, so too are the images the therapist chooses to use with the "audience," be it a teenager or a grandmother. Language should be age-appropriate and relevant. Asking a teenager to squeeze a lottery ticket between the knees to stimulate a strong, isometric adductor recruitment pattern may not work as well as if the therapist had used an image of squeezing a concert ticket between the knees.

Tone of voice can also make a difference. Depending on the outcome the therapist desires, the voice tone may be low or high, with pacing slow or fast.

Sensory Learning Styles
Day to day, we all use tactile, auditory, kinesthetic, or visual senses to automatically experience movement at work, activities of daily living, and athletics. While all these senses are used to some degree, each of us uses a primary sense to process information (8). Knowing whether a patient is more likely to respond to the use of imagery, touch, or voice can help practitioners choose a movement awareness teaching path that may or may not emphasize verbal imagery. As research has demonstrated, imagery doesn't work for everyone. Refer to Chapter 9 for more information about sensory learning.

Concentration and Practice
Discovering new ways of moving requires focus and mental practice. Focus implies concentration, a calm mind, and the ability to reduce or eliminate outside or unnecessary thoughts that may distract from the task at hand. Clinicians can offer imagery to affect movement change, but without the mover's concentration and mental practice over and over again, in a variety of settings, the effort can be for naught. As mentioned earlier, environment and body positioning can play a key role in providing a relaxing setting to foster success.

Teaching Settings
In some medical communities, physical therapy is delivered in a group setting. Examples of this include back care or prenatal exercise classes taught by physical therapists. Group lessons versus working one-on-one can influence the type and amount of imagery that is used. Initially, it is best to introduce one image at a time, adding images when appropriate or when the selected image isn't eliciting the desired response. An "imagery library" that is wide ranging and addresses the needs of many patients can be a

good resource once groups are accustomed to the inclusion of imagery in the lesson.

Moving From a Discussion Framework to Practical Application

Using imagery as a rehabilitation strategy is not fully demonstrated in the literature. This discussion advances imagery use to practical application, providing examples of ways to use imagery in common therapeutic movement patterns to help normalize muscle and joint function and improve effectiveness of movement. Here we suggest ways to enhance movement through imagery language that may focus on external, internal, or kinesthetic imagery suggested by Dahlkoetter.

Imagery to Facilitate Hip Flexion in Supine

The hip joint is a ball-and-socket joint composed of the femur and the pelvis, where the head of the femur is convex and the socket of the pelvis is concave. Hip flexion is a basic activity of daily living. We flex our hips to walk, sit, stand, or climb stairs. When the joint or the muscles around the joint are dysfunctional, physical therapists focus on restoring normal function to the hip and returning patients to activities of daily living at their optimal level. Using imagery to facilitate joint motion of the hip, first in supine, then in standing, may help enhance quality of motion and improve patient exercise compliance.

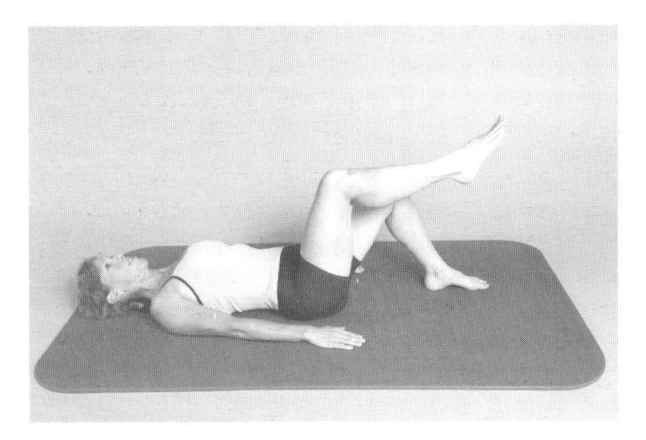

Cueing patients using kinesthetic imagery:

Lie on your back with your knees bent, feet flat on the floor. Lift your leg until your shin is parallel to the floor. Return the leg to the starting position. Repeat the same exercise, but this time pay attention to how the ball of your thighbone slides in the hip socket to facilitate flexing at the hip. Feel how the surfaces of the bones glide smoothly across each other. Feel how the weight of the thighbone changes as it lifts up and over the hip socket and then returns to the floor. Does the leg feel heavy? What other sensations do you feel? Practice this exercise in standing with the same imagery.

Cueing patients using external imagery:

Lie on your back with your knees bent, feet flat on the floor. Lift your leg until your shin is parallel to the floor. Return the leg to the starting position. Repeat the same exercise, but this time imagine that your knee is attached to a long string dangling from the ceiling. Imagine the string pulling the leg up and off the floor, guiding the knee to the point where it is hovering over the hip. Let the string guide your knee back to the floor. Does the leg feel light? What other sensations do you feel? Now practice this exercise in standing.

Finding Neutral Pelvis in Supine and Standing

In its position at the center of the body, the pelvis and the muscles that surround it are part of the powerhouse of the body. Moving with a stable pelvis is key to proper alignment of the spine and biomechanics, as is its position of neutral, which research shows maximizes muscular effort of the spine and minimizes stress to muscles and connective tissue. Many physical therapists are challenged to teach patients how to find neutral pelvis and how to apply the concept to activities of daily living, such as sitting at a desk at work, or how to lift on object using safe movement mechanics.

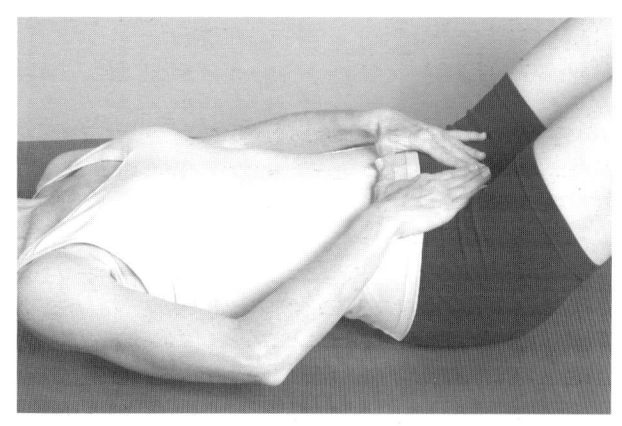

Cueing patients using internal imagery:

Lie on your back with your knees bent, feet flat on the floor. Create a triangle formed by your thumbs and index fingers (show triangle to your patient). Place the triangle on your pelvis, with the heels of your hands on your hipbones and your fingers on your symphysis pubis and pointing toward your legs. Ideally, the triangle will be parallel to the floor. Tip your pelvis forward and back—lengthwise—until you sense or feel that the triangle is parallel to the floor.

Cueing patients using external imagery:

Lie on your back with your knees bent, feet flat on the floor. Visualize that you have headlights sitting on top of your hipbones. Notice if the lights are shining up and over your head or down toward the floor. Adjust your pelvic position by rocking the pelvis back and forth lengthwise. Find the position where the lights are shining directly on the ceiling over your hips.

Once patients have mastered finding neutral in supine, where the body is most stable, challenge them by asking them to sit or stand and repeat the exercises. Advance learning by teaching patients to maintain a level pelvis while standing or walking.

Cueing patients using external imagery:

Stand with your feet placed underneath your hips. Visualize a carpenter's level on top of your pelvis and the air bubble inside located exactly in the middle. Tip your pelvis down to the left so that the bubble inside the level moves to the right. Tip your pelvis down to the right so that the bubble moves to the left. Position your pelvis so that the top of your pelvis is level again and the air bubble is in the middle. Now stand on one leg and try to keep the level balanced.

Bridge: Neuromuscular Reeducation or Strengthening of the Gluteus Maximus

For many patients, a weak gluteus maximus contributes to faulty movement patterns in activities of daily living, affecting gait and walking mechanics, stair climbing, or rising from a chair. Many physical therapists find themselves prescribing this essential exercise to help retrain or strengthen the gluteus maximus. Imagery can help facilitate normal muscle recruitment and proper joint mechanics of hip extension and flexion.

Bridge Start

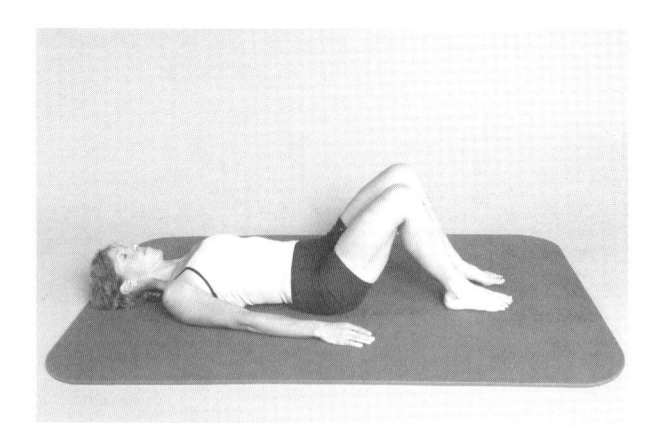

Bridge: Hips in Extension

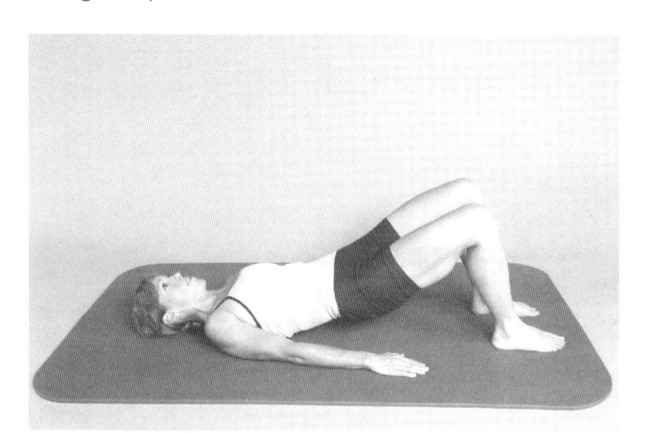

Cueing patients using kinesthetic imagery:

Lie on your back with your knees bent, your feet flat on the floor. Feel your back's pressure points on the floor. Where is your weight centered? Are there any pressure points or heaviness on your back that don't feel quite right? Next, turn your attention to your pelvis. Is the weight centered evenly side to side? Do you feel any discomfort? Now, keeping your body as still as you can, press your feet evenly into the floor and lift your hips and torso off the floor and up toward the ceiling as one unit, like you are unfolding an ironing board. Feel which muscles help do this and describe what you feel. Place your hips back on the floor. Repeat the same exercise, but this time feel as if you are unhinging at the hips, like opening a door, as you lift your hips toward the ceiling. Can you open the door a little farther without arching your back? Is any light shining in through the crack in the door?

Developing Your Imagery Library

The Principles, Core Muscle Facilitation, and Warm-up: Some Ideas

Developing your imagery library will not occur overnight. It's truly an evolutionary process. We attended many courses and observed other educators using imagery to advance our own. Keep in mind the line or plane of movement—sagittal, frontal, or transverse—and use imagery to inspire your intended outcome. Use the following ideas as starting points for your imagery exploration and look for opportunities to increase your "library."

Breathing

Use these images to increase awareness of proper breathing mechanics.

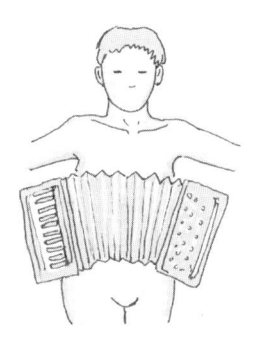

Expand the ribs out and in, like an accordian or balloon.

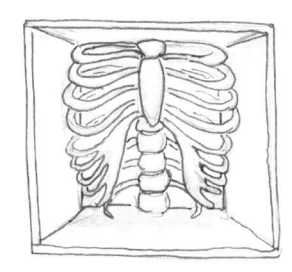

Imagine that the ribs are like a room. With your breath, expand the walls and floor of the room while keeping the ceiling still.

Neutral Pelvis

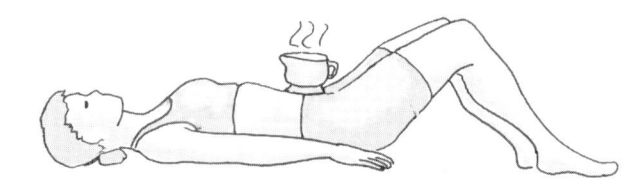

Use this image to teach normal pelvic motion and control of motion.

The hipbones and pubic bone create a triangle that is parallel to floor. Balance your favorite drink in the triangle.

Imprinted Pelvis

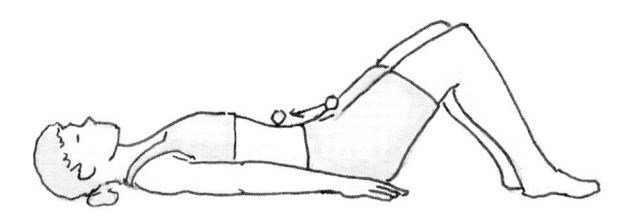

Use this image to teach normal pelvic motion and control of motion.

Imagine rolling a marble from your pubic bone to your belly button.

Pelvic Clock

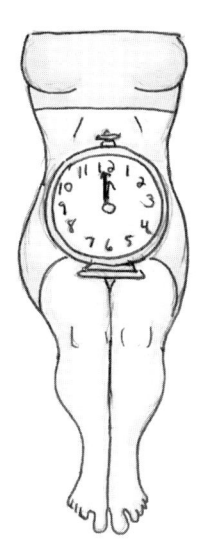

Use this image to teach normal pelvic motion and control of motion.

Imagine that a clock has been placed on your navel. Move south to find 6 o'clock, move north to find 12 o'clock, move east to find 3 o'clock, and move west to find 9 o'clock.

Recruiting Transversus Abdominis

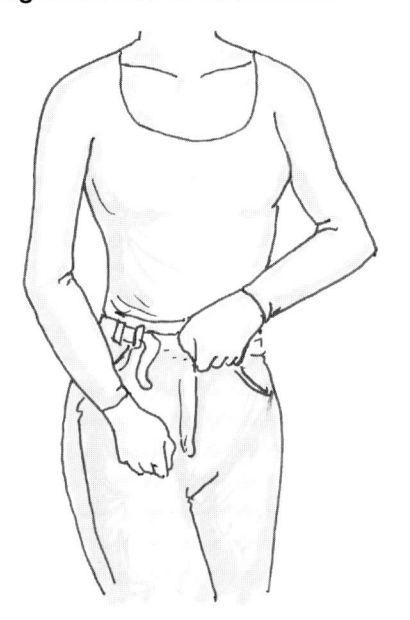

Use this image to encourage neuromuscular recruitment of deep muscles that are important to lumbo-pelvic stability.

Pretend you are zipping up a tight pair of pants from your pubic bone to your belly button. Or imagine your hip bones are like an elevator door. Feel the elevator doors closing across the pelvis as you slowly and gently press your belly button toward your spine.

Recruiting Pelvic Floor

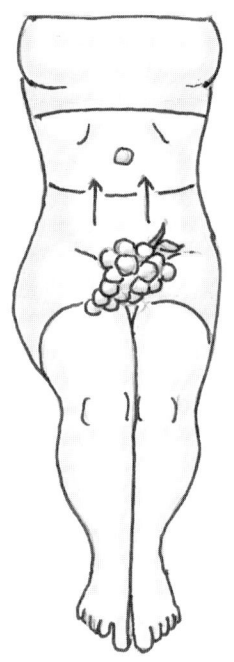

Use this image to encourage neuromuscular recruitment of deep muscles that are important to lumbo-pelvic stability.

Pull a grape up inside your pelvis. Or imagine sitting on a diamond composed of the following landmarks: ischial tuberosities, pubic bone, and tailbone. Pull all four points together and up with natural exhalation (5).

Scapular Depression

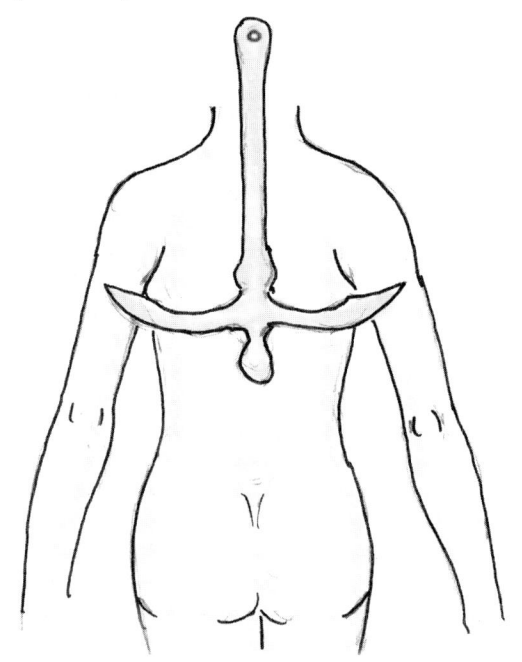

Use this image to teach the importance of scapular positioning in proper alignment.

Feel as if your shoulder blades are anchored on your back. Or slide your shoulder blades toward your back pockets.

Scapular Protraction/Retraction In Supine

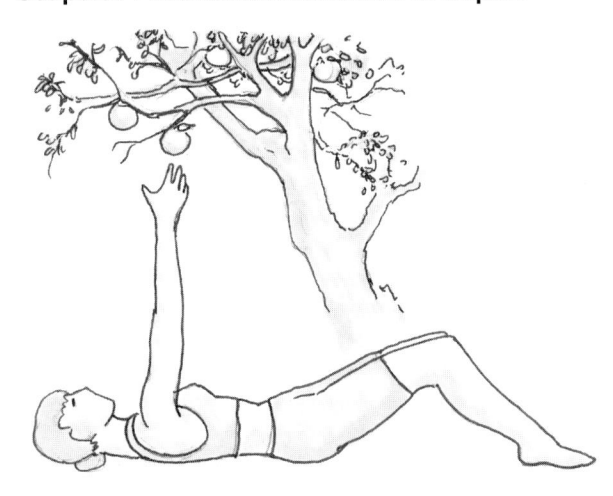

Use this image to teach the importance of scapular positioning in proper alignment.

Imagine reaching for an apple over your head and plucking it out of a tree. Or imagine that your shoulder blades are a nutcracker. Crack a nut by gently sliding your shoulder blades together; open the nutcracker by pulling your shoulders forward.

Rib Cage Positioning

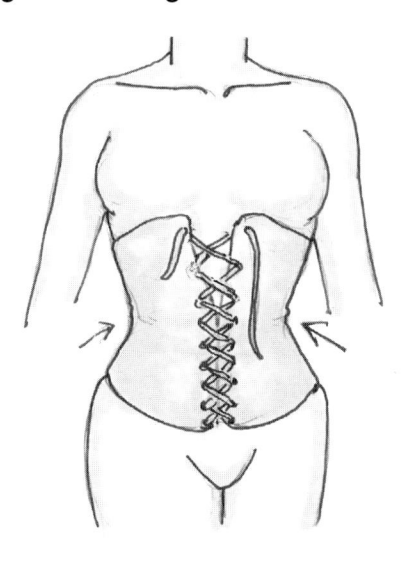

Use this image to facilitate abdominal recruitment and the importance of positioning with overhead and rotary movements.

Knit your ribs together as if you are wearing a corset. Or truss your ribs up like a turkey at Thanksgiving.

Head and Neck Positioning

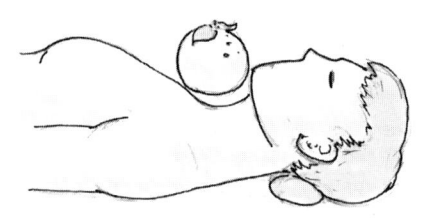

Use this image to teach the importance of head and neck positioning in proper alignment.

Hold orange between chin and chest.

Lengthening the Neck

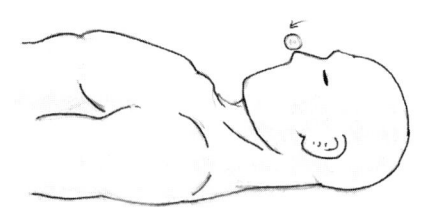

Use this image to teach what it feels likes to maintain neutral cervical spine.

Nod the length of a dime.

Eye Positioning

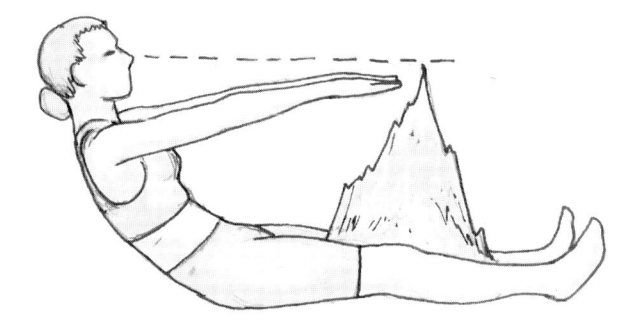

Use this image to teach the importance of eye positioning in proper body alignment.

Imagine your knees are a mountain top. Look over the top of the mountains.

Maintain Rib to Hip Connection

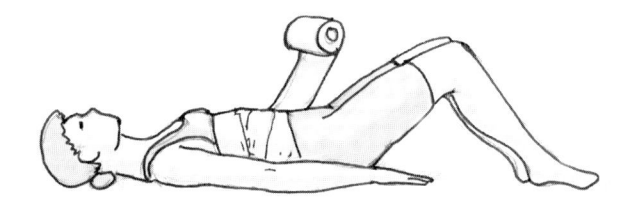

Use this image to encourage torso stabilization.

Imagine your torso is wrapped with duct tape.

Heel Slide

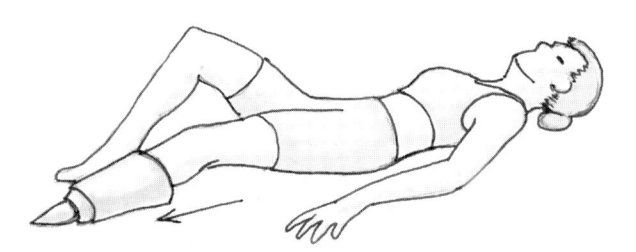

Use this image to encourage torso stabilization with hip extension and flexion.

Imagine that the heel is a magic marker. Draw a straight line with your marker as the heel slides away from body. Trace the line on the way back. Or, draw a line in the sand.

Bent Knee Fallout

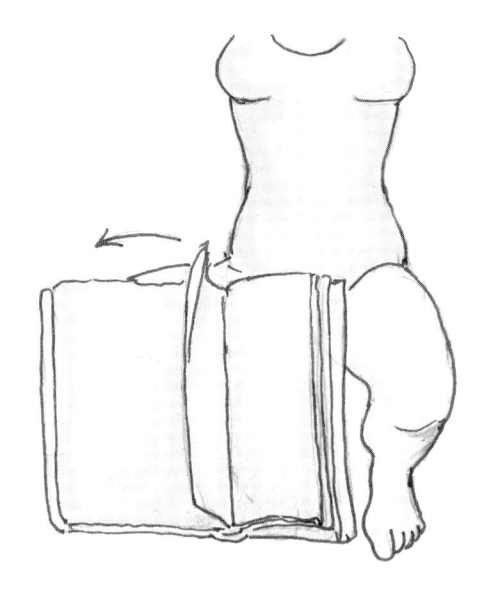

Use this image to encourage neutral pelvis with external rotation of the hip.

The hip is a book opening as the knee drops out and closing as the knee returns to the start position.

Spine Rolls

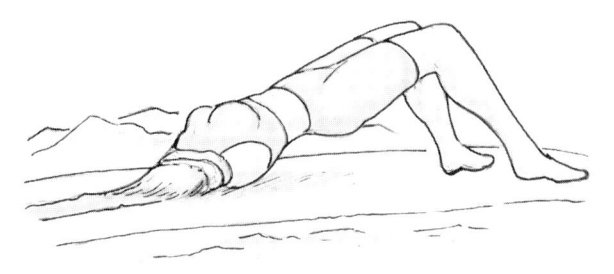

Use this image to encourage sequential articulation and mobilization of the spine.

Imagine painting a solid straight line on a highway with your spine.

Sitting

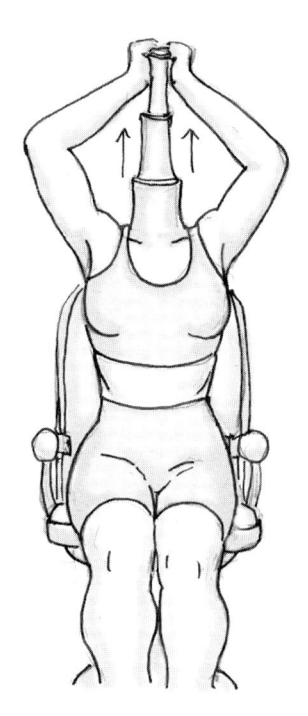

Use this image to encourage support from the muscles and joints in a weight-bearing position.

Imagine your spine is a telescope and lengthen it.

Standing

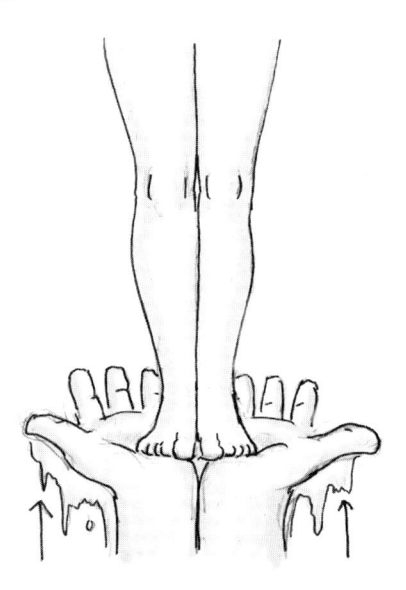

Use this image to encourage support from the muscles and joints in a weight-bearing position.

Feel the ground pushing up against the feet.

Sitting/Standing

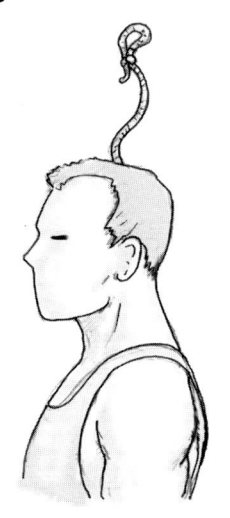

Use this image to encourage support from the muscles and joints in a weight-bearing position.

Imagine a string is coming out of your spine like a puppet, from the tailbone to the top of the head.

The Exercises
Spinal/Thoracic Flexion
Quarter Rollup

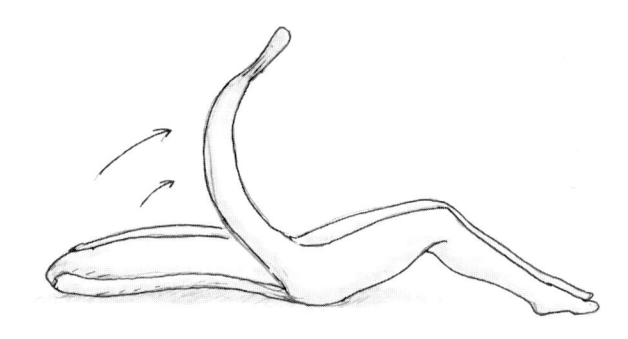

Use this image to encourage sequential articulation and mobilization of the spine.

Peel body off mat from top to bottom like a banana.

The Hundred

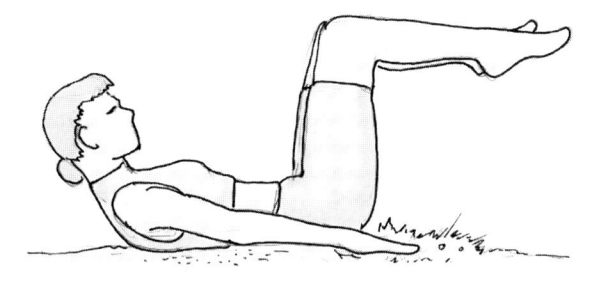

Use this image to encourage scapular stabilization and shoulder mobilization.

Imagine your arms as patting the sand.

Rolling Like a Ball

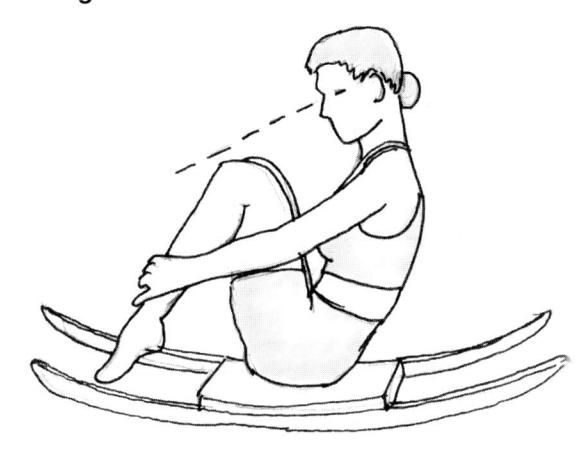

Use this image to encourage spinal stabilization via isometric contractions.

Roll as one unit as if you are a rocking chair.

Single Leg Stretch

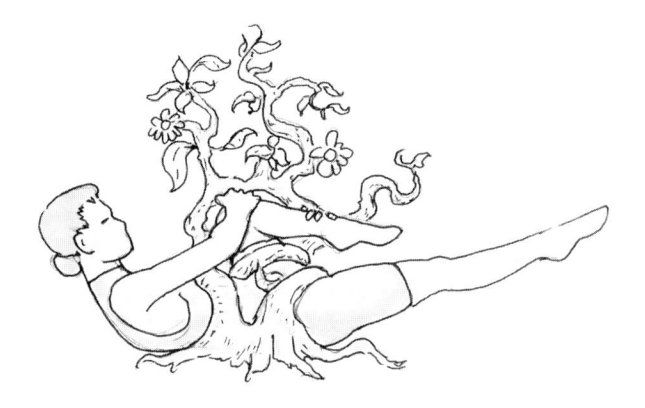

Use this image to encourage lumbo-pelvic stabilization.

Imagine that you have roots coming out of your spine.

Double Leg Stretch

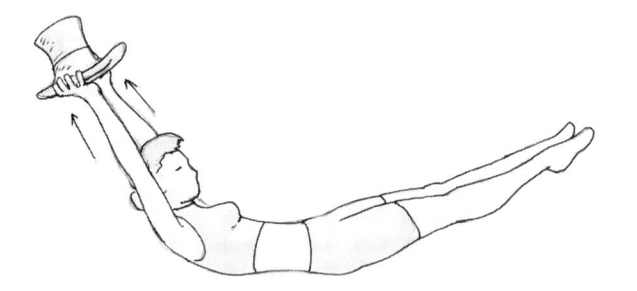

Use this image to encourage appropriate arm patterning.

Reach arms overhead like you're taking a hat off.

Spine Stretch

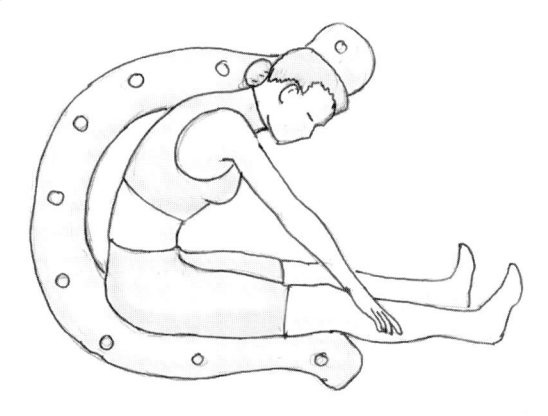

Use this image to teach spinal lengthening in flexion.

Create horse shoe shape with your spine.

Spinal/Thoracic Extension
Trunk Extension with Arm Patterns

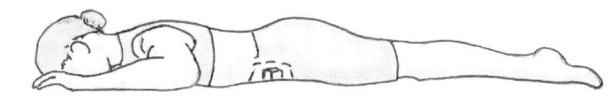

Use this image to teach abdominal and gluteal stabilization in spine extension.

Imagine that you are lying on an ice cube or snowball.

Swimming Progressions

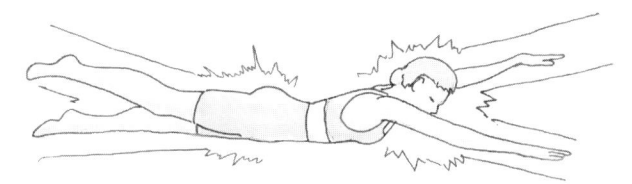

Use this image to encourage lengthening from the shoulder and hip joints, not the elbows, knees, wrists, or ankles.

Imagine ponts of light coming out of the shoulders and hips. Reach from the center of your body.

Torso Stabilization and Rotation
Spine Twist

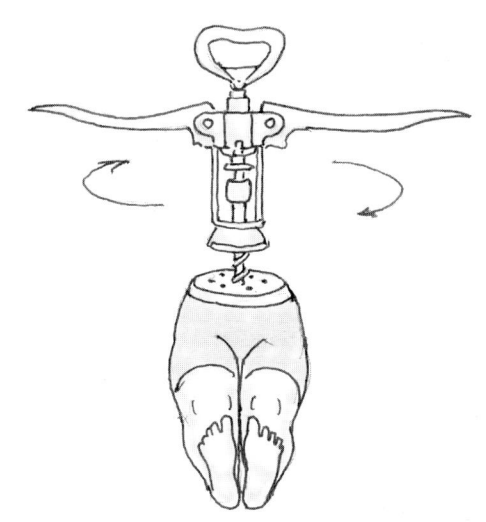

Use this image to teach torso stabilization with rotary movements.

Move as one unit, like a human blender. Or, imagine your spine is a corkscrew, unscrewing a bottle.

Criss Cross

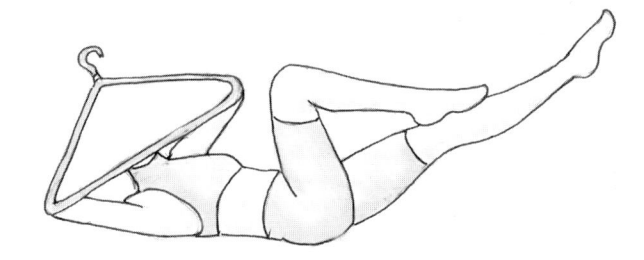

Use this image to encourage scapular and shoulder joint stabilization with rotary movement.

Imagine your arms form the shape of a coat hanger.

Hips: Joint Mobilization and Muscle Strengthening

One Leg Circle

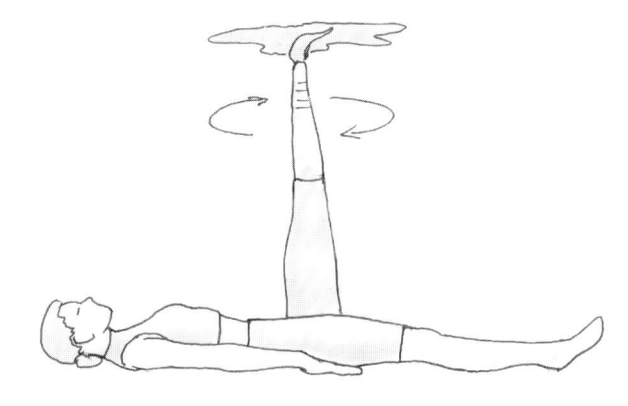

Use this image to encourage hip mobilization with torso stabilization.

Imagine your big toe as a paintbrush. Paint a circle on the ceiling.

Shoulder Bridge

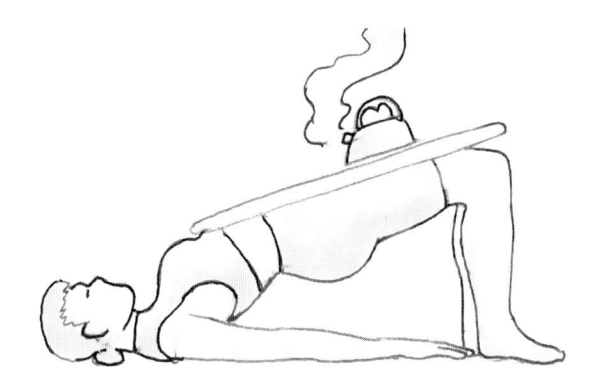

Use this image to teach torso stabilization with hip extension.

Keep your torso rigid like an ironing board, folding and unfolding at hips.

Hip Abduction/Adductor Progression

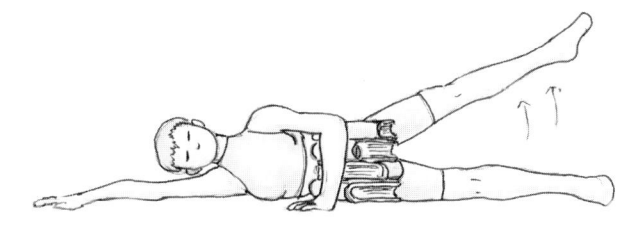

Use this image to encourage neutral pelvis in sidelying positions.

Stack your hips like a bookcase, with the hipbones aligned.

Upper Extremity Strengthening

Leg Pull Front Warm Up

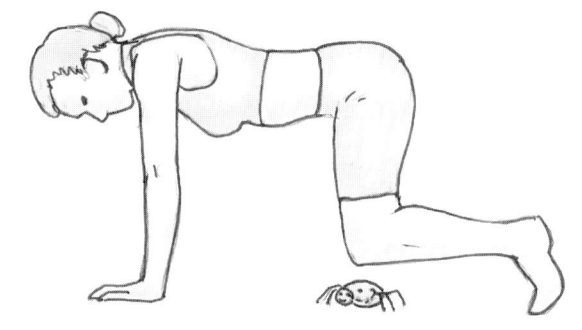

Use this image to instruct extent of movement from the floor.

Let a friendly bug crawl under your knees.

187

Pushups

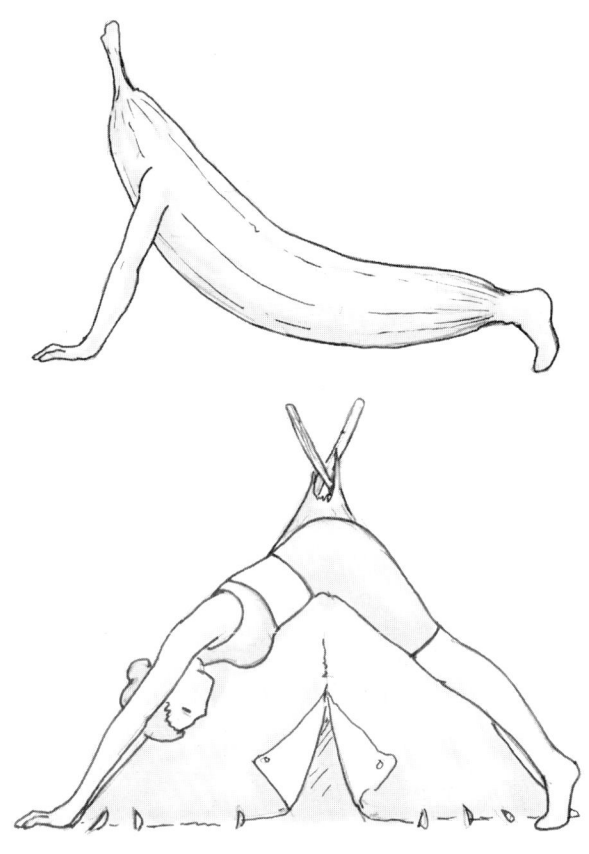

Use these images to encourage torso stabilization via lumbo-pelvic alignment in neutral.

Avoid a banana or teepee shape.

Imagery Success: In Conclusion

Imagery can be a successful tool in encouraging movement awareness and musculoskeletal movement in a therapeutic setting. Clinicians should keep in mind the line or plane of movement—sagittal, frontal, or transverse—and use imagery to inspire an intended patient outcome. Moreover, successful use requires that clinicians sharpen their communication skills, verbal to nonverbal, and combine the use of imagery with tactile and auditory sensory techniques.

Use of imagery in body and movement therapies is well documented and should be further examined for other musculoskeletal medical practices, such as physical therapy, to improve movement quality and function.

Chapter References

1. Sweigard, L.E. 1974. *Human Movement Potential: Its Ideokinetic Facilitation.* New York: Harper & Row.

2. Bakoulis, G. 2001. Examining Visualization: Does it really work? *Peak Running Performance* 10(1): 1-3.

3. Oishi, K., Maeshima, T. 2004. Autonomic nervous system activities during motor imagery in elite athletes. *Journal of Clinical Neurophysiology* 21(3): 170-179.

4. Gandevia, S.C. 1999. Mind, muscles and motoneurones. *Journal of Science and Medicine in Sport* 2(3): 167-180.

5. Yue, G., and Cole, K. 1992. Strength increases from the motor program: Comparison of training with maximal voluntary and imagined muscle contractions. *Journal of Neurophysiology* 67(5): 1114-1123.

6. Hodges, P. 2001. *Science of Stability: Clinical Application to Assessment and Treatment of Segmental Spinal Stabilization for Low Back Pain.* Course Manual, Northeast Seminars, East Hampstead, NH.

7. Franklin, E. 1996. *Dynamic Alignment Through Imagery.* Champaign, IL: Human Kinetics.

8. Sachs, L.D. 2003. Strategic communication. *Idea Health and Fitness Source*, February.

chapter 11

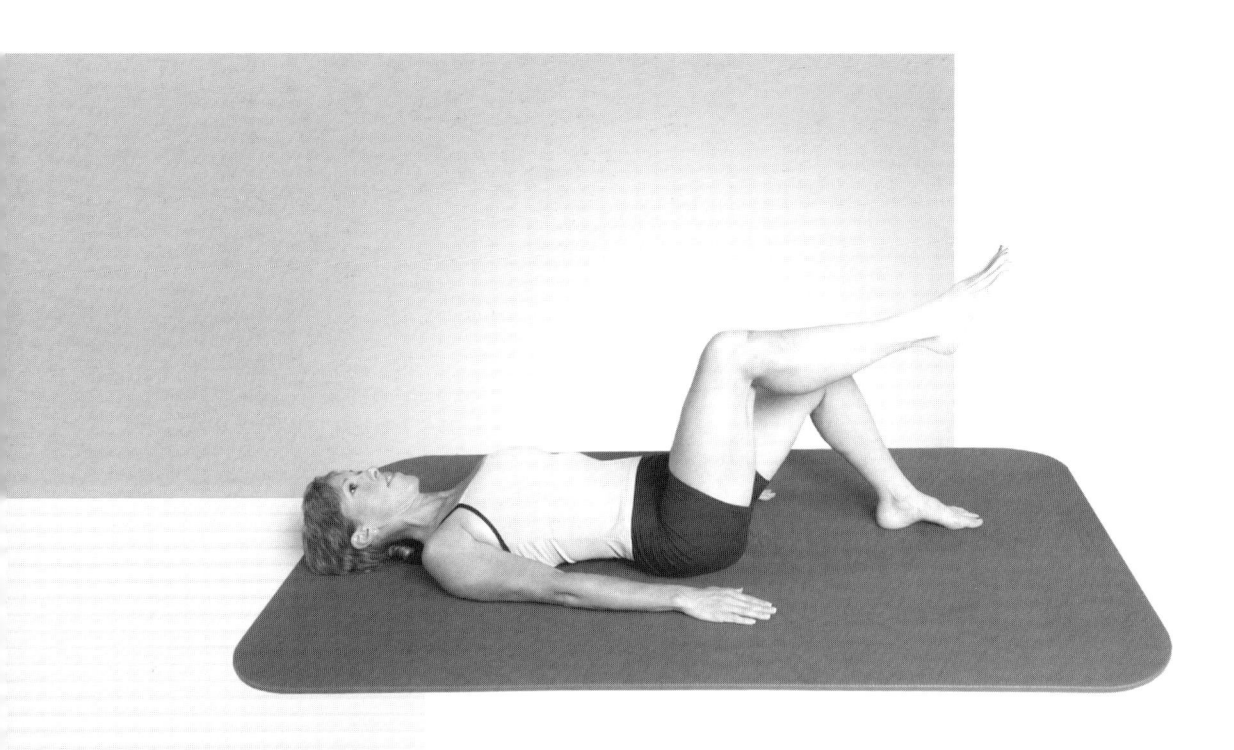

PATIENT FOCUS:
CASE STUDIES OF
PILATES APPLICATION
IN REHABILITATION

Numerous excellent Pilates resources are available on the market ranging from books to DVDs. However, bringing these resources into the clinical setting can be tricky. Some rehabilitation specialists have difficulty knowing when and how to apply them, how to modify a Pilates exercise, what to look for in a quality resource, or what are appropriate Pilates progressions.

This chapter is designed to help practitioners apply the exercises and ideas in this book to patient care. In this chapter, as throughout this book, we've given examples of patient populations that will benefit from a particular exercise(s) as an adjunct to conventional therapies. You are limited only by your own creativity. Consider using equipment to change the exercise or your perspective—try the exercises in sitting, standing, at the wall, or on an unstable surface.

Finding Quality Resources to Advance Your Knowledge

The popularity of Pilates has exploded in recent years. Sifting through books, videos, DVDs, workshops, and certification programs touting the best method can be overwhelming. Here are some ideas to consider and questions to ask when choosing resources to advance your knowledge.

Certification Programs and Courses

There are many certification programs and workshops from which to choose. The Pilates market is competitive, and savvy marketing programs targeting you abound. Let the buyer beware.

Select programs and courses where the instructor(s) is:

- Knowledgeable in musculoskeletal medicine, preferably a physical therapist, long-time fitness practitioner with a science-based education, or a combination of instructors, one of which is a physical therapist
- Using Pilates-based methodology in his or her clinical practice
- Using exercise modifications, progressions, and equipment as appropriate
- Operating from a musculoskeletal evidence base and is familiar with current literature
- Certified by a program whose educational requirements are rigorous and go beyond a weekend or week-long coursework. A number of programs offer a rehabilitation focus and would be appropriate for rehabilitation and advanced fitness practitioners.
- Up-to-date on annual continuing education, either Pilates-based or in related areas

Books, Audiovisual Aids

Books and audiovisuals aids are great sources of new ideas and exercises and help you stay current with Pilates trends. When we assess materials for purchase, we ask these questions:

- Is the product presented from an evidence base for rehabilitation?
- Does the instructor demonstrate good knowledge of musculoskeletal medicine?
- Does the instructor or author demonstrate modifications and progressions?
- Do the exercise models demonstrate good technique? Evaluate form and application of the correct movement patterns in key areas: cervical spine, scapula, and pelvis. Is there hyperflexion? Scapular winging? Anterior/posterior tilt?

Pilates and Posture

Pilates developed his unique method of exercise in part to counteract the effects of "technology" on posture. Considering today's version of technology, his foresight was amazing.

Here's the challenge: bringing modern-day science together with cutting-edge instinct birthed by Pilates. In Chapter 2, we discussed common faulty postures as identified by Florence Kendall. Here we pose some Pilates-based solutions to counteracting the modern-day symptoms and related results of a society overcome by technology and a sedentary lifestyle.

Pilates Exercise for Kyphotic and Lordotic Postures

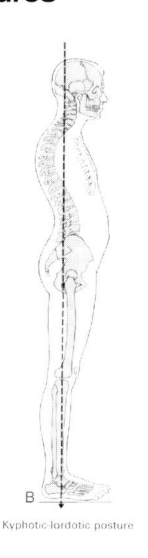

Kyphotic-lordotic posture

Posture characterizations (1):

Cervical spine: increased lordosis

Scapulae: abducted

Thoracic spine: increased kyphosis

Lumbar: increased lordosis

Pelvis: anterior tilt

Hip joints: flexed

Knees joints: hyperextended, slightly

Ankle joints: plantar flexed, slightly

Likely muscle imbalances:

Short and strong: neck extensors and hip flexors

Long and weak: neck flexors, upper back erectors, external obliques

Short: low back

Long and normal strength: hamstrings

Goals:

1. Deemphasize thoracic spinal flexion; anterior tilt/transitional movements; lumbar extension

2. Emphasize thoracic extension through concentric muscle contraction; lumbar flexion; eccentric contraction of the hip flexors and the pectoralis major; concentric contraction of the hip extensors; concentric contraction of the internal/external obliques; concentric contraction of the middle trapezius and rhomboid muscles

Types of exercises to consider:

- Neutral and/or posterior (imprinted) lumbar spine
- Exercises that enhance spinal mobility
- Closed chained upper extremity exercises
- Thoracic extension
- Hip extension
- Torso rotation

Exercises to limit but not avoid: Excessive repetitions of exercises that emphasize spinal flexion, such as Single-Leg Stretch, the Hundred, and Spine Stretch Forward

Equipment: A towel beneath the head to support neutral cervical alignment; a pad for the ASIS in prone lying positions if the patient is unable to support him-/herself in neutral pelvis, with the goal of progressing to no equipment

Suggested Exercises for Patients:

- *Quarter Rollup with Neutral Pelvis*
- *Rollup, keeping arms at sides*
- *One-Leg Circle, one leg bent, the other long (if neutral pelvis can be maintained)*
- *Spine Twist, preps and full*
- *Single-Leg Stretch, keep legs bent, posterior pelvic tilt*
- *Criss Cross, feet on the floor, neutral pelvis*
- *Double-Leg Stretch, feet on the floor, progressing to legs in tabletop*
- *Spine Stretch, provided hunched shoulders can be avoided*
- *Trunk Extension Progressions, emphasizing upper back and lumbo-pelvic stability*
- *Bridge/Shoulder Bridge Variations*
- *Hip Abduction/Adduction Progressions*
- *Swimming Progressions*
- *Leg Pull Front Warm-up*
- *Supine Knee Sways*
- *Hip Extension Preps/Full*
- *Leg Pull Front Warm-up*
- *Pushup*
- *Frog*
- *Clam in Sidelying/Standing*

Pilates Exercises for Flat Back Postures

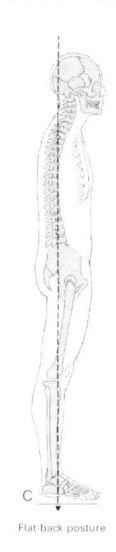

Flat-back posture

Posture characterizations (1):

Cervical spine: increased cervical lordosis

Thoracic spine: increased upper thoracic kyphosis; decreased lower thoracic kyphosis

Lumbar: decreased lordosis

Pelvis: posterior tilt

Hip joints: extended

Knee joints: extended

Ankle joints: slight plantar flexion

Likely muscle imbalances:

Short and strong: hamstrings

Long and weak: one-joint hip flexors

Goals:

1. Lower Extremities

   Deemphasize hamstrings and eccentric muscle contraction of the hip flexors

   Emphasize concentric muscle contraction of the hip flexors and low back extensors (if weak)

2. Upper Extremities

   Emphasize concentric contraction of the upper back extensors (Trunk Extension Patterns; Swimming Progressions)

Types of exercises to consider:

- Neutral spine
- Anterior tilt during transitional movements
- Imprint to neutral
- Exercises that enhance sequential, segmental mobility of the spine: Spine Stretch, Rollup, etc.
- Imprinted exercises: Criss Cross, legs in tabletop
- Closed chain training of upper extremities
- Torso rotation

Types of exercises to emphasize: Exercises that enhance segmental spinal articulation and mobility and open chain exercises with a posterior tilt, such as legs in tabletop with arm patterns

Exercises to limit: Frog; Hip Extension in Prone Preps/Full; Bridge Prep/Shoulder Bridge Variations; Swimming Progressions

Progress to the following as posture starts to change: Single-Leg Stretch, Criss Cross, Double-Leg Stretch

Equipment: May need a towel to support cervical alignment

Real-Life Application of Pilates Fundamental Exercises

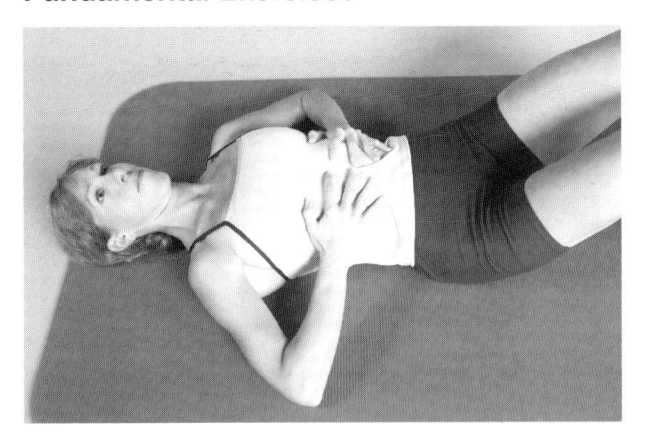

Breathing: Breathing initiates a chain of events that begins with contraction of the abdominals and rib mobility, increasing stability through contraction of the core muscles. Breathing also helps patients to focus on establishing a body-mind connection, decreases the likelihood of Valsalva during exercise, and promotes relaxation. Use proper, intentional breath to enhance flexibility and strengthening exercises, transitional movements, ADLs, work, and sport-specific drills.

The focus of breath for patients with low back dysfunction is to facilitate the deep core stabilizers with back stabilization exercises. The same thought process can be applied to exercise programming for the patient in need of shoulder strengthening. Breathing can also be used as an adjunct to manual therapy for myofascial restrictions of the diaphragm to restore normal breathing mechanics or to increase the mobility of hypomobile thoracic spine segment(s). Third, use breathing to retrain normal breathing mechanics when an altered breathing pattern is present. Health providers who work with women with pelvic floor dysfunction can use passive breathing to recruit the pelvic floor muscles via transversus abdominis contraction to co-activate those muscles. Teach proper breathing to patients who chronically experience nausea or light-headedness when performing exercises.

Real-Life Application: The principle of breathing is an essential element to include with exercise programming in every patient's rehabilitation. How you use breath will vary from patient to patient. Here are a few examples of how breathing can be used.

Bent-Knee Fallout

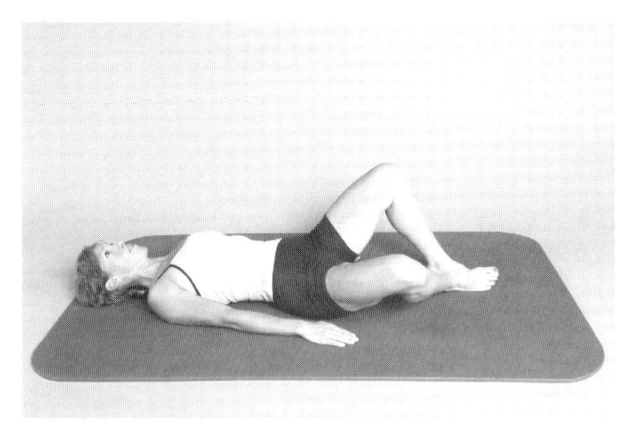

Use this movement pattern in training patients to isolate or dissociate the hip from the pelvis and spine in the transverse plane. Doing so helps to enhance neuromuscular control of the hip external rotators and/or hip adductors, increases the length of the hip adductors, and restores normal hip motion when deficient while maintaining pelvic stability. This exercise also increases your patient's awareness of how to move body parts independently.

Real-Life Application: The Bent-Knee Fallout has traditionally been used as a back stabilization exercise, but it can be used in other ways. For some patients, this exercise can be used as an adjunct to hip mobilization techniques for a tight anterior hip capsule to restore normal hip external rotation motion. For others, the focus may be to increase adductor length such as in rehabilitation of symphysis pubis dysfunction (i.e., pubic downslip). This is an excellent exercise to include in the early phase of hip adductor strain rehabilitation to facilitate neuromuscular reeducation of the hip adductors.

Single Leg in Tabletop

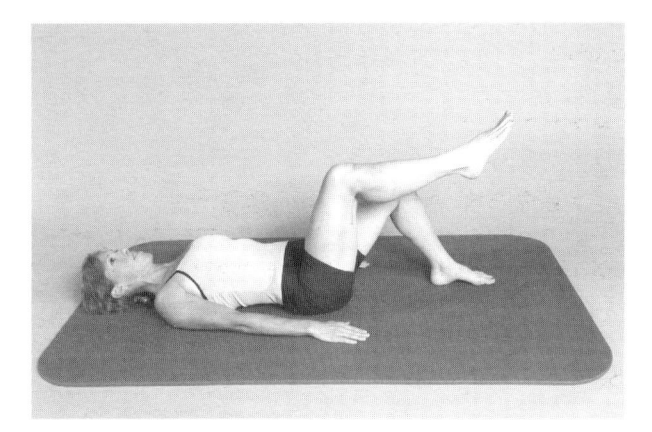

This exercise emphasizes open kinetic chain (OKC) training of the lower extremity while maintaining lumbo-pelvic stability and lower extremity alignment. The exercise helps strengthen the hip flexors while mobilizing the hip independent of the pelvis in the sagittal plane.

Real-Life Application: This exercise has also traditionally been considered a back stabilization exercise for rehabilitation of lumbar spine dysfunction. It can be used to restore hip flexion in patients after total hip replacement or as an adjunct to hip mobilization for a tight posterior/inferior hip capsule to enhance functional activities such as walking, transitioning to sitting on a toilet, climbing stairs, and/or dressing. It is an essential exercise to include in neuromuscular reeducation of the hip flexors with hip osteoarthritis and for patients with a flat back posture as defined by Kendall.

Trunk Extension

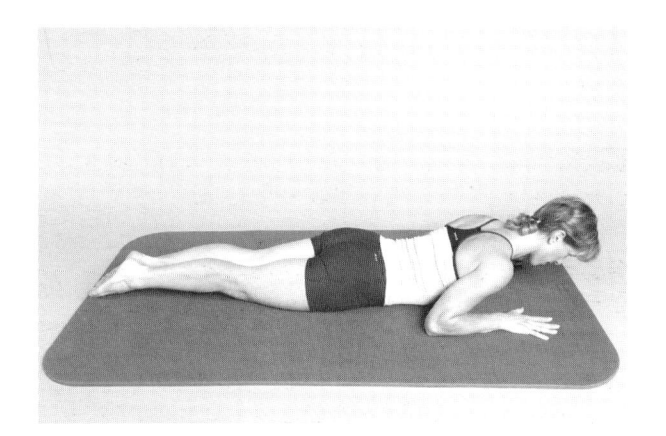

Use this exercise to enhance thoracic mobility and develop upper/mid-back erector spinae strength while maintaining pelvic stability and scapular/rib cage stabilization.

Real-Life Application: This exercise is excellent strengthening for osteoporotic and/or kyphotic patients. Use Trunk Extension as an adjunct to mobilization of thoracic spine to enhance spine mobility or muscle energy techniques for FRS dysfunction to encourage spinal extension.

Leg Pull Front Warm-up/Pushup Preparation:

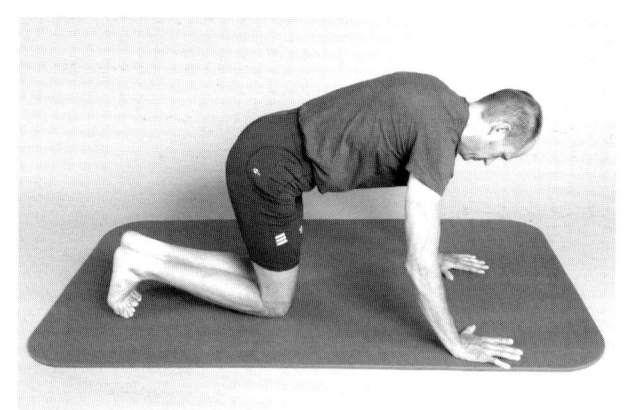

As mentioned in Chapter 7, this exercise provides closed kinetic chain (CKC) training of the upper extremity with emphasis on increasing joint approximation, stimulating joint proprioceptors, enhancing muscle co-activation patterns of the glenohumeral joint and scapulae, and decreasing glenohumeral joint translation.

Real-Life Application: This is an excellent exercise for shoulder instability and/or patients with scapular dysfunction that require stabilization in sports-related activities such as gymnastics, football (defensive/offensive linemen), and cycling. It also helps strengthen the upper fibers of the external obliques, helps reinforce torso stabilization via abdominal bracing, and provides isometric quadriceps strengthening and ankle mobilization.

Real-Life Case Studies

New Mom: Postpartum Female with Low Back Pain

Patient: A 32-year-old female client presents six months postpartum, post-Caesarean section. She has recurrent bilateral low back pain with prolonged standing and lifting. Back pain is presently intermittent. She would like to resume an exercise and strengthening program to regain her fitness and strength lost during pregnancy. She was working out a year prior to her pregnancy. What Pilates-based principles and exercises would complement your physical therapy program? Take a moment to make a few notes.

_____

_____

_____

_____

Significant findings:

Posture: Kyphotic/lordotic with anterior pelvic tilt

Right > left protracted scapula

Moderate genu recurvatum (hyperextended knees) bilaterally

Breathing: Upper chest breathing with poor L>R rib mobility noted with inhalation/exhalation

Lumbar range of motion: Within normal limits and pain free

Neurological exam: Unremarkable

Flexibility: Moderate tightness of one-/two-joint hip flexors, ITB, and TFL bilaterally

Manual muscle testing: Gluteus maximus: 4-/5 bilaterally; hip extension: 4-/5 bilaterally with compensatory hamstring firing bilaterally; lower trapezius: 3/5 (R), 3+/5 (L); middle trapezius: 4-/5 (R), 4/5 (L); rhomboids: 4-/5 (R), 4/5 (L); paraspinal extensors: 3+/5

Palpation: Scar well healed in pelvic area/horizontal incision, moderate decrease in mobility

Diastasis recti (negative)

Transversus abdominis recruitment: Abdominal popping noted bilaterally with attempting TrA contraction; bilateral TrA contraction noted with pelvic floor contraction and verbal cueing

Segmental mobility: Hypermobility noted L1-L5

Spine rotation: Compensatory L>R upper thoracic rotation with poor L>R IO and R>L EO activation with cueing

Functional assessment: Squat: genu recurvatum (starting position); increased lumbar lordosis with squat, poor kinesthetic awareness of neutral pelvis position with cueing

Pilates checklist:

☐ Complete a posture and functional assessment.

☐ Assess breathing and transversus abdominis muscle recruitment noting bilateral/unilateral asymmetries and address using Pilates and conventional physical therapy techniques.

☐ Choose Pilates principles and fundamental exercises appropriate for kyphotic/lordotic posture that emphasize concentric contractions of the thoracic and hip extensors; neutral/posterior tilt; concentric contraction of the internal/external obliques; and closed chain training of the upper extremities.

☐ Observe appropriate firing patterns of global and local abdominal/low back muscles.

Recommended Pilates-based exercises (in addition to conventional physical therapies):

1. Teach principles of core stabilization. First, normalize breathing mechanics. Next, train the TrA with pelvic floor contraction. Then advance to independent TrA contraction followed by abdominal bracing.

2. Enhance kinesthetic awareness by applying principles in weight-bearing movement with neutral pelvis, proper body mechanics, and lifting techniques relative to childcare.

3. Select Pilates-based exercises based on objective findings and compensatory strategies in the functional exam and patient goals that include resuming a resistance and exercise training program (for example, inability to maintain neutral pelvis with hip flexion, such as with a squat). Return to an exercise fundamental: supine Single Leg to Tabletop (Chapter 6).

- Pelvic Clock

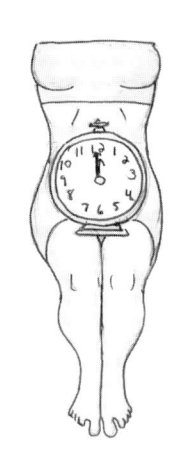

- Single Leg to Tabletop with progression to exercise in standing

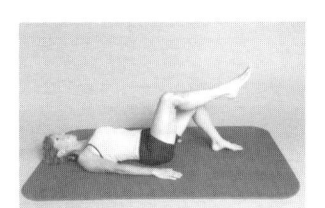

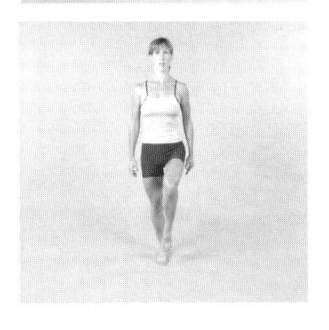

- Quarter Rollup with Neutral Pelvis

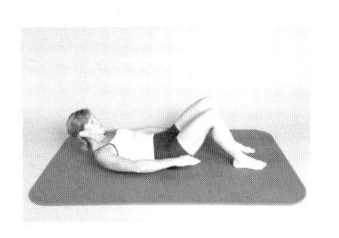

- Hundred with feet on the floor, progressing to legs in tabletop

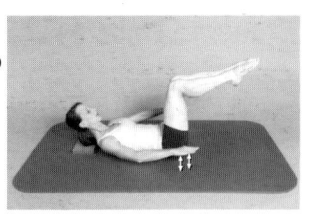

- One-Leg Circle with Two Knees Bent with progression to exercise in standing

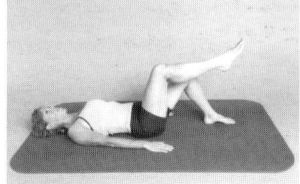

- Spine Twist with Legs Crossed with progression to exercise in standing

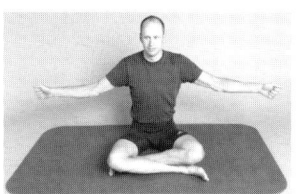

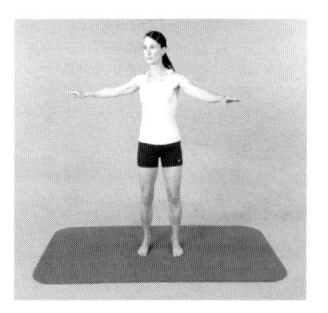

- Criss Cross with feet on the floor with progression to exercise in standing

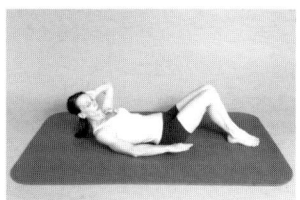

- Trunk Extension with Arm Patterns

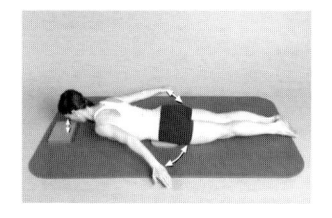

- Shoulder Bridge Prepatory Exercises, progressing to variations

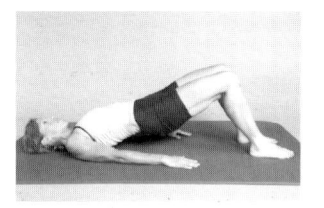

- Hip Abduction; Small Leg Circles with progression to exercise in standing

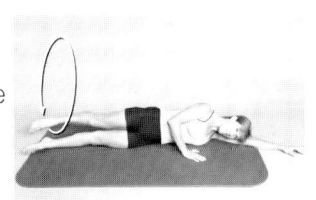

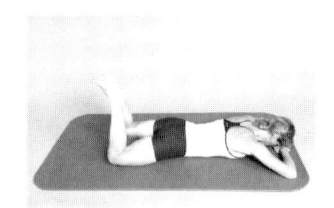

- Swimming Progressions

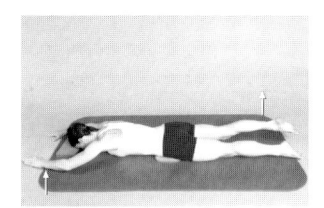

- Frog

- Leg Pull Front Warm-up

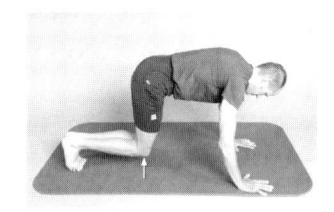

4. Advance patient once she has demonstrated appropriate breathing and stabilization techniques in beginner Pilates-based exercises.

Cross-Country Skier

Patient: A 37-year-old male cross-country skier presents with no complaints other than recurring unilateral low back pain (R). He has heard that Pilates, or core training, will help him to move into the coveted Elite Wave at the American Birkebeiner cross-country ski race held annually in February. In the course of his exercise and medical history, he tells you that he mountain bikes twice a week and works on the computer more than six hours a day.

Significant findings:

Posture: Kyphotic/lordotic

Mild left scoliosis, C-curve

Pelvic asymmetry, right hip high (reportedly due to adolescent sports-related injury)

Bilateral abducted/protracted scapulae

Lumbar range of motion: Within normal limits

Erector spinae hypertrophy, right side

Segmental mobility: Within normal limits

Ankle/foot: Pes planus, left side; neutral, right side

Flexibility: Moderate range of motion in hamstrings bilaterally; restricted rectus abdominis

Breathing: Normal breathing mechanics with noted poor rib mobility, right side

TrA recruitment: Normal

Abdominal Bracing: Normal

Functional assessment: Squat: increased lumbar lordosis with shoulder flexion at 180 degrees, weight transfer forward, reduced ankle range of motion secondary to soleus tightness, foot pronation L>R; Spine rotation: compensatory L>R upper thoracic rotation with poor L>R IO and R>L EO activation with cueing

Offer the patient some Pilates exercises to address his muscle imbalances and help him achieve his cross-country skiing goals.

Take a moment to make a few notes.

_____

_____

_____

_____

_____

Pilates checklist:

☐ Pilates should supplement this advanced athlete's dryland and weight training programs and work to counteract his training and desk work in a flexed position. Cross-country skiers require significant core strength and balance as well as strong latissimus dorsi, triceps, and other primary shoulder flexors/extensors. The hip abductors in particular must be conditioned for quick, powerful pushes as well as stabilization against the momentum of movement. Much time is spent in a spine-flexed position with emphasis on a slight posterior tilt of the pelvis. Scapular and shoulder stabilization is key to the technique with the scapulae slightly depressed and protracted.

☐ The sport requirements indicate a treatment plan that addresses this athlete's training needs while considering his unique muscle imbalances. A number of exercises should focus on lengthening the right lateral trunk muscles and hip adductors and strengthening of the same muscles on the left as well as his hip abductors. Exercises that help strengthen the posterior thoracic spine musculature should also be a focus.

☐ Given the number of training hours required to reach the Birkie's Elite Wave, special attention should be paid to counteracting anterior-focused concentric muscle contractions with concentric thoracic and hip extension exercises. Weight-bearing balance work warrants emphasis on pelvic symmetries in all planes of movement.

Recommended Pilates-based exercises:

- Teach principles of core stabilization

- Bent-Knee Fallout with Neutral Pelvis

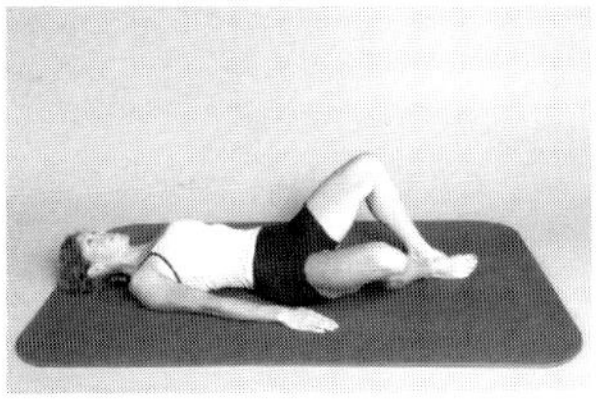

- Quarter Rollup in Neutral Pelvis with Shoulder Flexion/Extension (medicine ball in hands)

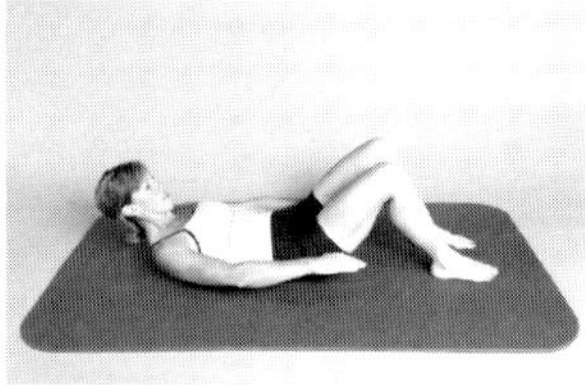

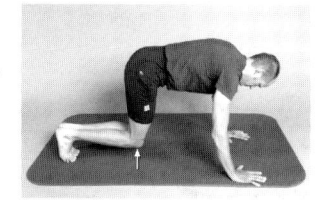

- Single-Leg Stretch, modified to 5 reps/release/5 reps to simulate concentric/eccentric sport demand

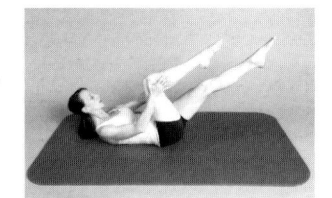

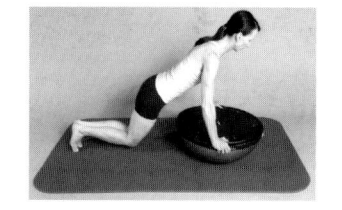

- Trunk Extensions, progressing to Diamond Window with rotation variation

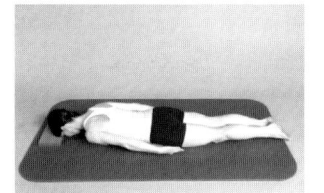

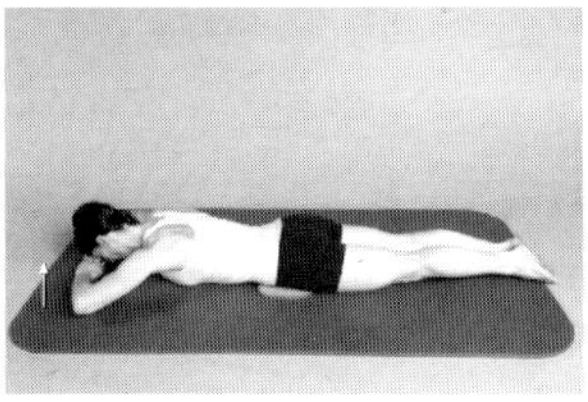

- Swimming Progressions with emphasis on shoulder stability

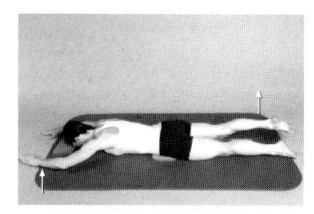

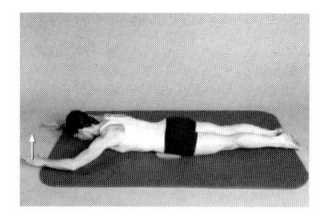

- Leg Pull Front Warm-up with emphasis on scapular stability

- Hip Abduction; Small to Large Leg Circles; advance to unilateral standing, unilateral standing on a balance board (Reebok Core Board® or BOSU®)

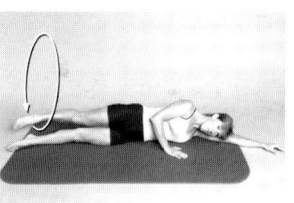

- Side Bend with emphasis on left side, advancing with body bar in sidelying; advance to weight-bearing with resistance

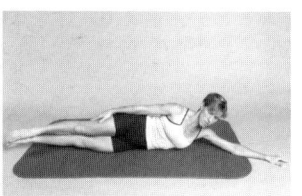

- Criss Cross in Standing, adding stability ball, advancing to medicine ball

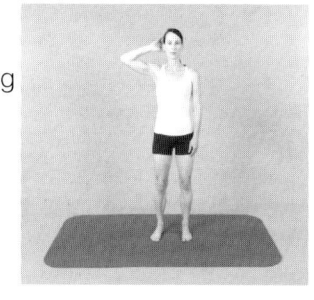

199

- Spine Twist crossed, advancing to Spine Twist in Standing and Lunge positions

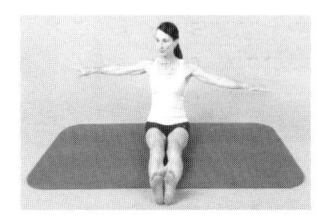

- Pushup with emphasis on torso and shoulder stability

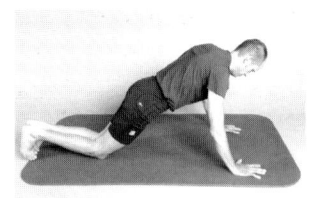

- Mermaid Stretch with emphasis on right side

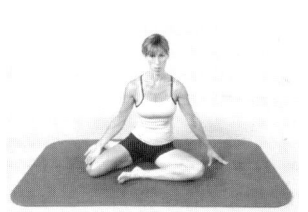

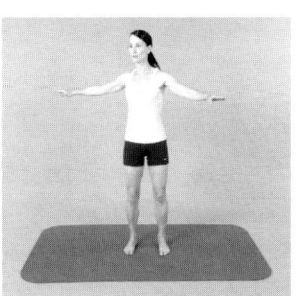

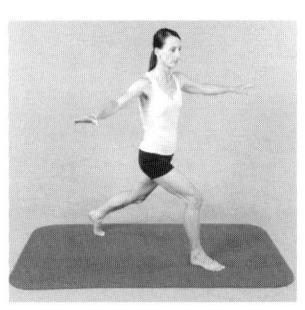

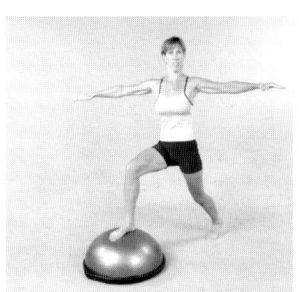

Patient with Hip Replacement

Patient: A 55-year-old male presents one month after total right hip replacement with complaints of right hip muscle fatigue and general discomfort when walking with a cane for long time periods, difficulty transitioning from sit to stand, and an inability to perform recreational walking. His short- and long-term goals include: 1) transitioning from sit to stand without difficulty in two and a half weeks; 2) walking without his cane in three to four weeks; and 3) walking a quarter mile three times per week in three months.

Significant findings:

Posture: Flat back, moderate L>R

Breathing: Upper chest breathing with poor rib cage mobility with exhalation

Hip active range of motion: Right hip flexion: 90 degrees; hip abduction: 30 degrees; and hip external rotation: 28 degrees

Manual muscle testing: Gluteus medius: 3-/5 (R), 4/5 (L); hip extension: 3-/5 (R), 4/5 (L); hip flexors: 3+/5 (R), 4/5 (L)

Palpation: Poor right lateral hip scar mobility (approximately 4 inches long) and moderate right gluteus medius atrophy present; poor right gluteus medius muscle firing with IM contraction

TrA recruitment: Compensatory firing of IO muscles bilaterally/posterior pelvic tilt secondary to gluteal firing

Functional assessment:

Gait: Moderate right Trendelenburg

Single-Leg Balance with hip flexion: Inability to dissociate right hip from pelvis (increased posterior tilt) with compensatory right trunk side bend.

Hip abduction: Increased right TFL firing, poor and delayed gluteus medius firing with compensatory posterior pelvic tilt and hip flexion

Squat: Inability to dissociate hips from pelvis (increased posterior tilt) and dynamic right knee valgus present

Hip extension: Compensatory hamstring firing with ability to dissociate hip from pelvis

Design an exercise program with consideration of the physician's guidelines using Pilates principles and mat exercises. Precautions for the first six weeks after total hip replacement include avoiding hip flexion beyond 90 degrees, hip adduction, and hip internal rotation to prevent hip dislocation. Take a moment to make a few notes.

_____

_____

_____

_____

_____

Pilates checklist:

☐ The overall goals are to enhance repatterning of muscle recruitment and quality of movement. Begin with principles of stabilization with specific focus on retraining breathing mechanics and TrA engagement.

☐ Next, select Pilates-based mat exercises that complement your treatment plan, including increasing hip range of motion, neuromuscular reeducation and strengthening of quadriceps, the gluteus medius and gluteus maximus muscles, scar tissue mobilization, and gait reeducation. Remember to select exercises that are within physician guidelines.

Recommended Pilates-based exercises include:

- Heel Slides

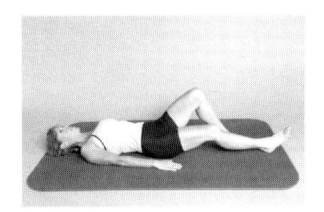

- Single Leg Tabletop with progression to standing when stabilization is mastered with Single-Leg Balance

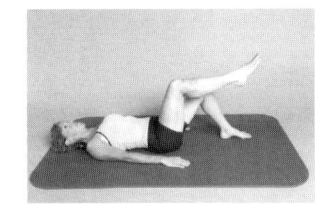

- Bent-Knee Fallout progressing to External Rotation with Knee Extension

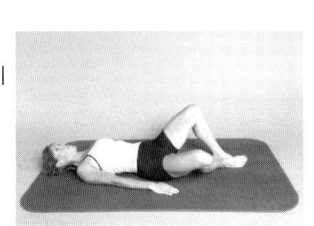

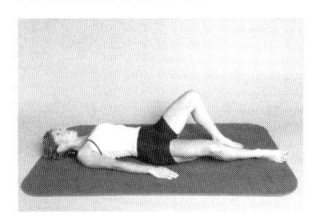

- Hip Abduction Progression 1 (pillow placed between the legs to avoid hip adduction)

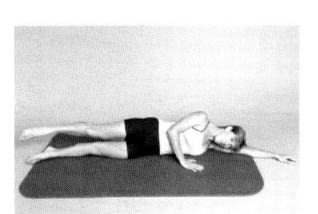

- Prone Hip Extension Preps/Variations with progression to standing to aid in gait reeducation

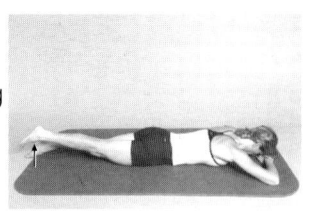

- Shoulder Bridge Prepatory Exercise 1

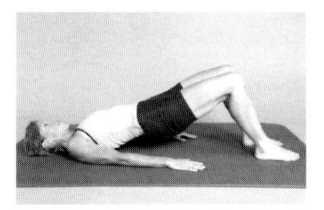

- One-Leg Circle (modify to circle out only and flex hip to starting position; avoid hip adduction)

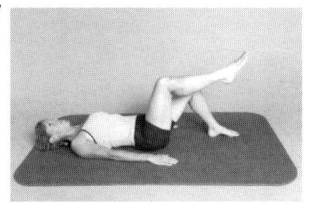

Apply principles to these traditional exercises:

- Squat
- Weight shift with progression to Single-Leg Balance
- Toe Raises
- Straight Leg Raise supine

Osteoporotic Female

Patient: A 50-year-old female presents with a five-year history of osteoporosis. Her status is currently osteopenia for the past three years. She is taking a bone-building medication prescribed by her primary care provider and is on a strengthening and aerobic conditioning program three to five times a week.

Medical History: Caesarean section and plantar fasciitis, right side

Significant findings:

Posture: Kyphotic, lordotic

Moderate bilaterally protracted shoulders L>R with poor postural awareness in sitting, standing, and with transitional movements

Genu valgus/recurvatum bilaterally

Excessive R>L foot pronation

Protruded abdomen

Gluteal atrophy bilaterally

Breathing: abdominal breathing

Lumbar range of motion: Within normal limits and pain free

Strength: Lower trapezius: 2+/5 (L), 3-/5 (R); middle trapezius: 3+/5(L), 4-/5 (R); rhomboids: 4-/5 (L), 4/5 (R); serratus anterior: 4-/5 (L), 4/5 (R); back extensors: 2/5; gluteus medius: 4/5 (R), 4+/5 (L); gluteus maximus: 4-/5 (bilaterally)

Flexibility: Moderate L>R pectoralis major and minor, moderate L>R upper trapezius/levator scapula, moderate bilateral hip flexor/quadriceps muscle tightness; gastrocnemius length: 0 degrees (R), 3 degrees (L)

TrA recruitment: Absent TrA recruitment pattern; bilateral TrA contraction via pelvic floor contraction

Palpation: Myofascial diaphragm restrictions bilaterally

Functional assessment:

Gait: Excessive R>L foot pronation

Single-Leg Balance: 5 seconds (R), 8 seconds (L)

Squat: Inability to dissociate hip from pelvis (increased anterior tilt) with dynamic right knee valgus present with increased R>L foot pronation

Transition from sit to stand: Increased anterior pelvic tilt, dynamic right knee valgus, excessive R>L foot pronation

Hip Extension: Compensatory hamstring firing bilaterally with increased lumbar lordosis

Bridge: Compensatory posterior pelvic tilt at beginning and end of exercise; posterior pelvic tilt initiated via gluteal muscles

Design a program using Pilates principles and exercises that will complement your conventional physical therapy treatment. What areas do you want to emphasize and deemphasize? Take a moment to make a few notes.

_____

_____

_____

_____

_____

Pilates checklist:

☐ Contraindications for individuals with a diagnosis of osteoporosis include spinal flexion and rotation due to the compressive forces on the spine. Assess breathing and note dysfunction, if present. Because the patient is osteopenic, proceed with a conservative treatment plan.

☐ Assess the transversus abdominis and lumbar multifidus and note asymmetries. The treatment goals include normalizing breathing mechanics, normalizing the TrA recruitment pattern, progressing to abdominal bracing and core strength, increasing proprioception, and enhancing the quality of functional movement. Design a Pilates-based program that will complement the patient's current training program, build core strength, and help her improve her current status of osteopenia.

☐ Choose exercises that work the muscles around joints known to be fracture sites: lumbar spine, wrist, and hip.

☐ Initially, the treatment focus is to enhance breathing mechanics, which include myofascial release of the diaphragm and pectoral muscles, reeducation of breathing mechanics, and use of equipment as an option to provide feedback for posterolateral rib cage expansion. Next, introduce TrA training via pelvic floor contraction with progression to isolated contraction and then abdominal bracing. Scapular stabilization and rib cage placement training are important principles to review for optimizing torso stabilization. Once these principles are mastered, emphasize movement patterns that include thoracic and hip extension; limit but don't avoid spine-flexed and rotated positions.

Recommended Pilates-based exercises:

- Teach principles of core stabilization with emphasis on retraining breathing and normalize TrA recruitment with progression to abdominal bracing

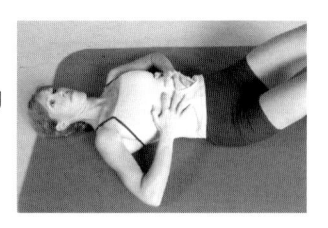

- Pelvic Tilt and Pelvic Clock with focus on limited gluteal substitution

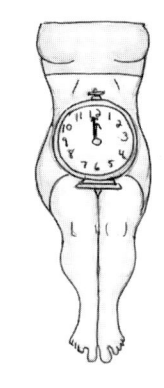

- Quarter Rollup with Neutral Pelvis

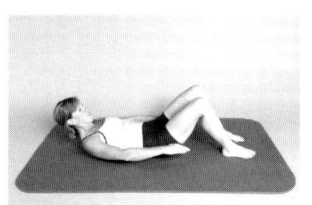

- Trunk Extension with Arm Patterns, advancing when ready

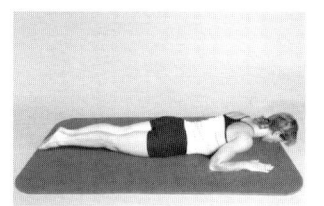

- Spine Twist with legs crossed, emphasis on limited ROM

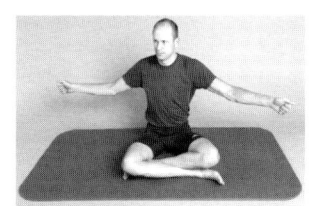

- Single-Leg Stretch with knees flexed, head on floor

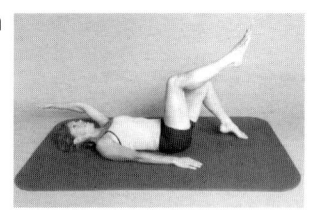

- Criss Cross, feet on floor and one hand behind the head, emphasis on limited ROM

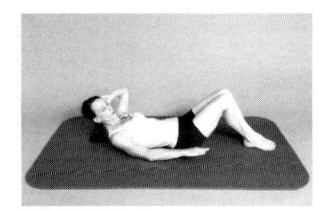

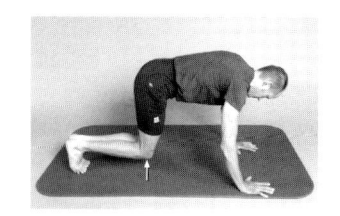

- Prone Hip Extension preps with progression to full exercise

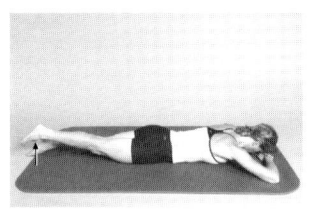

- Swimming

Progressions

- Hip Abduction/

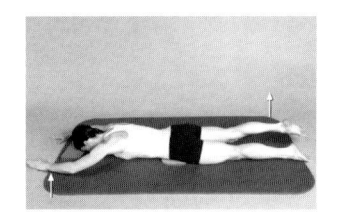

Adduction Progressions

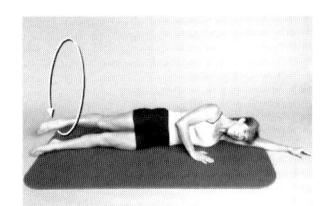

- Leg Pull Front Warm-up

- Pushup

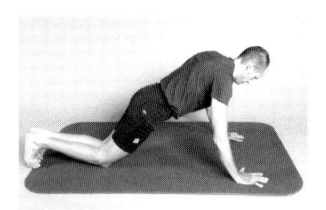

Apply principles to the following traditional exercises:

- Squat
- Weight shift with progression to Single-Leg Balance
- Weight training program
- ADLs (i.e., transition from sit to stand)

ACL Reconstruction in a Young Athlete

An 18-year-old male college basketball center is three weeks post right anterior cruciate ligament reconstruction with patellar tendon allograft. His major complaints include limping with walking and ascending and descending stairs one at a time.

Significant findings:

Knee active range of motion: 0-125 degrees

Strength: Quadriceps IM contraction: good in long/short sit, fair in standing with compensatory gluteal firing (R); hamstring: 4/5 (R), 5/5 (L)

TrA assessment: Normal TrA recruitment pattern bilaterally

Abdominal bracing: Normal

Flexibility: Hamstring: 70 degrees (R), 85 degrees (L)

Swelling: Suprapatellar (mild)

Functional assessment:

Gait: Ambulates with slight extensor lag (R)

Knee Bends: Fair quadriceps muscle recruitment and eccentric control with compensatory anterior pelvic tilt and lateral shifting to the left

Single-Leg Balance: 5 seconds (R) with poor body alignment (anterior pelvic tilt/protracted scapula), fair quadriceps control (dynamic knee valgus), 30 seconds (L)

What Pilates principles could you use to enhance gait reeducation, Knee Bends, and proprioceptive training during this phase of rehabilitation based on the objective and functional assessment findings? Take a moment to make a few notes.

_____

_____

_____

_____

_____

To support these important components of rehabilitation and set the foundation for functional training, it is essential to include the principles of core stabilization in conventional therapeutic exercises. The principles complement treatment to assist in normalizing the quadriceps/hamstring length-tension relationship of the knee and hip joints via neutral pelvis positioning, using breath to engage the deep core stabilizers and challenge stabilization with range of motion and strengthening exercises, and enhancing torso stabilization with knee motion and strengthening exercises. For example:

- Quadriceps reeducation: IM in standing with the ability to stabilize the torso with the primary and secondary stabilizers and increasing challenge with the addition of breath. Progress to Knee Bends once a normal quadriceps recruitment pattern and torso stabilization are demonstrated.
- Knee Bends: Challenge lumbo-pelvic and scapular stabilization as well as breathing while mobilizing and strengthening the hips and knees
- Single-Leg Balance: Challenge lumbo-pelvic and scapular stabilization while maintaining even pressure throughout the foot with a slightly flexed knee

Recommended Pilates-based mat exercises:

- Heel Slides

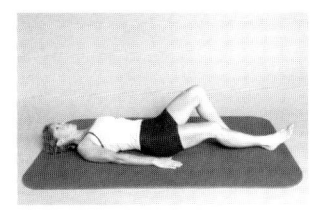

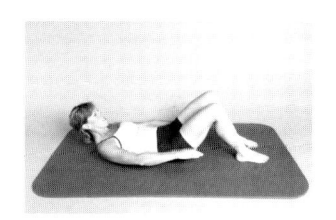

- Single Leg in Tabletop

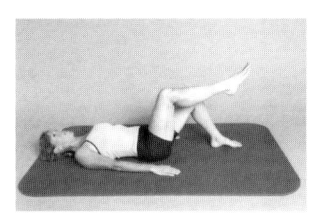

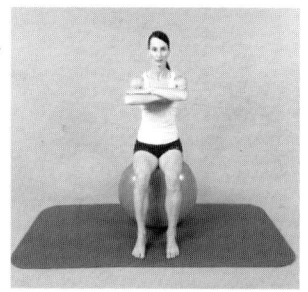

- Prone Hip Extension

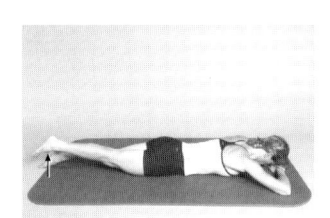

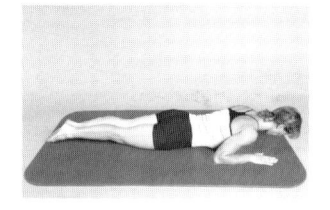

- Hip Abduction Progression 1

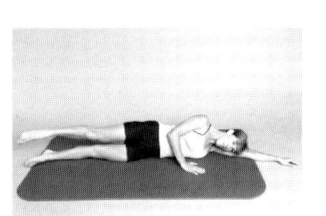

- Quarter Rollup in Neutral Pelvis

- Spine Twist in a Chair, advancing to a stability ball

- Trunk Extension Prepatory Exercises 1-3

Chapter References

1. Kendall, F.P., McCreary, E.K., Provance, P.G. 1993. *Muscles, Testing and Function, Posture and Pain*, Fourth Edition. Baltimore, MD: Williams and Wilkins.

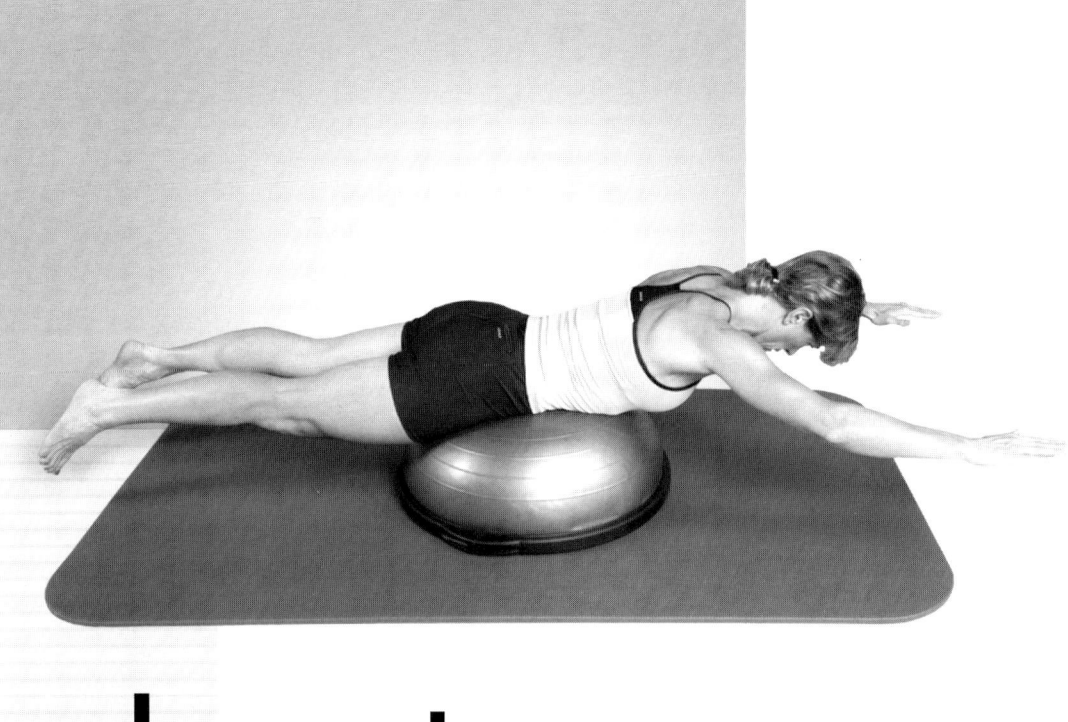

chapter 12

Fitness Training for Athletes: Rehabilitation and Return to Play

Today's athletic training programs increasingly include Pilate-based principles of stabilization and exercises. As a method of dynamic training, Pilates can help increase strength, power, and control of the body's midsection through movement patterns that focus on precision.

What's the secret of Pilates relative to sport? The Pilates method of conditioning allows for efficient transfer of energy from the core to the lower and upper extremities, allowing the athlete to meet the demands and challenges of sport with better control of sport-specific momentum, rotary movement, balance, reaction time, and coordination.

Pilates also benefits the athlete in creating a more balanced body. It is no surprise that even the strongest of athletes have muscle imbalances. With the high level of training and repetitive movements occurring within particular sports, some muscles become too strong and some too tight. The result can be acute or chronic injuries.

Strengthening core muscles develops torso stability and muscle balance, allowing joints to work maximally through their range. This is critical for efficient movement of the upper and lower extremities (1). Pilates also helps athletes increase awareness of their muscle imbalances and understand the impact of core training on their torso.

Athletic Rehabilitation: Using Pilates to Affect Patient Outcomes

Unfortunately, many of today's treatment protocols do not take advantage of core stabilization training when rehabilitating the injured athlete. While it is an essential component for rehabilitation of lumbar spine dysfunctions, it isn't as common to rehabilitation of an athlete's upper or lower extremity injuries.

We believe that Pilates principles and exercises are critical to the orthopaedic rehabilitation of any athletic injury. Athletes benefit from improved core strength, identification of faulty movement patterns, reduced compensatory strategies, a more stable base of support, and restored biomechanics with the long-term goal of enhanced performance.

In Chapter 4, practitioners learned how to develop a customized Pilates rehabilitation program based on information gathered from a patient's medical history, musculoskeletal assessment, functional assessment, and goals. Taken a step further, we've created an outline for a Pilates-based athletic program that addresses sport-specific demands, injury factors relative to sport, and integration of Pilates into the athlete's injury rehabilitation.

Examining the Demands of Sport

Every sport is unique in the demands placed on the athlete's body. Sport-dependent, the physiological demands range from anaerobic, aerobic, or a combination of both. Sprinting, kicking, throwing, jumping, landing, pivoting, direction changes, acceleration, deceleration, and balance and coordination of upper and lower extremities symmetrically or asymmetrically are common elements in sport. Movements may be closed or open kinetic chain, rotational, compressive, uniplanar, multiplanar, multidirectional, explosive, ballistic, or combinations thereof (2).

A good starting point in getting the athlete back to play is to analyze his or her sport, identifying the physiological demands and the different types of movement. How does that athlete's body respond to these demands? In some sports, it is critical to look at the requirements within a sport. For example, the demands for a football quarterback will be different than those for a running back; a sprinter's requirements will be different than a marathoner's.

1. ***Analyze the demands of your patient's sport.***
   What are the predominant movement patterns and actions of the extremities and spine? Is movement explosive or compressive? Is movement primarily in the sagittal, frontal, or transverse plane, or a combination of all?

Examples:

- The demands for sprinting require torso stabilization to allow efficient transfer of energy of the upper and lower extremities with maintenance of acceleration and speed during linear motion (2).

- The demands for road biking require the ability to maintain a slight posterior tilt, even weight on the ischial tuberosities, and scapular control to avoid upper body tension.
- The demands of golf require stabilization of the pelvis in neutral while coordinating spinal rotation with movement of the upper and lower extremities (2).

2. **Observe pelvic control.** Is the position of the pelvis important for core stabilization? Yes. Do all sports require neutral pelvis with athletic movements? No. While it's true that neutral spine is the strongest training position from a lumbo-pelvic perspective, some sports require a slight posterior tilt (i.e., skating technique for cross-country skiing) for maximum efficiency and others require an anterior tilt (i.e., gymnastics). To be efficient, running requires both anterior and posterior tilting within the running cycle. (3)

- The important take-away for practitioners is that athletes must be: 1) aware of their pelvis position and 2) have the ability to control it for their sport via muscle strength and coordination.

3. **Observe scapular control.** Is scapular stabilization important for core stabilization? Yes. Do all sports require scapular stabilization with athletic movements? Yes; however, the position in which the scapulae are stabilized is dependent on an athlete's sport. The scapulae may be stabilized in a protracted position for some sports such as cross-country skiing (i.e., skate and classic) or overhead throwing, or stabilized in retraction and depression for other sports such as swimming (i.e., backstroke), or a combination of both, as in pitching a baseball.

4. **What are the target muscles and their role in the sport?** What are the predominant muscles and actions for an athlete's particular sport? The athlete's body is constantly moving and requires core stabilization to support the spine while multiple muscle synergies of the upper and lower extremities occur simultaneously. Core stabilization is not just about strengthening the abdominal muscles. Other critical muscles of the core include the gluteals and low back to develop balanced core strength on the front and back of the body. These muscles must also assist in force absorption and help decelerate the body against motion and gravity.

5. **Analyze the abdominals.** The abdominals have two functions: as spinal stabilizers and spinal mobilizers. The TrA acts as a stabilizer of the lumbo-pelvic region. The rectus abdominis and the internal and external oblique muscles have dual functions as stabilizers and mobilizers of the spine. Together, all work synergistically to stabilize the spine in the sagittal, frontal, and/or transverse planes via isometric contractions and to mobilize the spine in flexion, rotation, and lateral flexion according to their specific roles.

6. **Observe the gluteals.** The gluteals are both stabilizers and mobilizers. In closed chain unilateral weight-bearing movement, the gluteus medius provides a stable base of support via its role as a stabilizer (2). In open chain activity, the gluteus medius is a mobilizer via hip abduction (2). The gluteus maximus acts as a mobilizer with hip extension and partners with the abdominals to maintain neutral pelvis with movement of the upper extremities.

7. **Test the low back.** The remaining core stabilizers of the lumbar spine include the lumbar multifidus and the erector spinae. While they are not discussed as often as the abdominals and gluteals, they are just as important. The multifidus stabilizes via its connections to the lumbar spine, resists rotation with sagittal and frontal plane movement via isometric contractions, and acts as a mobilizer in spine extension, lateral flexion, and contralateral rotation. The erector spinae muscles act as a mobilizer of the spine in extension with bilateral muscle contraction and lateral flexion with unilateral contraction. They also stabilize frontal plane movement of the trunk.

8. **Observe the primary movers.** In addition to the core muscles, look at the primary movers of the upper and lower extremities within the athlete's sport. Ask: What are the movement requirements? What type of muscle contractions? Eccentric, concentric, co-activation patterns, or a combination? Is the normal muscle recruitment sequence, strength, and flexibility of muscle(s) altered as identified in your musculoskeletal exam affecting sport performance?

A Weak Core: Relating Sport and Injury

We all recognize that the demands of an athlete's sport can lead to injury, but how many of us have related a sports injury to weak core muscles or lack of torso stabilization capabilities?

Compensatory movement patterns occur for a variety of reasons. One of those may be a weak core. Research is lacking in this area relative to athletic injury; however, there is anecdotal evidence that supports core muscle imbalances and athletic injuries. For example, an injury might occur to the arm of a baseball pitcher if he or she fails to bring the muscles of the trunk into the throwing action, thereby placing excessive strain on the shoulder muscles (4). Decreased core strength for the runner may result in decreased pelvic and torso stabilization and affect performance (1) and/or contribute to injuries of the low back, pelvis, knee, and hip.

So, where do you start? Here are some guidelines for getting athletes back to play.

1. Identify faulty movement patterns.

The basic functional movement assessment in Chapter 4 may be adequate for practitioners to identify compensatory strategies with specific elements of a sport and relate it to their musculoskeletal assessment findings. Video analysis is another option. It is a comprehensive tool used to assess an athlete's sport biomechanics and faulty movement mechanics.

The biomechanical faults need to be correlated to the practitioner's findings. For example, the runner with a weak gluteus medius may demonstrate any of the following biomechanical faults with a video analysis assessment (5):

- Excessive unilateral side bend
- Wide arm carriage
- Wide base of support
- Contralateral hip drop
- Foot crossover with heel strike

If video analysis is not available, use the athlete's coach or trainer as a resource to gather information about an athlete's mechanics with sport. You will be surprised what a coach can tell you about your athlete's technique and movement quality. Relate your objective findings to identified faulty techniques.

2. Create a Pilates-based rehabilitation program.

When creating a Pilates-based core training program and/or integrating Pilates-based principles in conventional exercise programs for the injured athlete, selected exercises should mimic movement associated with the athlete's sport. The program can be broken into three phases:

- Developing stability
- Isolated-integration
- Sport-specific skills training

Each of these phases is integrated into the more conventional rehabilitation stages: acute, recovery, and functional (6). A portion of the Pilates-based program may parallel conventional rehabilitation programming. The length of each of these stages and phases is dependent on the athlete's injury, associated musculoskeletal deficiencies, and ability to demonstrate Pilates-based principles of core stabilization with precision and control. The table below provides an overview of our Pilates-based approach.

Three-Phase Pilates-Based Rehabilitation Program

Phases	Goal 1	Goal 2: Rehab-based	Goal 3: Pilates-based
Phase 1	Develop stability	Regain pain-free motion, decrease pain and inflammation, increase neuromuscular control, reduce muscle atrophy (6).	Introduce Pilates principles of torso stabilization.
Phase 2	Integrated isolation	Increase joint range of motion, improving muscle strength, enhancing neuromuscular control (6)	Introduce uniplanar and unijoint movement patterns in supine, progressing to weight bearing as appropriate. Introduce basic torso stabilization principles with fundamental lower/upper extremity motion.
Phase 3	Sport-specific skills training	Introduce sport-specific movement patterns, plyometrics.	Introduce multiplanar, multijoint movement patterns in supine, progressing to weight bearing with emphasis on torso stabilization with sport-specific movement patterns of arms and legs and plyometrics. Introduce equipment to challenge Pilates-based principles of torso stabilization.

Phase 1: Developing stability. The first phase will probably be the most difficult for the injured athlete. Why? The athlete starts out at the same level as everyone else. For athletes who are used to performing exercises at a high level, the experience can cause frustration because he or she may not experience the typical workout sensations of fatigue and challenge.

It can also be humbling for some to experience muscles such as the TrA contract for the first time and experience muscles such as the serratus anterior quivering and fatiguing with just a few repetitions. Use this opportunity to educate the athlete about target muscles that he or she needs to develop and why this is an essential building block to improve function for a balanced body. This approach will set the tone for advanced phases of training.

In this phase, the focus is developing core stability via the Pilates-based principles of stabilization to create a foundation for the remaining phases of core training. What does this mean to the athlete? The focus is core strengthening to promote stabilization before introduction of movement of the upper and lower extremities, which will challenge stabilization (7). The athlete must be able to perform Pilates-based principles of stabilization in isolation and in combination before proceeding to the next level.

This phase is concurrent with the acute phase of rehabilitation where the focus is regaining pain-free range of motion, reducing muscle atrophy, increasing neuromuscular control, decreasing pain and inflammation of the injured area, and maintaining cardiovascular fitness and the strength of uninvolved extremities (6). Once the principles of core stabilization are mastered and the injury has healed adequately, the athlete can be advanced to the next phase of training.

Phase 2: Isolated-integration. In this phase, lumbo-pelvic stabilization is challenged by introducing uniplanar and unijoint movements of the upper and/or lower extremities. This phase can occur during the acute and recovery stages of rehabilitation. The goals for the recovery stage of rehabilitation include increasing joint range of motion, enhancing neuromuscular control, and improving muscle strength of the injured area (6).

Remember that Pilates-based exercise selection is based on the clinician's assessment, physician protocols (nonsurgical and surgical), identified muscle imbalances, joint hypomobilities and hypermobilities, and key muscle actions and movement patterns that are specific to the patient's sport. Maintain or improve cardiovascular fitness.

Phase 3: Sport-specific skills training. In this stage of functional rehabilitation, sport-specific movement patterns and plyometrics are introduced. These patterns will challenge the athlete's ability to stabilize and effectively mobilize specific joints in a controlled environment to develop muscle stamina and power and kinesthetic awareness (6).

Based on your knowledge base, Pilates-based exercises can be modified or enhanced to meet the goals of the injured athlete during this stage in the following ways:

- Progressing exercises to multiplanar and multijoint sport-specific movement patterns.
- Using equipment such as a stability ball, Reebok Core Board®, or BOSU® to simulate unstable surfaces in both weight-bearing and semi-weight-bearing positions, effectively challenging balance and dynamic movement of an athlete's sport. The BOSU® can be an effective tool in teaching athletes to control the forces of acceleration/deceleration.
- Increase speed of movement with the focus of precision and control of the pelvis and scapulae against the rhythm of movement.
- Functional training using resistance, such as a medicine ball, to challenge stabilization of the core and extremities and simulate concentric/eccentric phases of movement, and use of equipment with sport movements.

Sample Program 1: Pilates-based ACL Reconstruction Rehabilitation Program

Here is an example of how practitioners can enhance a conventional post-ACL reconstruction program with Pilates-based principles and mat exercises.

Phase I (Acute ROM/Neuromuscular Control)

Conventional exercise: Heel Slides

Principles to use: Breathing, neutral pelvic position

Purpose: To challenge lumbo-pelvic stabilization and restore pain-free knee range of motion

Compensatory strategies: Inability to maintain pelvic position; abdominal popping; hip hiking, observed either in the involved extremity with knee flexion or in the uninvolved extremity with knee extension; upper body tension; Valsalva

Quadriceps/Hamstring Sets (Co-contraction)

Principles to use: Breathing, neutral pelvic position

Purpose: To develop lumbo-pelvic stabilization and neuromuscular control of the quadriceps and hamstrings with muscles in the optimal length training position

Compensatory strategies: Inability to maintain pelvic position; compensatory gluteal firing; abdominal popping; upper body tension; Valsalva

Straight Leg Raise (Supine)

Principles to use: Breathing, neutral pelvic position, and scapular control

Purpose: To challenge lumbo-pelvic stabilization, isometric quadriceps muscle strengthening at the knee joint, concentric/eccentric contraction of the hip flexors, and hip mobilization

Compensatory strategies: Inability to maintain pelvic position; compensatory gluteal firing; abdominal popping; pressing the uninvolved foot into the mat; using momentum

Conventional exercise: Straight Leg Raise (Abduction)

Pilates-based exercise: Hip Abduction 1

Principles to use: Breathing, neutral pelvic position scapular control

Purpose: To challenge lumbo-pelvic stabilization, isometric quadriceps strengthening and concentric/eccentric strengthening of the gluteal muscles, and hip mobilization; hyperextended knee

Compensatory strategies: Inability to maintain pelvic position; abdominal popping; trunk side bend; upper body tension; Valsalva

Conventional exercise: Straight Leg Raise (Extension)

Pilates-based exercise: Prone Hip Extension

Principles to use: Breathing, neutral pelvic position, scapular control, cervical spine alignment

Purpose: To challenge lumbo-pelvic stabilization, concentric/eccentric strengthening of gluteal/hamstring muscles, and hip mobilization.

Compensatory strategies: Inability to maintain pelvic position; abdominal popping; weight shifting unilaterally; segmental hinging (T12-L1); upper body tension; Valsalva

Prone Knee Flexion

Principles to use: Breathing, neutral pelvic position, scapular control, and cervical spine alignment

Purpose: To challenge lumbo-pelvic stabilization, concentric/eccentric strengthening of the hamstring muscles, and knee mobilization

Compensatory strategies: Inability to maintain pelvic position; abdominal popping; hip flexion; upper body tension; Valsalva

Weight Shifting In Standing

Principles to use: Breathing, neutral pelvic position, scapular control, and cervical spine alignment

Purpose: First exercise to introduce closed kinetic chain training to develop lumbo-pelvic stabilization in standing; co-activation of hip adductors, gluteals, hamstrings, and quadriceps muscles; excellent tool for gait training

Compensatory strategies: Inability to maintain pelvic position; abdominal popping; knee hyperextension; trunk side bend; upper body tension; Valsalva

Phase II (Recovery: ROM/Neuromuscular Control/Strength)

Knee Bends

Principles to use: Breathing, neutral pelvic position, scapular placement, and cervical spine alignment

Purpose: To challenge lumbo-pelvic stabilization; concentric/eccentric strengthening of the quadriceps, hamstrings, and gluteal muscles; mobilize the knee/hip; and develop a foundation for advanced CKC training

Compensatory strategies: Inability to maintain pelvic position; abdominal popping; heel rise secondary to decreased soleus flexibility and/or ankle joint mobility; upper body tension; Valsalva; knee hyperextension; knees coming forward to toes; lateral weight shifting

Wall Slides

Principles to use: Breathing, neutral pelvic position, scapular control, and cervical spine alignment

Purpose: Advanced closed kinetic training to challenge lumbo-pelvic stabilization; concentric/eccentric strengthening of the quadriceps, hamstrings, and gluteal muscles; develop endurance of the quadriceps, hamstrings, and gluteal muscles; hip joint mobilization.

Compensatory strategies: Inability to maintain pelvic position; abdominal popping; hip internal/external rotation; upper body tension; Valsalva; knee hyperextension; inability to fire the quadriceps muscles leading to compensatory gluteal and soleus firing; knees coming forward of ankles

Single-Leg Balance

Principles to use: Breathing, neutral pelvic position, scapular placement, and cervical spine alignment

Purpose: To challenge lumbo-pelvic stabilization; increase the strength of the hip, knee, and ankle with co-activation muscle synergies; develop proprioception

Compensatory strategies: Trunk side bend; inability to maintain pelvic position; knee hyperextension; foot pronation/supination

Knee Bend with Weight Shift

Principles to use: Breathing, neutral pelvic position, scapular placement, and cervical spine alignment

Purpose: To challenge lumbo-pelvic stabilization, increase weight bearing on the involved leg in preparation for unilateral CKC strengthening/foundation for functional training; concentric/eccentric strengthening of the quadriceps, hamstrings, and gluteal muscles; mobilize the knee/hip; knee hyperextension

Compensatory strategies: Trunk side bend; inability to maintain pelvic position

Phase III (Functional Strength, Power and Endurance)

Bilateral Supported Hopping

Principles to use: Breathing, neutral pelvic position, scapular placement, and cervical alignment

Purpose: To challenge lumbo-pelvic stabilization with sport-specific movements and plyometrics; increase weight bearing on the involved leg in preparation for unilateral CKC strengthening/ foundation for functional training; concentric/ eccentric strengthening of the quadriceps, hamstrings, and gluteal muscles; mobilize the knee/hip

Compensatory strategies: Trunk side bend; inability to maintain pelvic position; hyperextended knees; landing flat-footed or heavily

Sample Program 2: Case Scenario—ACL Reconstruction

The patient is an 18-year-old male basketball center with an identified swayback posture who is four weeks post right anterior cruciate ligament reconstruction. He has 0 degrees of right knee extension but continues to ambulate with a slight extensor lag. A compensatory anterior pelvic tilt and fair quadriceps eccentric control are noted with Knee Bends. He is able to perform a Single-Leg Balance for 10 seconds, but poor alignment presents.

1. What Pilates-based principles could you use to improve form during Knee Bends and Single-Leg Balance exercises?

2. What faulty movement patterns would you expect with other traditional exercises during this phase of ACL rehab?

Recommendations:

a. Use the Pilates-based principles of breathing and pelvis and rib cage positioning to help improve the athlete's quality of movement and neuromuscular control, correct faulty movement patterns, and develop a foundation for sport-specific training.

b. Because compensatory anterior pelvic tilt was noted with Knee Bends, the principle of pelvic stabilization is the first focus area. By stabilizing the pelvis, the quadriceps muscle/length tension relationship between hip and knee joint will be optimal and will facilitate a better neuromuscular training pattern. Start to integrate other principles of stabilization once the patient is able to demonstrate lumbo-pelvic stabilization with Knee Bends. It is also critical to assess the quadriceps recruitment pattern with Knee Bends. There may be compensatory firing of such muscles as the gluteals, and additional cueing may be needed to facilitate a normal firing sequence.

c. If poor alignment presents with the Single-Leg Balance and stabilization is not achieved with principles of stabilization, modify this exercise to weight shifting as noted in Phase I with emphasis on neutral body alignment and increase the time on the uninvolved leg. Also check the quadriceps and gluteus medius recruitment patterns as the patient shifts weight to the involved leg. The patient needs to demonstrate appropriate alignment and lumbo-pelvic stabilization with the Single-Leg Balance starting position to progress to the full exercise.

Expect to see an inability to dissociate hip movement from the pelvis in most exercises and ensuing compensatory strategies, particularly in the trunk. Use Pilates-based exercises such as Prone Hip Extension Preps and Full, Hip Abduction 1, and Heel Slide exercises to support your gait reeducation efforts.

Returning Your Athlete to Play: The Demands of Basketball

Your basketball player is now six months postsurgery and would like a sport-specific Pilates-based strengthening program to work on core strength. In considering the athlete's return to play, what are the demands of the sport? What functional movement patterns would you assess, and what faulty movement patterns will you be looking for?

Besides cardiovascular fitness, key elements of basketball include jumping, landing, sprinting, passing, dribbling, shooting, acceleration, deceleration, directional changes (forward, backward, lateral, vertical), pivoting, and cutting.

The predominant movement patterns include closed/open kinetic chain lower extremity, open chain upper extremity, and symmetrical–asymmetrical upper and lower extremities, uniplanar to multidirectional.

Start with the Musculoskeletal and Functional Movement Assessments

As in Chapter 4, complete the musculoskeletal assessment first to establish baseline measurements and then perform a functional movement assessment. Assess sport-specific movement patterns that mimic the sport of basketball, such as squatting, lunging, and rotary movements or a combination thereof. Look for the patient's ability to dissociate hip movement from the pelvis, control the quadriceps muscle eccentrically in CKC patterns, torso rotation and stabilization, and overall quality of movement (i.e., coordination, timing).

Assess the following movement patterns for principles of stabilization and control:

- Knee Bends
- Single-Leg Balance
- Lunge
- Spinal rotation (Spine Twist)
- Jumping (takeoff/landing mechanics), running, and layups

Program Design

Given noted swayback posture, exercises should emphasize neutral pelvis, spinal articulation, and concentric contraction of the hip flexors, external obliques, upper back extensors, and neck flexors. Also take into account the findings of your functional assessment, such as lack of eccentric quadriceps muscle control and hyperextended knees with knee bends.

Start with the Pilates-based principles of stabilization. Progress to Pilates exercises as noted below:

- Quarter Rollup with Neutral Pelvis
- Beginner Trunk Extensions
- One-Leg Circle
- Spine Twist, progressing from preps to full
- Double-Leg Stretch, feet on floor, progressing to full
- Single-Leg Stretch
- Shoulder Bridge
- Hip Abduction/Adduction Progressions
- Leg Pull Front Warm-up
- Pushups

How would you advance this athlete to a more sport-specific Pilates-based core training program?

Advanced Sport-Specific Core Program

Start with the Pilates-based principles of stabilization. Progress to the following exercises:

- Quarter Rollup with overhead basketball lift
- Trunk Extensions over BOSU® in neutral starting position
- One-Leg Circle with exercise band
- Spine Twist in squat, lunge, and standing positions with use of a medicine ball or with foot (feet) on a BOSU®
- Double-Leg Stretch with basketball in hands, with a focus on rib cage positioning
- Single-Leg Stretch on the Reebok Core Board®
- Shoulder Bridge on stability ball and Shoulder Bridge with leg press on stability ball
- Hip Abduction/Adduction on BOSU® or Reebok Core Board®
- Leg Pull Front Warm-up on stability ball
- Pushups on BOSU® or Reebok Core Board®

Chapter References

1. Kissane, J. 2001. The importance of core strength for the runner. *Running Times*, December, pp. 16-19.

2. Elphinston, E., Pook, P. 1999. *The Core Workout*, Second Edition. Hong Kong, China: Core Workout.

3. Schache, A.G., Bennell, K.L., Blanch, P.D., Wrigley, T.V. 1999. The coordinated movement of the lumbo-pelvic-hip complex during running: A literature review. *Gait and Posture* 10: 30-47.

4. Bruce, S.L. 2001. Shouldering pain. *Advance for Directors in Rehabilitation*, November, pp. 25-28.

5. Schleck, L., Smith, E. 1998. Video Analysis and Assessment of Runners. Robbinsdale, MN: Institute for Athletic Medicine, Case studies 12, 13, 14.

6. Kibler, W.B., Herring, S.A., Press, J.M. 1998. *Functional Rehabilitation of Sports and Musculoskeletal Injuries.*. Gaithersburg, MD: Aspen.

7. Foran, B. 2001. *High Performance Sports Conditioning*. Champaign, IL: Human Kinetics.

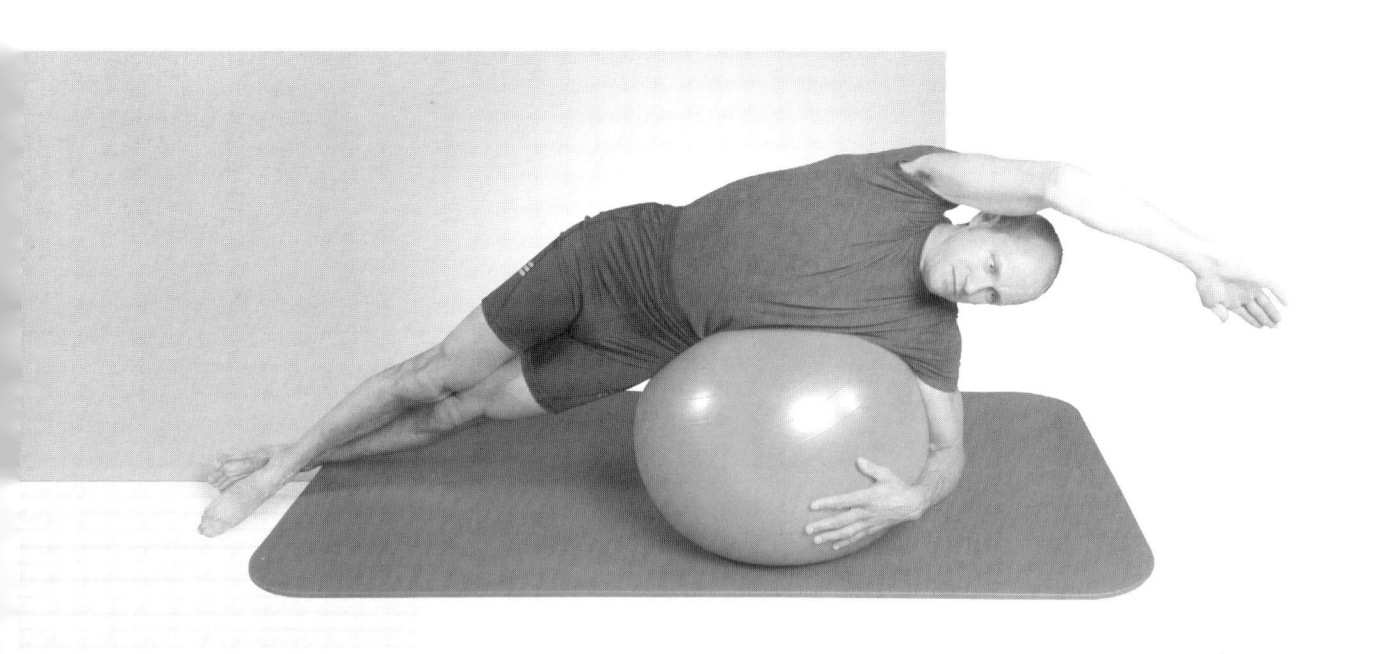

chapter 13

References and Resources

Other Helpful Resources

There are many resources available to you in addition to the references we've listed at the end of each chapter. Here are some we have found helpful in advancing our knowledge base over the years. We encourage you to sample from an array of products and select those you feel best meet your patient's needs.

Printed Resources

American College of Sports Medicine. 2001. *ACSM's Resource Manual: Guidelines for Exercise Testing and Prescription*, Fourth Edition. Baltimore, MD: Lippincott Williams & Wilkins.

Calais-Germain, B. 1993. *Anatomy of Movement*. Seattle, WA: Eastman Press.

Craig, C. 2001. *Pilates on the Ball*. Rochester, VT: Healing Arts Press.

Craig, C. 2003. *Abs on the Ball*. Rochester, VT: Healing Arts Press.

Sieg, K.W., Adams, S.P. 1996. *Illustrated Essentials of Musculoskeletal Anatomy*, Third Edition. Gainesville, FL: Mega Books.

Siler, B. 2000. *The Pilates Body*. New York: Broadway Books.

Ungaro, A. 2002. *Pilates Body in Motion*. New York: Borling Kindersley Publishing.

Audiovisual Resources (Videos, DVDs, etc.)

Balanced Body	www.pilates.com
Polestar Education	www.polestareducation.com
STOTT Pilates	www.stottpilates.com
Pilates Method Alliance	www.pilatesmethodalliance.com

About the Authors

Elizabeth Smith, P.T., A.T.C., ACSM Health/Fitness Instructor

Elizabeth Smith is a physical therapist and certified athletic trainer with certifications from the Academy of Orthopedic Medicine in manual therapy of the spine and STOTT Pilates in mat and Reformer. She brings more than 15 years of physical therapy experience in outpatient orthopaedic and sports medicine rehabilitation, with specializations in spine care, women's health, running injuries, and core training, and is a clinic supervisor in the Minneapolis-based Institute for Athletic Medicine. She is president of Body in Balance, Inc., which offers personal training, consulting, and Pilates-based continuing education courses for health professionals. She is a certified American College of Sports Medicine Health/Fitness Instructor and brings more than five years of experience teaching fitness classes, including Pilates, Reebok Core Board®, and fitness yoga. She is co-author of numerous book chapters and publications on the topics of aging and sport. Exercise has always been part of her life. Her passions include Pilates, volleyball, cross-country skiing, mountain biking, running, and hiking.

Kristin Smith, C.F.T., ACSM Health/Fitness Instructor

Fitness trainer Kristin Smith brings more than 20 years of movement expertise to her Twin Cities-based fitness training practice and creates programs that help people improve their quality of movement and performance through self-awareness. As president of KAS Fitness Training, she provides personal training in one-to-one and group settings where she specializes in postrehabilitation, sports performance, core stabilization, and Pilates-based continuing education courses for health professionals. She is a certified STOTT Pilates instructor in mat and Reformer and teaches wide-ranging fitness classes that include Reebok Core Board®, BOSU®, Pilates, and weight training. She is a certified personal trainer by the American Council on Exercise and a certified American College of Sports Medicine Health/Fitness Instructor. She is a frequent lecturer on Pilates, mind-body, and fitness topics and has authored numerous articles on the same. An outdoor enthusiast, she enjoys cross-country skiing, biking, and running.